# Learning Cognitive-Behavior Therapy

## An Illustrated Guide

*Second Edition*

# Learning Cognitive-Behavior Therapy

## An Illustrated Guide

*Second Edition*

Jesse H. Wright, M.D., Ph.D.
Professor and Gottfried and Gisela Kolb Endowed Chair in Outpatient Psychiatry; Director, University of Louisville Depression Center, University of Louisville School of Medicine, Louisville, Kentucky

Gregory K. Brown, Ph.D.
Research Associate Professor of Clinical Psychology in Psychiatry, Perelman School of Medicine, University of Pennsylvania, Philadelphia, Pennsylvania

Michael E. Thase, M.D.
Professor of Psychiatry, Perelman School of Medicine, University of Pennsylvania and the Corporal Michael J. Crescenz Veterans Affairs Medical Center, Philadelphia, Pennsylvania

Monica Ramirez Basco, Ph.D.
Associate Director Science Policy, Planning, and Analysis, National Institutes of Health, Office of Research on Women's Health, Bethesda, Maryland

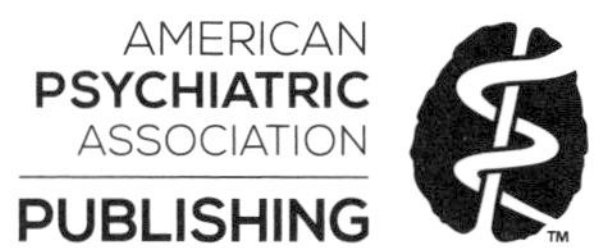

Manufactured in the United States of America on acid-free paper
23 22 6 5 4 3
Second Edition

American Psychiatric Association Publishing
800 Maine Avenue SW
Suite 900
Washington, DC 20024-2812
www.appi.org

**Library of Congress Cataloging-in-Publication Data**
Names: Wright, Jesse H., author. | Brown, Gregory K., 1959– author. | Thase, Michael E., author. | Basco, Monica Ramirez, author.
Title: Learning cognitive-behavior therapy : an illustrated guide / by Jesse H. Wright, Gregory K. Brown, Michael E. Thase, Monica Ramirez Basco.
Other titles: Core competencies in psychotherapy.
Description: Second edition. | Arlington, VA : American Psychiatric Association Publishing, [2017] | Series: Core competencies in psychotherapy | Includes bibliographical references and index.
Identifiers: LCCN 2016052314 (print) | LCCN 2016052881 (ebook) | ISBN 9781615370184 (alk. paper) | ISBN 9781615371259 (ebook)
Subjects: | MESH: Cognitive Therapy—methods | Behavior Therapy—methods | Mental Disorders—therapy
Classification: LCC RC489.C63 (print) | LCC RC489.C63 (ebook) | NLM WM 425.5.C6 | DDC 616.89/1425—dc23
LC record available at https://lccn.loc.gov/2016052314

**British Library Cataloguing in Publication Data**
A CIP record is available from the British Library.

# Contents

## List of Learning Exercises

## List of Troubleshooting Guides



## List of Videos

# Preface

In writing this second edition of *Learning Cognitive-Behavior Therapy: An Illustrated Guide*, we have been especially mindful of the transformative work of our principal mentor and teacher, Aaron T. Beck, M.D. When he began his studies on cognitive processing over 50 years ago, there were no evidence-based psychosocial treatments for mental disorders. Now there is abundant evidence that cognitive-behavior therapy (CBT) is effective for a wide range of psychiatric conditions. And CBT has become a first-line treatment method that is bringing symptom relief to many thousands of patients throughout the world. This book is an outgrowth of his contributions in proposing the core principles of CBT, leading and inspiring a decades-long research effort, and imparting wisdom in a career lasting through very old age.

We also are indebted to our other teachers and colleagues for their ideas that are incorporated into this second edition of *Learning Cognitive-Behavior Therapy*. The concepts described in this book are the product of the dedicated work of legions of researchers and clinicians who have added to the knowledge base of CBT. Our students have also played a large role in our development as educators in CBT. This book is based in part on the courses we have been teaching at the University of Louisville and the University of Pennsylvania, and our presentations at meetings of professional organizations. The feedback and suggestions we've received from our students and coworkers have enriched our knowledge of how to help others become successful practitioners of CBT.

Our goals in writing this book have been to provide an easy-to-use guide to learning the essential skills of CBT and to assist readers in achieving competence in this treatment method. We begin by tracing the origins of the CBT model and giving an overview of core theories and techniques. Next we describe the therapeutic relationship in CBT, explain how to conceptualize a case with the CBT model, and detail effective ways to structure sessions. If you understand these basic features of CBT, you should have a solid platform for learning the specific procedures for changing cognitions and behaviors that are described in the middle chapters of the book (e.g., methods for modifying automatic thoughts; behavioral strategies for treating low energy, lack of interest, and avoidance; and interventions for revising maladaptive core beliefs). The last group of chapters in *Learning Cognitive-Behavior Therapy* moves beyond basic skills to help you learn about CBT strategies for treating complex and severe disorders, in addition to methods for reducing suicide risk. Since publication of the first edition of this book, there has been growing evidence for the effectiveness of CBT in suicidal patients. We want readers to be able to implement these methods that have life-saving potential (see Chapter 9, "Cognitive-Behavior Therapy to Reduce Suicide Risk").

Another development since the first edition is increased interest in therapies that are related to CBT but utilize alternate, and complementary, treatment methods. Such approaches include dialectical behavior therapy, mindfulness-based cognitive therapy, and well-being therapy. Although a full grounding in these approaches can't be accomplished in this book, Chapter 10, "Treating Chronic, Severe, or Complex Disorders," orients readers to alternate methods as they are applied to conditions such as personality disorders and chronic or recurrent depression, and gives suggestions for further reading and study. The final chapter of the book is devoted to recommendations and tips for gaining competence in CBT, avoiding or coping with burnout, and continuing to build knowledge and experience as a cognitive-behavior therapist.

Specific competencies for performing CBT have been described by the American Association of Directors of Psychiatric Residency Training (AADPRT). These competencies are discussed in Chapter 11, "Building Competence in Cognitive-Behavior Therapy." However, we elected not to organize the book around these competencies because we wanted to write a guide that would be useful to a broad range of readers, including practicing clinicians and trainees from multiple disciplines. Nonetheless, the book does provide background information and learning exercises that should help psychiatry residents and others acquire the skills described in the AADPRT competencies.

We've found that the best way to grasp the essence of CBT is to combine readings and didactic sessions with opportunities to see therapy being conducted—whether in videos, role-plays, or observations of actual sessions. This book includes 23 video illustrations of clinician interactions with patients (see the Video Guide just after this Preface for information about the videos and how to access them). The next step is to practice the methods with patients, ideally with careful supervision from a trained cognitive-behavior therapist. To help you build skills in CBT, we've included a variety of learning exercises and troubleshooting guides. The learning exercises are designed to enhance your ability to implement key cognitive and behavioral methods. And the troubleshooting guides will help you find solutions for challenging treatment situations.

When we describe the histories used in the video illustrations, we present them as if they were actual cases. In fact, they are simulations based on amalgams of the clinicians' experiences in treating persons with similar problems. We use the convention of describing patients as if they were real throughout the book because of the ease of writing and reading case material with this style of communication. When case material is used, we change genders, background information, and other data so the identities of patients whom we or our colleagues have treated are obscured. Also, to avoid the cumbersome phrasing of "he or she," we alternate the genders of personal pronouns when we are not writing about specific cases.

Implementation of CBT can be enhanced by the use of worksheets, checklists, thought records, and other written exercises. Therefore, we have included a number of these helpful forms for you to use in planning or performing CBT. Examples are provided in the text and in Appendix 1, "Worksheets and Checklists." Appendix 1 is also available as a free download in its entirety and in larger format on the American Psychiatric Association Publishing Web site: https://www.appi.org/wright.

Learning experiences for becoming skilled in CBT can be quite stimulating and productive. Reading about the rich history of CBT can help anchor your treatment interventions to a broad philosophical, scientific, and cultural framework. Studying the theories that underlie the cognitive-behavioral approach can expand your understanding of the psychology of psychiatric disorders and can provide valuable guidance for the practice of psychotherapy. And learning the methods of CBT can give you pragmatic, empirically tested tools for a wide range of clinical problems.

We hope that you will find this book a valuable companion in your work on learning CBT.

*Jesse H. Wright, M.D., Ph.D.*
*Gregory K. Brown, Ph.D.*
*Michael E. Thase, M.D.*
*Monica Ramirez Basco, Ph.D.*

# Video Guide

This second edition of *Learning Cognitive-Behavior Therapy: An Illustrated Guide* has been designed to help you learn CBT in three major ways: reading, seeing, and doing. Toward that goal, the videos that accompany this book illustrate key features of CBT.

These video illustrations feature the work of volunteer clinicians who agreed to demonstrate commonly used CBT methods. Videos were filmed in a simple, naturalistic style, because our intent was to show methods that clinicians might use in actual sessions, not to produce slick or professional videos with paid actors following scripts. We wanted to illustrate realistic interventions that have the types of strengths and imperfections characteristic of real treatment sessions. Therefore, we asked clinicians from varied disciplines to role-play scenarios based on their experiences in treating patients with CBT. A nurse practitioner, Catherine Batscha, D.N.P., plays a patient with anxiety disorder (interviewed by the principal author, J.H.W.); a psychiatry resident, Gerry-Lynn Wichmann, M.D., plays a pregnant woman with depression (interviewed by another psychiatry resident, Meredith Birdwhistell, M.D.); a psychologist, Eric Russ, Ph.D., plays a young man with depression who has difficulty grasping CBT and making needed changes (interviewed by G.K.B., a coauthor of the book); Francis Smith, D.O., a psychiatry resident, plays a man with low self-esteem and depression triggered by a move from his hometown (interviewed by a leading expert in CBT, Donna Sudak, M.D.); a retired English professor, Millard Dunn, Ph.D., plays an older man who is struggling with depression (interviewed by Lloyd Kevin Chapman, Ph.D., an experienced cognitive-behavior therapist who is in private practice); Maria Jose Lisotto, M.D., another psychiatry resident, plays a woman with obsessive-compulsive disorder (interviewed by a psychologist, Elizabeth Hembree, Ph.D.); and Delvin Barney plays a student with suicidal thinking (interviewed by coauthor G.K.B.).

Instead of showing an entire session for each case, we asked the clinicians to produce brief vignettes that demonstrate key CBT methods such as the collaborative therapeutic relationship, agenda setting, identifying automatic thoughts, examining the evidence, exposure to feared stimuli, and modifying core beliefs. This format was chosen because we wanted to illustrate specific points when they occurred in the book and to directly link explanations of core methods with video illustrations.

The videos are intended to be watched in sequence as they appear in the book and at the time you are reading about the specific topic. For example, the first two videos are designed to accompany Chapter 2, "The Therapeutic Relationship: Collaborative Empiricism in Action." **We recommend that you wait until you have read the text that explains the methods demonstrated in the videos before viewing them.**

We also suggest that you supplement the videos accompanying this book by viewing other recorded sessions so that you can see a diverse sample of techniques and styles. Sources for acquiring videos of entire sessions conducted by master cognitive-behavior therapists (e.g., A.T. Beck, Christine Padesky, Jacqueline Persons) are listed in Appendix 2, "Cognitive-Behavior Therapy Resources."

The clinical cases portrayed in this book and corresponding videos are fictional. Any resemblance to real persons is purely coincidental. The videos feature the work of volunteers who agreed to demonstrate the featured interview techniques.

## Video Access

Video cues provided in the text identify the video illustrations by name and approximate running time, as shown in the following example:

> **Video 1.** Getting Started—CBT in Action: Dr. Wright and Kate (12:17)

The video illustrations are streamed via the Internet and can be viewed online by navigating to **https://www.appi.org/wright** and using the embedded video player. The videos are optimized for most current operating systems, including mobile operating systems.

# Videos Discussed by Chapter

## Chapter 2: The Therapeutic Relationship: Collaborative Empiricism in Action

**Video 1.** Getting Started—CBT in Action:
Dr. Wright and Kate (12:17)
**Video 2.** Modifying Automatic Thoughts:
Dr. Wright and Kate (8:48)

## Chapter 4: Structuring and Educating

**Video 3.** Agenda Setting: Dr. Wichmann and Meredith (3:16)
**Video 4.** Difficulty Setting an Agenda:
Dr. Brown and Eric (2:50)
**Video 1.** Getting Started—CBT in Action:
Dr. Wright and Kate (12:17)

## Chapter 5: Working With Automatic Thoughts

**Video 5.** Eliciting Automatic Thoughts:
Dr. Sudak and Brian (9:09)
**Video 6.** Difficulty With Thought Recording:
Dr. Brown and Eric (6:31)
**Video 7.** Using Imagery to Uncover Automatic Thoughts:
Dr. Brown and Eric (6:44)
**Video 8.** Examining the Evidence:
Dr. Sudak and Brian (11:58)
**Video 2.** Modifying Automatic Thoughts:
Dr. Wright and Kate (8:48)
**Video 9.** Developing Rational Alternatives:
Dr. Sudak and Brian (8:50)
**Video 10.** Difficulty Finding Rational Alternatives:
Dr. Brown and Eric (10:37)
**Video 11.** Cognitive Rehearsal:
Dr. Wright and Kate (9:31)

## Chapter 6: Behavioral Methods I: Improving Mood, Increasing Energy, Completing Tasks, and Solving Problems

**Video 12.** Behavioral Action Plan:
Dr. Wichmann and Meredith (3:34)
**Video 13.** Activity Scheduling:
Dr. Wichmann and Meredith (9:32)
**Video 14.** Difficulty Completing an Activity Schedule:
Dr. Chapman and Charles (8:03)
**Video 15.** Developing a Graded Task Assignment:
Dr. Chapman and Charles (7:43)

## Chapter 7: Behavioral Methods II: Reducing Anxiety and Breaking Patterns of Avoidance

**Video 16.** Breathing Training for Panic Attacks:
Dr. Wright and Kate (7:48)
**Video 17.** Exposure Therapy for Anxiety:
Dr. Wright and Kate (10:00)
**Video 18.** Imaginal Exposure for OCD:
Dr. Hembree and Mia (9:39)
**Video 19.** In Vivo Exposure Therapy for OCD:
Dr. Hembree and Mia (8:37)

## Chapter 8: Modifying Schemas

**Video 20.** Uncovering a Maladaptive Schema:
Dr. Sudak and Brian (12:22)
**Video 21.** Changing a Maladaptive Schema:
Dr. Sudak and Brian (12:26)
**Video 22.** Putting a Revised Schema Into Action:
Dr. Sudak and Brian (10:48)

## Chapter 9: Cognitive-Behavior Therapy to Reduce Suicide Risk

**Video 23.** Safety Planning: Dr. Brown and David (8:37)

# Acknowledgments

Developing a book with video illustrations required a great deal of support from our colleagues and friends. We owe a special note of gratitude to the people who volunteered to play the therapists and patients in the videos: Catherine Batscha, D.N.P., Gerry-Lynn Wichmann, M.D., Meredith Birdwhistell, M.D., Eric Russ, Ph.D., Francis Smith, D.O., Donna Sudak, M.D., Millard Dunn, Ph.D., Lloyd Kevin Chapman, Ph.D., Maria Jose Lisotto, M.D., Elizabeth Hembree, Ph.D., and Delvin Barney. These individuals made a major contribution to this book by agreeing to demonstrate CBT skills to a broad audience of readers. The videos were filmed with great care by Ron Harrison and Michael Peak from the University of Louisville, and Ries Video Productions in Philadelphia. Ron Harrison edited the videos in collaboration with the authors.

Production of this book with its combination of text, video, learning exercises, and worksheets was possible only with the inspired assistance of Carol Wahl from the University of Louisville. A person with formidable expertise in manuscript preparation, plus remarkable equanimity, she was our chief problem solver as we brought this project to completion.

## Disclosures

Jesse H. Wright, M.D., Ph.D., has an equity interest in *Good Days Ahead*, a computer program described in this book. He has received federal grants (R21-MH57470, R41-MH62230, RO1-MH082762, and

R18-HSO24047) for development of this software and testing of computer-assisted CBT. His conflict of interest pertaining to research on *Good Days Ahead* is managed with a plan with the University of Louisville. He has stock ownership in Empower Interactive and Mindstreet, and he receives book royalties from Simon & Schuster, Guilford Press, and American Psychiatric Association Publishing. Gregory K. Brown, Ph.D., and Michael E. Thase, M.D., participated with Dr. Wright in research on computer-assisted CBT (RO1-MH082762), and Monica Ramirez Basco, Ph.D., participated in research supported by R21-MH57470, but all coauthors (Drs. Brown, Thase, and Basco) have no equity interest or other financial interest in *Good Days Ahead*.

# 1

# Basic Principles of Cognitive-Behavior Therapy

Cognitive-behavior therapy (CBT) is based on a set of well-developed principles that are used to formulate treatment plans and guide the actions of the therapist. This opening chapter focuses on explaining these core concepts and illustrating how the basic cognitive-behavioral model has influenced the development of specific techniques. We begin with a brief overview of the historical background of CBT. The fundamental principles of CBT have been linked to ideas that were first described thousands of years ago (Beck et al. 1979; D.A. Clark et al. 1999).

## Origins of CBT

CBT is a commonsense approach that is based on two central tenets: 1) our cognitions have a controlling influence on our emotions and behavior; and 2) how we act or behave can strongly affect our thought patterns and emotions. The cognitive elements of this viewpoint were recognized by the Stoic philosophers Epictetus, Cicero, Seneca, and others two millennia before the introduction of CBT (Beck et al. 1979). For example, the Greek Stoic Epictetus wrote in the *Enchiridion*, "Men are disturbed not by the things which happen, but by the opinions about the things" (Epictetus 1991, p. 14). Also, in Eastern philosophical traditions, such as Taoism and Buddhism, cognition is regarded as a primary force in determining human behavior (Beck et al. 1979; Campos 2002). In his book *Ethics for the New Millennium*, the Dalai Lama (1999) noted, "If we can reorient our thoughts and emotions, and reorder our behavior, not only can we learn to cope with suffering more easily, but we can prevent a great deal of it from starting in the first place" (p. xii).

The perspective that developing a healthy style of thinking can reduce distress or give a greater sense of well-being is a common theme across many generations and cultures. The ancient Persian philosopher Zoroaster based his teachings on three main pillars: thinking well, acting well, and talking well. Benjamin Franklin, one of the founding fathers of the United States, wrote extensively on the development of constructive attitudes, which he believed would favorably influence behavior (Isaacson 2003). During the nineteenth and twentieth centuries, European philosophers—including Kant, Heidegger, Jaspers, and Frankl—continued to develop the idea that conscious cognitive processes play a fundamental role in human existence (D.A. Clark et al. 1999; Wright et al. 2014). For example, Frankl (1992) concluded that finding a sense of meaning in life helps serve as an antidote to despair and disillusionment.

Aaron T. Beck was the first person to fully develop theories and methods for using cognitive and behavioral interventions for emotional disorders (Beck 1963, 1964). Although Beck departed from psychoanalytic concepts, he noted that his cognitive theories were influenced by the work of several post-Freudian analysts, such as Adler, Horney, and Sullivan. Their focus on distorted self-images presaged the development of more systematized cognitive-behavioral formulations of psychiatric disorders and personality structure (D.A. Clark et al. 1999). Kelly's (1955) theory of personal constructs (core beliefs or self-schemas) and Ellis's rational-emotive therapy also contributed to the development of cognitive-behavioral theories and methods (D.A. Clark et al. 1999; Raimy 1975).

Beck's early formulations were centered on the role of maladaptive information processing in depression and anxiety disorders. In a series of papers published in the early 1960s, he described a cognitive conceptualization of depression in which symptoms were related to a negative thinking style in three domains: self, world, and future (the "negative cognitive triad"; Beck 1963, 1964). Beck's proposal for a cognitively oriented therapy targeted at reversing dysfunctional cognitions and related behavior was then tested in a large number of outcome studies (Cuijpers et al. 2013; Wright et al. 2014). The theories and methods outlined by Beck and many other contributors to CBT have been extended to a wide array of conditions, including depression, anxiety disorders, eating disorders, schizophrenia, bipolar disorder, chronic pain, personality disorders, and substance abuse. Hundreds of controlled studies of CBT have been completed for a variety of psychiatric disorders (Bandelow et al. 2015; Butler and Beck 2000; Cuijpers et al. 2013).

The behavioral components of the CBT model had their beginnings in the 1950s and 1960s, when clinical researchers began to apply the ideas of Pavlov, Skinner, and other experimental behaviorists (Rachman 1997). Joseph Wolpe (1958) and Hans Eysenck (1966) were pioneers in exploring the potential of behavioral interventions such as desensitization (graded contact with feared objects or situations) and relaxation training. Many of the early approaches to using behavioral principles for psychotherapy paid limited attention to the cognitive processes involved in psychiatric disorders. Instead, the focus was on shaping measurable behavior with reinforcers and extinguishing fearful responses with exposure protocols.

As research on behavior therapy expanded, a number of prominent investigators—such as Meichenbaum (1977) and Lewinsohn and associates (1985)—began to incorporate cognitive theories and strategies into their treatment programs. They noted that the cognitive perspective added context, depth, and understanding to behavioral interventions. In applying Lewinsohn's behavioral theory, Addis and Martell (2004) observed that patients with depression often do not get enough positive reinforcement from their environment to maintain adaptive behavior. As patients become less active, they become more severely depressed. A lack of interest in pleasurable or mastery activities can lead to additional depressive symptoms, such as sadness, fatigue, and anhedonia, which, in turn, result in greater inactivity. Over time, this pattern can create a vicious cycle that can spiral downward into severe depression. Also, Beck advocated the inclusion of behavioral methods from the outset of his work because he recognized that these tools are effective in reducing symptoms and because he conceptualized a close relationship between cognition and behavior. Although there are still some purists who may debate the merits of using a cognitive or behavioral approach alone, most pragmatically oriented therapists consider cognitive and behavioral methods to be effective partners in both theory and practice.

A good illustration of the coming together of cognitive and behavioral theories can be found in the work of D.M. Clark (1986; D.M. Clark et al. 1994) and Barlow (Barlow and Cerney 1988; Barlow et al. 1989) on treatment programs for panic disorder. They have observed that patients with panic disorder typically have a constellation of cognitive symptoms (e.g., catastrophic fears of physical calamities or loss of control) and be-

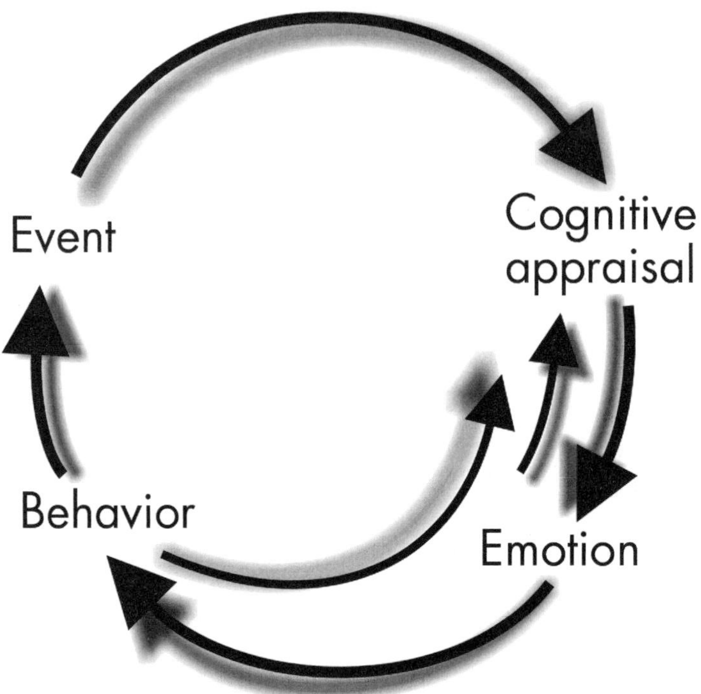


**Figure 1–1.** Basic cognitive-behavioral model.

havioral symptoms (e.g., escape or avoidance). Extensive research has demonstrated the efficacy of a combined approach that uses cognitive techniques (to modify fearful cognitions) along with behavioral methods, including exposure therapy, breathing training, and relaxation (Barlow et al. 1989; D.M. Clark et al. 1994; Wright et al. 2014).

## The Cognitive-Behavioral Model

The principal elements of the cognitive-behavioral model are diagrammed in Figure 1–1. Cognitive processing is given a central role in this model because humans appraise the significance of events in the environment around and within them (e.g., stressful events, feedback or lack of feedback from others, memories of events from the past, bodily sensations), and cognitions are often associated with emotional reactions. For example, Richard, a man with a social anxiety disorder, was preparing to attend a party in his neighborhood and had the following thoughts: "I won't know what to say.…Everyone will know I'm nervous.…I'll look like a misfit.…I'll clutch and want to leave right away." The emotions and physiological responses that were stimulated by these maladaptive

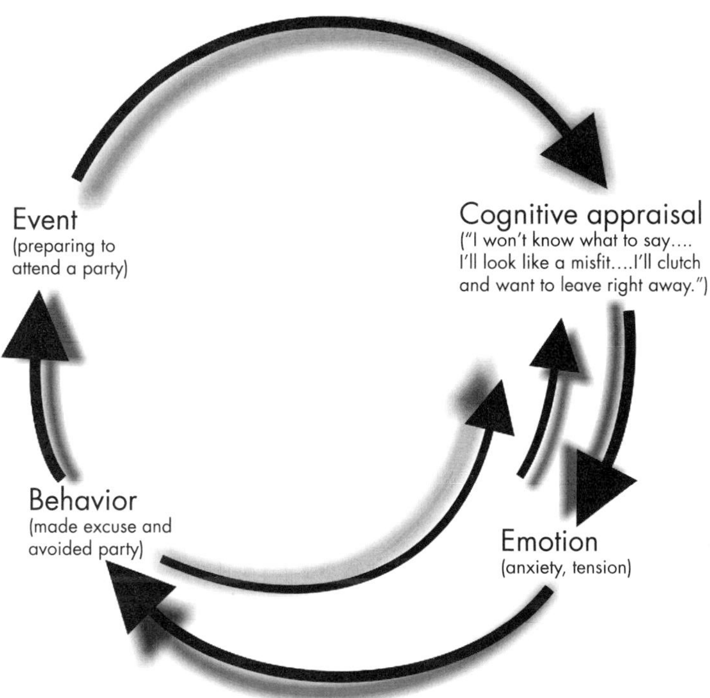


**Figure 1–2.** Basic cognitive-behavioral model: example of a patient with social phobia.

cognitions were predictable: severe anxiety, physical tension, and autonomic arousal. He began sweating, felt "butterflies" in his stomach, and had a dry mouth. His behavioral response was also problematic. Instead of facing the situation and attempting to gain skills in mastering social situations, he called to tell the host that he had the flu.

Avoidance of the feared situation reinforced Richard's negative thinking and became part of a vicious cycle of thoughts, emotions, and behavior that deepened his problem with social anxiety. Each time he maneuvered to escape from social situations, his beliefs about being incapable and vulnerable were strengthened. These fearful cognitions then amplified his emotional discomfort and made it less likely that he would engage in social activities. Richard's cognitions, emotions, and actions are diagrammed in Figure 1–2.

In treating problems like Richard's, cognitive-behavior therapists can draw from a variety of methods that are targeted at all three areas of pathological functioning identified in the basic CBT model: cognitions, emotions, and behaviors. For example, Richard might be taught how to recognize and change his anxiety-ridden thoughts, use relaxation or imagery to reduce anxious emotions, implement a step-by-step hierarchy to break the pattern of avoidance, and build social skills.

Before describing theories and methods of CBT in more detail, we want to explain how the model outlined in Figure 1–1 is used in clinical practice and how it relates to broader concepts of the etiology and treatment of psychiatric disorders. The basic CBT model is a construct used to help clinicians conceptualize clinical problems and implement specific CBT methods. As a working model, it is purposefully simplified to direct the attention of the clinician to the relationships among thoughts, emotions, and behaviors and to guide treatment interventions.

Cognitive-behavior therapists also recognize that there are complex interactions among biological processes (e.g., genetics, brain functioning, neuroendocrine systems, inflammation), environmental and interpersonal influences, and cognitive-behavioral elements in the genesis and treatment of psychiatric disorders (Wright 2004; Wright and Thase 1992). The CBT model assumes that cognitive and behavioral changes are modulated through biological processes and that psychotropic medications and other biological treatments influence cognitions (Wright et al. 2014). Recent research has supported this position by showing that pharmacotherapy and CBT may target different regions in the brain and, when effective, can have complementary effects on brain circuitry (e.g., see McGrath et al. 2013).

Research on combined pharmacotherapy and psychotherapy has provided additional support for considering biological influences in implementing the CBT model. Combined treatment with CBT and medication can improve efficacy, especially for severe conditions such as chronic or treatment-resistant depression, schizophrenia, and bipolar disorder (Hollon et al. 2014; Lam et al. 2003; Rector and Beck 2001). However, high-potency benzodiazepines such as alprazolam may impair the effectiveness of CBT (Marks et al. 1993).

To provide overall direction for treatment, an integrated, fully detailed formulation that includes cognitive-behavioral, biological, social, and interpersonal considerations is strongly recommended. Methods for developing multifaceted case conceptualizations are discussed and illustrated in Chapter 3, "Assessment and Formulation." The remainder of this chapter is devoted to introducing the core theories and methods of CBT.

## Basic Concepts

### Levels of Cognitive Processing

Three primary levels of cognitive processing have been identified by Beck and his colleagues (Beck et al. 1979; D.A. Clark et al. 1999; Dobson and

Shaw 1986). The highest level of cognition is *consciousness,* a state of awareness in which decisions can be made on a rational basis. Conscious attention allows us to 1) monitor and assess interactions with the environment, 2) link past memories with present experiences, and 3) control and plan future actions (Sternberg 1996). In CBT, therapists encourage the development and application of adaptive conscious thought processes such as rational thinking and problem solving. The therapist also devotes considerable effort to helping patients recognize and change maladaptive thinking at two additional levels of cognition: *automatic thoughts* and *schemas* (Beck et al. 1979; D.A. Clark et al. 1999; Wright et al. 2014), both characterized by relatively autonomous information processing:

- *Automatic thoughts* are cognitions that stream rapidly through our minds when we are in the midst of situations (or are recalling events). Although we may be subliminally aware of the presence of automatic thoughts, typically these cognitions are not subjected to careful rational analysis.
- *Schemas* are core beliefs that act as templates or underlying rules for information processing. They serve a critical function in allowing humans to screen, filter, code, and assign meaning to information from the environment.

In contrast to psychodynamically oriented therapy, CBT does not posit specific structures or defenses that block thoughts from awareness (D.A. Clark et al. 1999). Instead, CBT emphasizes techniques designed to help patients detect and modify automatic thoughts and schemas, especially those that are associated with emotional symptoms such as depression, anxiety, or anger. CBT teaches patients to "think about their thinking" to reach the goal of bringing autonomous cognitions into conscious awareness and control.

## Automatic Thoughts

A large number of the thoughts that we have each day are part of a stream of cognitive processing that is just below the surface of the fully conscious mind. These automatic thoughts are typically private or unspoken and occur in a rapid-fire manner as we evaluate the significance of events in our lives. D.A. Clark and colleagues (1999) used the term *preconscious* in describing automatic thoughts, because these cognitions can be recognized and understood if our attention is drawn to them. Persons with psychiatric disorders such as depression or anxiety often experience floods of automatic thoughts that are maladaptive or distorted. These thoughts can generate painful emotional reactions and dysfunctional behavior.

One of the most important clues that automatic thoughts might be occurring is the presence of strong emotions. The relationship between

| Event | Automatic thoughts | Emotions |
|---|---|---|
| My mother calls and asks why I forgot my sister's birthday. | "I messed up again."<br>"There's no way I will ever please her."<br>"I can't do anything right."<br>"What's the use?" | Sadness, anger |
| Thinking about a big project that is due at work. | "It's too much for me."<br>"I'll never get it done in time."<br>"I won't be able to face my boss."<br>"I'll lose the job and everything else in my life." | Anxiety |
| My husband complains that I'm irritable all the time. | "He's really down on me."<br>"I'm failing as a wife."<br>"I don't enjoy anything."<br>"Why would anyone want to be around me?" | Sadness, anxiety |

**Figure 1–3.** Martha's automatic thoughts.

events, automatic thoughts, and emotions is illustrated by an example from the treatment of Martha, a woman experiencing major depression (Figure 1–3).

In this example, Martha's automatic thoughts demonstrate the common finding of negatively biased cognitions in depression. Although she was depressed and was having problems with her family and her work, she was actually functioning much better than was apparent from her overly critical automatic thoughts. A large body of research has confirmed that persons with depression, anxiety disorders, and other psychiatric conditions have a high frequency of distorted automatic thoughts (Blackburn et al. 1986; Haaga et al. 1991; Hollon et al. 1986). In depression, automatic thoughts often center on themes of hopelessness, low self-esteem, and failure. Persons with anxiety disorders usually have automatic thoughts that include predictions of danger, harm, uncontrollability, or inability to manage threats (D.A. Clark et al. 1990; Ingram and Kendall 1987; Kendall and Hollon 1989).

Everyone has automatic thoughts; they do not occur exclusively in people with depression, anxiety, or other emotional disorders. By recognizing their personal automatic thoughts and employing other cognitive-behavioral processes, clinicians can improve their understanding of basic concepts, increase their empathy with patients, and deepen awareness of their own cognitive and behavioral patterns that could influence the therapeutic relationship.

Throughout this book, we suggest exercises that we believe will help you learn the core principles of CBT. Most of these learning exercises involve practicing CBT interventions with patients or in role-play exercises with a colleague, but in some you will be asked to examine your own thoughts and feelings. The first exercise is to write down an example of automatic thoughts. Try to do this for a situation from your own life. If a personal example does not come to mind, you can use a vignette from a patient you have interviewed.

**Learning Exercise 1–1.** Recognizing Automatic Thoughts: A Three-Column Thought Record

1. Draw three columns on a sheet of paper and label them "Event," "Automatic thoughts," and "Emotions."
2. Now think back to a recent situation (or a memory of an event) that seemed to stir up emotions such as anxiety, anger, sadness, physical tension, or happiness.
3. Try to imagine being back in this situation, just as it happened.
4. What automatic thoughts were occurring in this situation? Write down the event, the automatic thoughts, and the emotions on the three-column thought record.

Sometimes automatic thoughts can be logically sound and can be an accurate reflection of the reality of the situation. For example, it could be true that Martha is in danger of losing her job or that her husband is making critical comments about her behavior. CBT does not involve glossing over actual problems. If a person is facing significant difficulties, the clinician should show understanding and empathy while using cognitive and behavioral methods to help the person cope with the situation. However, in people with psychiatric disorders, there are usually excellent opportunities to spot errors in reasoning and other cognitive distortions that can be modified with CBT interventions.

## Cognitive Errors

In his initial formulations, Beck (1963, 1964; Beck et al. 1979) theorized that there are characteristic errors in logic in the automatic thoughts and other cognitions of persons with emotional disorders. Subsequent research has confirmed the importance of cognitive errors in pathological styles of information processing. For example, cognitive errors have been found to occur substantially more frequently in depressed persons than in control subjects (Lefebvre 1981; Watkins and Rush 1983). Beck and coworkers (1979; D.A. Clark et al. 1999) described six main categories of cognitive errors: selective abstraction, arbitrary inference, overgeneralization, magnification and minimization, personalization, and absolutistic (all-or-nothing) thinking. Definitions and examples of each of these cognitive errors are provided in Table 1–1.

As you probably noticed from reviewing the examples in Table 1–1, there can be a good deal of overlap between cognitive errors. Dan, the person who was using absolutistic thinking, was also ignoring the evidence of his own strengths and minimizing his friend Ed's problems. The man who fell victim to selective abstraction (ignoring the evidence) after not receiving a holiday card had additional cognitive errors such as all-or-nothing thinking ("Nobody cares about me anymore"). In implementing CBT methods for reducing cognitive errors, therapists typically teach patients that the most important aim is simply to recognize that one is making cognitive errors—not to identify each and every error in logic that is occurring.

## Schemas

In cognitive-behavioral theory, schemas are defined as basic templates or rules for information processing that underlie the more superficial layer of automatic thoughts (D.A. Clark et al. 1999; Wright et al. 2014). Schemas are enduring principles of thinking that start to take shape in early childhood and may be influenced by genetics and a multitude of life experiences, including parental teaching and modeling, formal and informal educational activities, peer experiences, traumas, and successes.

Bowlby (1985) and others observed that humans need to develop schemas to manage the large amounts of information that they encounter each day and to make timely and appropriate decisions. For example, if a person has a basic rule of "always plan ahead," it is unlikely that she will spend much time debating the merits of going into a new situation without advance preparation. Instead, she will automatically begin to lay the groundwork for successfully managing the situation.

It has been suggested by D.A. Clark and colleagues (1999) that there are three main groups of schemas:

1. **Simple schemas**

   *Definition:* Rules about the physical nature of the environment, practical management of everyday activities, or laws of nature that may have little or no effect on psychopathology.

   *Examples:* "Be a defensive driver"; "A good education pays off"; "Take shelter during a thunderstorm."

**Table 1–1.** Cognitive errors

**Selective abstraction (sometimes called *ignoring the evidence* or *the mental filter*)**

*Definition:* A conclusion is drawn after looking at only a small portion of the available information. Salient data are screened out or ignored in order to confirm the person's biased view of the situation.

*Example:* A depressed man with low self-esteem does not receive a holiday card from an old friend. He thinks, "I'm losing all my friends; nobody cares about me anymore." He ignores the evidence that he has received cards from other friends, his old friend has sent him a card every year for the past 15 years, his friend has been busy this past year with a move and a new job, and he still has good relationships with other friends.

**Arbitrary inference**

*Definition:* A conclusion is reached in the face of contradictory evidence or in the absence of evidence.

*Example:* A woman with a fear of elevators is asked to predict the chances that an elevator will fall if she rides in it. She replies that the chances are 10% or more that the elevator will fall to the ground and that she will be injured. Many people have tried to convince her that the chances of a catastrophic elevator accident are negligible.

**Overgeneralization**

*Definition:* A conclusion is made about one or more isolated incidents and then is extended illogically to cover broad areas of functioning.

*Example:* A depressed college student gets a B on a test. He considers this unsatisfactory. He is overgeneralizing when he has automatic thoughts such as "I'm falling short everywhere in my life; I can't do anything right."

**Magnification and minimization**

*Definition:* The significance of an attribute, event, or sensation is exaggerated or minimized.

*Example:* A woman with panic disorder starts to feel light-headed during the onset of a panic attack. She thinks, "I'll faint; I might have a heart attack or a stroke."

**Personalization**

*Definition:* External events are related to oneself when there is little or no basis for doing so. Excessive responsibility or blame is taken for negative events.

*Example:* There has been an economic downturn, and a previously successful business is now struggling to meet the annual budget. Layoffs are being considered. A host of factors have led to the budget crisis, but one of the managers thinks, "It's my fault; I should have seen this coming and done something about it; I've failed the company."

**Table 1–1.** Cognitive errors *(continued)*

| |
|---|
| Absolutistic (or *all-or-nothing*) thinking |
| *Definition:* Judgments about oneself, personal experiences, or others are placed into one of two categories (e.g., all bad or all good, total failure or total success, completely flawed or completely perfect). |
| *Example:* Dan, a man with depression, compares himself with Ed, a friend who appears to have a good marriage and whose children are doing well in school. Although the friend has a fair amount of domestic happiness, his life is far from ideal. Ed has troubles at work, financial strains, and physical ailments, among other difficulties. Dan is engaging in absolutistic thinking when he tells himself, "Ed has everything going for him; I have nothing." |

2. **Intermediary beliefs and assumptions**

   *Definition:* Conditional rules such as if-then statements that influence self-esteem, emotional regulation, and behavior.

   *Examples:* "I must be perfect to be accepted"; "If I don't please others all the time, they will reject me"; "If I work hard, I can succeed."
3. **Core beliefs about the self**

   *Definition:* Global and absolute rules for interpreting environmental information related to self-esteem.

   *Examples:* "I'm unlovable"; "I'm stupid"; "I'm a failure"; "I am a good friend"; "I can trust others."

In our clinical practice, we typically do not try to explain the different levels of schemas (e.g., intermediary assumptions vs. core beliefs) to patients. We have found that most patients benefit more from recognizing the general concept that schemas or core beliefs (we use these terms interchangeably) have a strong influence on self-esteem and behavior. We also teach patients that all people have a mixture of adaptive (healthy) schemas and maladaptive core beliefs. Our goal in CBT is to identify and build up the adaptive schemas while attempting to modify or reduce the influence of maladaptive schemas. A short list of adaptive and maladaptive schemas is presented in Table 1–2.

The relationship between schemas and automatic thoughts has been detailed in the *stress-diathesis hypothesis.* Beck and others have suggested that in depression and other conditions, maladaptive schemas may remain dormant, or have reduced salience, until a stressful life event occurs that activates the core belief (Beck et al. 1979; D.A. Clark et al. 1999; Miranda 1992). The maladaptive schema is then strengthened to the point that it stimulates and drives the more superficial stream of negative auto-

**Table 1–2.** Adaptive and maladaptive schemas

| Adaptive schemas | Maladaptive schemas |
|---|---|
| No matter what happens, I can manage somehow. | If I choose to do something, I *must* succeed. |
| If I work at something, I can master it. | I'm stupid. |
| I'm a survivor. | I'm a fake. |
| Others can trust me. | I can never be comfortable around others. |
| I'm lovable. | Without a man (woman), I'm nothing. |
| People respect me. | I must be perfect to be accepted. |
| If I prepare in advance, I usually do better. | No matter what I do, I won't succeed. |
| There's not much that can scare me. | The world is too frightening for me. |

*Source.* Adapted from Wright et al. 2014.

matic thoughts. This phenomenon is illustrated in the treatment of Mark, a middle-aged man who became depressed after being laid off from a job.

Mark was not depressed before losing his job, but he began to have many self-doubts after he had trouble finding new work. When Mark looked at the employment section of his local newspaper, he was riddled with automatic thoughts such as "They won't want me"; "I'll never get a job as good as the last one"; "Even if I get an interview, I'll clutch and not know what to say." After starting CBT, the therapist was able to help Mark uncover several deeply held schemas about competence that had hovered below the surface for many years. One of these was "I'm never good enough," a core belief that had been quiescent in better times but was now stimulating a cascade of negative automatic thoughts every time he tried to find a job.

## Information Processing in Depression and Anxiety Disorders

In addition to the theories and methods for automatic thoughts, schemas, and cognitive errors, a number of other important contributions have influenced the development of cognitively oriented treatment interventions. We briefly describe some of these research findings on depression and anxiety disorders to provide an expanded theoretical background for treatment methods detailed in later chapters. The key features of patho-

**Table 1–3.** Pathological information processing in depression and anxiety disorders

| Predominant in depression | Predominant in anxiety disorders | Common to both depression and anxiety disorders |
|---|---|---|
| Hopelessness<br>Low self-esteem<br>Negative view of environment<br>Automatic thoughts with negative themes<br>Misattributions<br>Overestimates of negative feedback<br>Impaired performance on cognitive tasks requiring effort or abstract thinking | Fears of harm or danger<br>Increased attention to information about potential threats<br>Overestimates of risk in situations<br>Automatic thoughts associated with danger, risk, uncontrollability, incapacity<br>Underestimates of ability to cope with feared situations<br>Misinterpretations of bodily stimuli | Heightened automatic information processing<br>Maladaptive schemas<br>Increased frequency of cognitive errors<br>Reduced cognitive capacity for problem solving<br>Increased attention to self, especially perceived deficits or problems |

*Source.* Adapted from Wright et al. 2014.

logical information processing in depression and anxiety disorders are summarized in Table 1–3.

## The Link Between Hopelessness and Suicide

One of the most clinically relevant findings from research on depression is the association between hopelessness and suicide. A number of studies have demonstrated that depressed persons are likely to have high levels of hopelessness and that lack of hope raises the risk of suicide (Beck et al. 1975, 1985, 1990; Fawcett et al. 1987). Hopelessness was found to be the most important predictor of suicide in depressed inpatients who were followed up for 10 years after discharge (Beck et al. 1985). Similar findings were described in a related study with outpatients (Beck et al. 1990). Putting these observations to work, Brown, Beck, and colleagues (2005) found that cognitive therapy resulted in a lower rate of suicide attempts when compared to usual clinical care. This treatment included specific suicide prevention strategies such as conducting a narrative interview of recent suicidal crises to help guide treatment, developing a safety plan, identifying reasons for living, constructing a hope kit, and engaging patients in a guided imagery task to practicing using their skills during suicidal crises. Because we think that CBT methods for reducing suicide risk should be a basic clinical skill, we include a chapter on this topic later in the book (see Chapter 9, "Cognitive-Behavior Therapy to Reduce Suicide Risk").

## Attributional Style in Depression

Abramson et al. (1978) and others proposed that depressed persons assign meanings (attributions) to life events that are negatively distorted in three domains:

1. **Internal versus external.** Depression is associated with a tendency to make attributions to life events that are biased in an internal direction. Thus, depressed individuals commonly take excessive blame for negative events. In contrast, nondepressed persons are more likely to view noxious happenings as being due to external forces such as bad luck, fate, or the actions of others.
2. **Global versus specific.** Instead of viewing negative events as having only isolated or limited significance, people with depression may conclude that these occurrences have far-reaching, global, or all-encompassing implications. Persons who are not depressed have a better capacity to wall off negative events and prevent them from having a pervasive effect on self-esteem and behavioral responses.
3. **Fixed versus changeable.** In depression, negative or troubling situations may be viewed as being unchangeable and unlikely to improve in the future. A healthier style of thinking is observed in nondepressed persons, who more often believe that negative conditions or circumstances will recede with time (e.g., "This too will pass").

Research on attributional style in depression has been criticized because early studies were performed with students and nonclinical populations, and other investigations have produced inconsistent results. Nevertheless, the weight of evidence supports the concept that attributions can be distorted in depression and that CBT methods can be helpful in reversing this type of biased cognitive processing. In our clinical work, we have found that many depressed patients can readily grasp the concept that their thinking style is skewed in the direction of internal, global, and fixed attributions.

## Distortions in Response to Feedback

A series of investigations on responses to feedback have revealed differences between depressed and nondepressed persons that have significant implications for therapy. Depressed subjects have been found to underestimate the amount of positive feedback that is given and to expend less effort on tasks after they have been told that they have performed poorly. Nondepressed control subjects have shown patterns that may indicate a *positive self-serving bias*—they may hear more positive feedback than is actually given or downplay the significance of negative feedback (Alloy and Ahrens 1987).

Because a goal of CBT is to help patients develop an accurate and rational style of information processing, therapists need to recognize and address possible feedback distortions. One of the principal methods of doing this—providing and asking for detailed feedback in therapy sessions—is described in Chapter 2, "The Therapeutic Relationship: Collaborative Empiricism in Action," and Chapter 4, "Structuring and Educating." These techniques utilize the therapy experience as a learning opportunity for appropriately hearing, responding to, and giving feedback.

## Thinking Style in Anxiety Disorders

Persons who experience anxiety disorders have been shown to have several characteristic biases in information processing (see Table 1–3). One of these areas of dysfunction is a heightened level of attention to information in the environment about potential threats. For example, the woman with the elevator phobia described in Table 1–1 may hear sounds in an elevator that make her worry about its safety. A person who did not have this fear would probably pay little or no attention to these stimuli. People with anxiety disorders also commonly view the triggers for their fear as being unrealistically dangerous or likely to cause harm. Many individuals with panic disorder have fears that the panic attacks—or the situations that induce them—may cause catastrophic damage, perhaps even heart attacks, strokes, and death.

Other studies of information processing have shown that patients with anxiety disorders often have a diminished estimate of their ability to manage or cope with fear-laden situations; a sense of uncontrollability; and a high frequency of negative self-statements, misinterpretations of bodily stimuli, and overestimates of the risk for future calamities. Awareness of these different types of biased information processing can help clinicians plan and implement treatment for anxiety disorders.

## Learning, Memory, and Cognitive Capacity

Depression is often associated with significant impairments in ability to concentrate and in performance of challenging, effortful, or abstract learning and memory functions (Weingartner et al. 1981). Reductions in problem-solving capacity and task performance have also been observed in both depression and anxiety disorders (D.A. Clark et al. 1990). In CBT, these cognitive performance deficits are addressed with specific interventions (e.g., structuring, psychoeducational methods, and rehearsal) designed to enhance learning and assist patients in improving their problem-solving skills (see Chapter 4, "Structuring and Educating").

## Overview of Therapy Methods

When clinicians are beginning to learn CBT, they sometimes make the error of viewing this approach as just a collection of techniques or interventions. In doing so, they bypass some of the most important ingredients of CBT and go directly to the implementation of techniques such as thought recording, activity scheduling, or exposure therapy. It is easy to fall into this trap because CBT is well known for its effective interventions, and patients often like to get involved in specific exercises. However, if you focus prematurely or too heavily on implementing techniques, you will miss the essence of CBT.

Before choosing and applying techniques, you will need to develop an individualized conceptualization that directly ties cognitive-behavioral theories with the patient's unique psychological makeup and constellation of problems (see Chapter 3, "Assessment and Formulation"). The case conceptualization is an essential guide for the work of cognitive-behavior therapists. Other core features of CBT include a highly collaborative therapeutic relationship, artful application of Socratic questioning methods, and effective structuring and psychoeducation (Table 1–4). This book is designed to help you acquire crucial general skills in CBT, in addition to learning specific interventions for common psychiatric conditions. As a prelude to the detailed descriptions in later chapters, we provide a brief overview of treatment methods here.

### Therapy Length and Format

CBT is a problem-oriented therapy that is often delivered in a short-term format. Treatment for uncomplicated depression or anxiety disorders typically lasts from 5 to 20 sessions. However, longer courses of CBT may be necessary if there are comorbid conditions or if the patient has had chronic or treatment-resistant symptoms. CBT for personality disorders, psychosis, or bipolar disorder may need to be extended beyond 20 sessions. In addition, patients with chronic or recurrent illnesses may benefit

**Table 1–4.** Key methods of cognitive-behavior therapy (CBT)

| |
|---|
| Problem-oriented focus |
| Individualized case conceptualization |
| Collaborative empirical therapeutic relationship |
| Socratic questioning |
| Use of structuring, psychoeducation, and rehearsal to enhance learning |
| Eliciting and modifying automatic thoughts |
| Uncovering and changing schemas |
| Behavioral methods to reverse patterns of helplessness, self-defeating behavior, and avoidance |
| Building CBT skills to help prevent relapse |

from a therapy design in which most of the CBT is front-loaded (i.e., there are weekly or biweekly visits) in the first months of treatment, but the clinician continues to see the patient for intermittent booster sessions for longer periods of time. Psychiatrists who are experienced in this method may use CBT combined with pharmacotherapy in short sessions during the maintenance phase of recurrent depression, bipolar disorder, or other chronic illnesses.

In its traditional format, CBT is usually delivered in sessions lasting 45–50 minutes. However, there are opportunities for customizing the length of sessions to meet patient needs, improve the efficiency of treatment, and/or enhance outcome. For example, longer sessions, 90 or more minutes, have been successfully implemented for rapid treatment of patients with anxiety disorders (Öst et al. 2001) and may be especially useful for patients with posttraumatic stress disorder (McLean and Foa 2011) or obsessive-compulsive disorder (Foa 2010). Sessions of less than 50 minutes are usually recommended for inpatients, persons with psychosis, and others with severe symptoms that substantially interfere with concentration (Kingdon and Turkington 2004; Stuart et al. 1997; Wright et al. 2009). Also, as detailed in Chapter 4, "Structuring and Educating," brief sessions have been shown to be effective for treatment of depression if combined with use of a skill-building computer program for CBT (Thase et al. 2017; Wright 2016; Wright et al. 2005).

Another format for abbreviated therapy sessions can be used by psychiatrists or nurse practitioners who are experienced in CBT. Brief sessions may be employed, along with medications and treatment adjuncts such as computer-assisted therapy and self-help books, as an alternative to the traditional "50-minute hour." The two psychiatrists (J.H.W. and M.E.T.) who are authors of this volume use the brief-session format with a portion of their patients, and have coauthored another book, *High-Yield Cognitive-Behavior Therapy for Brief Sessions: An Illustrated Guide* (Wright et al. 2010), for clinicians who want to learn about alternative delivery methods. We recommend that trainees and other students of CBT first learn how to implement treatment in the traditional 45- to 50-minute format. A solid grounding in basic methods is needed as a foundation prior to attempts to reduce the length of sessions.

## Focus on the "Here and Now"

A "here and now" problem-oriented approach is emphasized because attention to current issues helps stimulate the development of action plans to counter symptoms such as hopelessness, helplessness, avoidance, and procrastination. Also, cognitive and behavioral responses to recent events are more accessible and verifiable than responses to occurrences in the distant past. An additional benefit of working primarily on current functioning is a reduction in dependence and regression in the therapeutic relationship.

Although CBT interventions are typically focused on present events, thoughts, emotions, and behaviors, a longitudinal perspective—including consideration of early childhood development, family background, traumas, positive and negative formative experiences, education, work history, and social influences—is critical to fully understanding the patient and planning treatment.

## Case Conceptualization

When we are in CBT sessions and are doing our best work, we sense that the case conceptualization is directly guiding each question, each nonverbal response, each intervention, and the myriad adjustments we make in therapy style to enhance communication with the patient. In other words, we have a carefully thought out strategy and are not doing therapy by the seat of our pants. As you learn to become an effective cognitive-behavior therapist, you will need to practice developing formulations that bring together information from the diagnostic assessment, observations on the unique background of the patient, and cognitive-behavioral theory in a detailed treatment plan. Case conceptualization methods are explained in Chapter 3, "Assessment and Formulation."

## Therapeutic Relationship

A number of the features of helpful therapeutic relationships are shared between CBT, psychodynamic therapy, nondirective therapies, and other common forms of psychotherapy. These attributes include understanding, kindness, and empathy. Like all good therapists, practitioners of CBT should have the ability to generate trust and demonstrate equanimity under pressure. However, in comparison to other well-known therapies, the therapeutic relationship in CBT differs in being oriented toward a high degree of collaboration, a strongly empirical focus, and the use of action-oriented interventions.

Beck and associates (1979) coined the term *collaborative empiricism* to describe the patient-therapist relationship in CBT. The patient and therapist work together much as an investigative team, developing hypotheses about the accuracy or coping value of a variety of cognitions and behaviors. They then collaborate on developing a healthier style of thinking, building coping skills, and reversing unproductive patterns of behavior. Cognitive-behavior therapists are typically more active than those who practice other forms of therapy. They help structure sessions, give feedback, and coach patients on how to build CBT skills.

Patients are also encouraged to assume significant responsibility in the treatment relationship. They are asked to give the therapist feedback, to help set the agenda for therapy sessions, and to work on practicing CBT interventions in everyday life situations. Overall, the therapeutic relationship in CBT is characterized by openness in communication and a work-oriented, pragmatic, team-oriented approach to managing problems.

## Socratic Questioning

The style of questioning used in CBT is consistent with a collaborative empirical relationship and the goal of helping patients recognize and change maladaptive thinking. *Socratic questioning* involves asking the patient questions that stimulate curiosity and inquisitiveness. Instead of a didactic presentation of therapy concepts, the clinician tries to get the patient involved in the learning process. A specialized form of Socratic questioning is *guided discovery,* in which the therapist asks a series of questions to reveal dysfunctional thought patterns or behavior.

## Structuring and Psychoeducation

CBT uses structuring methods such as agenda setting and feedback to maximize the efficiency of treatment sessions, help patients organize their efforts toward recovery, and enhance learning. An effort is made to state therapy agendas in terms that give clear direction for the session and permit measurement of progress. For example, well-articulated agenda items might be "develop a plan to get back to work"; "reduce the tension in my relationship with my son"; or "find ways to get over the divorce."

During the session, the therapist guides the patient in using the agenda to productively explore important topics and tries to avoid digressions that have little chance of helping achieve treatment goals. However, therapists have considerable latitude to deviate from the agenda if important new topics or ideas are identified or if staying with the current agenda is not producing the desired results. Regular feedback is given and received by both patient and therapist to check on understanding and to shape the direction of the session.

A variety of psychoeducational methods are used in CBT. Teaching experiences in sessions typically involve using situations from the patient's life to illustrate concepts. Usually the therapist gives brief explanations and follows them with questions that promote the patient's involvement in the learning process. A number of tools are available to assist therapists in providing psychoeducation. Examples are readings in self-help books, handouts, rating scales, and computer programs. A full description of these tools is provided in Chapter 4, "Structuring and Educating."

## Cognitive Restructuring

A large part of CBT is devoted to helping the patient recognize and change maladaptive automatic thoughts and schemas. The most frequently used method is Socratic questioning. Thought records are also heavily utilized in CBT. Capturing automatic thoughts on a written form can often kindle a more rational style of thinking.

Other commonly used methods include identifying cognitive errors, examining the evidence (pro-con analyses), reattribution (modifying attributional style), listing rational alternatives, and cognitive rehearsal. The latter technique involves practicing a new way of thinking by imagery or role-play. This may be done in treatment sessions with the therapist's assistance. Or, after patients gain experience in using rehearsal methods, they can carry out assignments to practice on their own at home.

The overall strategy of cognitive restructuring is to identify automatic thoughts and schemas in therapy sessions, teach patients skills for changing cognitions, and then have patients perform a series of homework exercises designed to extend therapy lessons to real-world situations. Repeated practice is usually needed before patients can readily modify ingrained, maladaptive cognitions.

## Behavioral Methods

The CBT model emphasizes that the relationship between cognition and behavior is a two-way street. The cognitive interventions described above, if successfully implemented, are likely to have salutary effects on behavior. Likewise, positive changes in behavior are typically associated with an improved outlook or other desired cognitive modifications.

Most behavioral techniques used in CBT are designed to help people 1) increase participation in activities that improve mood, 2) change patterns of avoidance or helplessness, 3) gradually face feared situations, 4) build coping skills, and 5) reduce painful emotions or autonomic arousal. In Chapter 6, "Behavioral Methods I: Improving Mood, Increasing Energy, Completing Tasks, and Solving Problems," and Chapter 7, "Behavioral Methods II: Reducing Anxiety and Breaking Patterns of Avoidance," we detail effective behavioral methods for depression and anxiety disorders. Some of the most important interventions that you will learn are behavioral activation, hierarchical exposure (systematic desensitization), graded task assignments, activity and pleasant events scheduling, breathing training, and relaxation training. These techniques can provide you with powerful tools for helping to reduce symptoms and promote positive change.

## Building CBT Skills to Prevent Relapse

One of the bonuses of the CBT approach is the acquisition of skills that can reduce the risk for relapse. Learning how to recognize and change automatic thoughts, use common behavioral methods, and implement the other interventions described earlier in this chapter can help patients manage future triggers for the return of symptoms. For example, a person who learns to recognize cognitive errors in automatic thoughts may be better able to avoid catastrophic thinking in stressful situations encountered after therapy ends. During the later phases of CBT, the therapist often focuses specifically on relapse prevention by helping the patient identify potential problems that have a high likelihood of causing difficulty. Then rehearsal techniques are used to practice effective ways of coping.

To illustrate the CBT approach to relapse prevention, consider the case of a person who is being discharged from an inpatient unit after a suicide attempt. Although the individual may be much improved and not currently suicidal, a good cognitive-behavioral treatment plan would include discussion of the possible challenges of return to home and work, followed by coaching on ways to respond to these challenges. CBT with this patient also would include the development of a specific safety plan.

## Summary

CBT is one of the most widely practiced forms of psychotherapy for psychiatric disorders. This treatment approach is based on precepts about the role of cognition in controlling human emotion and behavior that have been traced to the writings of philosophers from ancient times to the present. The constructs that define CBT were developed by Aaron T. Beck and other influential psychiatrists and psychologists beginning in the 1960s. CBT is distinguished by the large amount of empirical research that has examined its basic theories and has demonstrated the efficacy of treatment.

The learning process for becoming a skilled cognitive-behavior therapist involves studying basic theories and methods, viewing examples of CBT interventions, and practicing this treatment approach with patients. In this chapter, we introduced the core concepts of CBT, such as the cognitive-behavioral model, the importance of recognizing and modifying automatic thoughts, the influence of schemas in information processing and psychopathology, and the key function of behavioral principles in designing treatment interventions. The chapters that follow give detailed explanations and illustrations of how to put the basic principles of CBT to work.

## References

Abramson LY, Seligman MEP, Teasdale JD: Learned helplessness in humans: critique and reformulation. J Abnorm Psychol 87(1):49–74, 1978 649856

Addis ME, Martell CR: Overcoming Depression One Step at a Time: The New Behavioral Activation Approach to Getting Your Life Back. Oakland, CA, New Harbinger, 2004

Alloy LB, Ahrens AH: Depression and pessimism for the future: biased use of statistically relevant information in predictions for self versus others. J Pers Soc Psychol 52(2):366–378, 1987 3559896

Bandelow B, Reitt M, Röver C, et al: Efficacy of treatments for anxiety disorders: a meta-analysis. Int Clin Psychopharmacol 30(4):183–192, 2015 25932596

Barlow DH, Cerney JA: Psychological Treatment of Panic. New York, Guilford, 1988

Barlow DH, Craske MG, Cerney JA, et al: Behavioral treatment of panic disorder. Behav Ther 20:261–268, 1989

Beck AT: Thinking and depression. Arch Gen Psychiatry 9:324–333, 1963 14045261

Beck AT: Thinking and depression, II: theory and therapy. Arch Gen Psychiatry 10:561–571, 1964 14159256

Beck AT, Kovacs M, Weissman A: Hopelessness and suicidal behavior: an overview. JAMA 234(11):1146–1149, 1975 1242427

Beck AT, Rush AJ, Shaw BF, et al: Cognitive Therapy of Depression. New York, Guilford, 1979

Beck AT, Steer RA, Kovacs M, Garrison B: Hopelessness and eventual suicide: a 10-year prospective study of patients hospitalized with suicidal ideation. Am J Psychiatry 142(5):559–563, 1985 3985195

Beck AT, Brown G, Berchick RJ, et al: Relationship between hopelessness and ultimate suicide: a replication with psychiatric outpatients. Am J Psychiatry 147(2):190–195, 1990 2278535

Blackburn IM, Jones S, Lewin RJP: Cognitive style in depression. Br J Clin Psychol 25 (Pt 4):241–251, 1986 3801730

Bowlby J: The role of childhood experience in cognitive disturbance, in Cognition and Psychotherapy. Edited by Mahoney MJ, Freeman A. New York, Plenum, 1985, pp 181–200

Brown GK, Ten Have T, Henriques GR, et al: Cognitive therapy for the prevention of suicide attempts: a randomized controlled trial. JAMA 294(5):563–570, 2005 16077050

Butler AC, Beck JS: Cognitive therapy outcomes: a review of meta-analyses. Journal of the Norwegian Psychological Association 37:1–9, 2000

Campos PE: Special series: integrating Buddhist philosophy with cognitive and behavioral practice. Cogn Behav Pract 9:38–40, 2002

Clark DA, Beck AT, Stewart B: Cognitive specificity and positive-negative affectivity: complementary or contradictory views on anxiety and depression? J Abnorm Psychol 99(2):148–155, 1990 2348008

Clark DA, Beck AT, Alford BA: Scientific Foundations of Cognitive Theory and Therapy of Depression. New York, Wiley, 1999

Clark DM: A cognitive approach to panic. Behav Res Ther 24(4):461–470, 1986 3741311

Clark DM, Salkovskis PM, Hackmann A, et al: A comparison of cognitive therapy, applied relaxation and imipramine in the treatment of panic disorder. Br J Psychiatry 164(6):759–769, 1994 7952982

Cuijpers P, Berking M, Andersson G, et al: A meta-analysis of cognitive-behavioural therapy for adult depression, alone and in comparison with other treatments. Can J Psychiatry 58:376–385, 2013 23870719

Dalai Lama: Ethics for the New Millennium. New York, Riverhead Books, 1999

Dobson KS, Shaw BF: Cognitive assessment with major depressive disorders. Cognit Ther Res 10:13–29, 1986

Epictetus: Enchiridion. Translated by George Long. Amherst, NY, Prometheus Books, 1991

Eysenck HJ: The Effects of Psychotherapy. New York, International Science Press, 1966

Fawcett J, Scheftner W, Clark D, et al: Clinical predictors of suicide in patients with major affective disorders: a controlled prospective study. Am J Psychiatry 144(1):35–40, 1987 3799837

Foa EB: Cognitive behavioral therapy of obsessive-compulsive disorder. Dialogues Clin Neurosci 12:199–207, 2010 20623924

Frankl VE: Man's Search for Meaning: An Introduction to Logotherapy. Boston, MA, Beacon Press, 1992

Haaga DA, Dyck MJ, Ernst D: Empirical status of cognitive theory of depression. Psychol Bull 110(2):215–236, 1991 1946867

Hollon SD, Kendall PC, Lumry A: Specificity of depressotypic cognitions in clinical depression. J Abnorm Psychol 95(1):52–59, 1986 3700847

Hollon SD, DeRubeis RJ, Fawcett J, et al: Effect of cognitive therapy with antidepressant medications vs antidepressants alone on the rate of recovery in major depressive disorder: a randomized clinical trial. JAMA Psychiatry 71(10):1157–1164, 2014 25142196

Ingram RE, Kendall PC: The cognitive side of anxiety. Cognit Ther Res 11:523–536, 1987

Isaacson W: Benjamin Franklin: An American Life. New York, Simon & Schuster, 2003

Kelly G: The Psychology of Personal Constructs. New York, WW Norton, 1955

Kendall PC, Hollon SD: Anxious self-talk: development of the Anxious Self-Statements Questionnaire (ASSQ). Cognit Ther Res 13:81–93, 1989

Kingdon DG, Turkington D: Cognitive Therapy of Schizophrenia. New York, Guilford, 2004

Lam DH, Watkins ER, Hayward P, et al: A randomized controlled study of cognitive therapy for relapse prevention for bipolar affective disorder: outcome of the first year. Arch Gen Psychiatry 60(2):145–152, 2003 12578431

Lefebvre MF: Cognitive distortion and cognitive errors in depressed psychiatric and low back pain patients. J Consult Clin Psychol 49(4):517–525, 1981 6455451

Lewinsohn PM, Hoberman HM, Teri L, et al: An integrative theory of depression, in Theoretical Issues in Behavior Therapy. Edited by Reiss S, Bootzin R. New York, Academic Press, 1985, pp 331–359

Marks IM, Swinson RP, Basoglu M, et al: Alprazolam and exposure alone and combined in panic disorder with agoraphobia: a controlled study in London and Toronto. Br J Psychiatry 162:776–787, 1993 8101126

McGrath CL, Kelley ME, Holtzheimer PE, et al: Toward a neuroimaging treatment selection biomarker for major depressive disorder. JAMA Psychiatry 70(8):821–829, 2013 23760393

McLean CP, Foa EB: Prolonged exposure therapy for post-traumatic stress disorder: a review of evidence and dissemination. Expert Rev Neurother 11(8):1151–1163, 2011 21797656

Meichenbaum DH: Cognitive-Behavior Modification: An Integrative Approach. New York, Plenum, 1977

Miranda J: Dysfunctional thinking is activated by stressful life events. Cognit Ther Res 16:473–483, 1992

Öst LG, Alm T, Brandberg M, Breitholtz E: One vs five sessions of exposure and five sessions of cognitive therapy in the treatment of claustrophobia. Behav Res Ther 39(2):167–183, 2001 11153971

Rachman S: The evolution of cognitive behavior therapy, in Science and Practice of Cognitive Behavior Therapy. Edited by Clark DM, Fairburn CG. New York, Oxford University Press, 1997, pp 3–26

Raimy V: Misunderstandings of the Self. San Francisco, CA, Jossey-Bass, 1975

Rector NA, Beck AT: Cognitive behavioral therapy for schizophrenia: an empirical review. J Nerv Ment Dis 189(5):278–287, 2001 11379970

Sternberg RJ: Cognitive Psychology. Fort Worth, TX, Harcourt Brace, 1996

Stuart S, Wright JH, Thase ME, Beck AT: Cognitive therapy with inpatients. Gen Hosp Psychiatry 19(1):42–50, 1997 9034811

Thase ME, Wright JH, Eells TD, et al: Improving efficiency and reducing cost of psychotherapy for depression: computer-assisted cognitive-behavior therapy versus standard cognitive-behavior therapy. Unpublished paper submitted for publication; data available on request from authors. Philadelphia, PA, January 2017

Watkins JT, Rush AJ: Cognitive Response Test. Cognit Ther Res 7:125–126, 1983

Weingartner H, Cohen RM, Murphy DL, et al: Cognitive processes in depression. Arch Gen Psychiatry 38(1):42–47, 1981 7458568

Wolpe J: Psychotherapy by Reciprocal Inhibition. Stanford, CA, Stanford University Press, 1958

Wright JH: Integrating cognitive-behavioral therapy and pharmacotherapy, in Contemporary Cognitive Therapy: Theory, Research, and Practice. Edited by Leahy RL. New York, Guilford, 2004, pp 341–366

Wright JH: Computer-assisted cognitive-behavior therapy for depression: progress and opportunities. Presented at National Network of Depression Centers Annual Conference, Denver, Colorado, September, 2016

Wright JH, Thase ME: Cognitive and biological therapies: a synthesis. Psychiatr Ann 22:451–458, 1992

Wright JH, Wright AS, Albano AM, et al: Computer-assisted cognitive therapy for depression: maintaining efficacy while reducing therapist time. Am J Psychiatry 162(6):1158–1164, 2005 15930065

Wright JH, Turkington D, Kingdon DG, Basco MR: Cognitive-Behavior Therapy for Severe Mental Illness: An Illustrated Guide. Washington, DC, American Psychiatric Publishing, 2009

Wright JH, Sudak DM, Turkington D, Thase ME: High-Yield Cognitive-Behavior Therapy for Brief Sessions: An Illustrated Guide. Washington, DC, American Psychiatric Publishing, 2010

Wright JH, Thase ME, Beck AT: Cognitive-behavior therapy, in The American Psychiatric Publishing Textbook of Psychiatry, 6th Edition. Edited by Hales RE, Yudofsky SC, Roberts L. Washington, DC, American Psychiatric Publishing, 2014, pp 1119-1160

# 2

# The Therapeutic Relationship

## Collaborative Empiricism in Action

One of the appealing features of cognitive-behavior therapy (CBT) is the collaborative, straightforward, and action-oriented style of the therapeutic relationship that it employs. Although the relationship between therapist and patient is not considered to be the principal mechanism for change as in some other forms of psychotherapy, a good working alliance is a critically important part of treatment (Beck et al. 1979). Just like clinicians who use other major forms of psychotherapy, cognitive-behavior therapists seek to provide a treatment environment with a high degree of genuineness, warmth, positive regard, and accurate empathy—the common qualities of all effective therapies (Beck et al. 1979; Keijsers et al. 2000; Rogers 1957). In addition to these nonspecific features of the therapeutic relationship, CBT is characterized by a specific type of working alliance, *collaborative empiricism*, that is geared toward promoting cognitive and behavioral change.

Research on the therapeutic relationship in multiple types of psychotherapy has repeatedly shown a powerful association between treatment outcome and the strength of the therapist-patient bond (Beitman et al. 1989; Klein et al. 2003; Wright and Davis 1994). A review of investigations of the therapeutic relationship in CBT also revealed that the quality of the cognitive-behavioral therapeutic alliance influences the results of treatment (Keijsers et al. 2000). Thus, there is substantial evidence that efforts to build therapeutic CBT relationships have a strong impact on the course of treatment.

Learning to forge the most effective therapist-patient relationships is a career-long journey. All clinicians start the process with basic building blocks from their experiences in prior relationships. Among the typical reasons that people choose therapy as a profession is that they have the innate ability to understand others and to discuss emotionally charged topics with considerable sensitivity, kindness, and equanimity. However, learning to maximize these talents usually requires substantial amounts of clinical experience, along with case supervision and personal introspection. As an introduction to the therapeutic relationship in CBT, we briefly discuss the nonspecific features of treatment and then turn to the main focus of this chapter: the collaborative empirical working alliance.

## Empathy, Warmth, and Genuineness

From a cognitive-behavioral perspective, accurate empathy involves the capacity to place yourself in the position of patients so you can sense what they are feeling and thinking while retaining objectivity for sorting out possible distortions, illogical reasoning, or maladaptive behavior that may be contributing to the problem. Beck and coworkers (1979) emphasized that it is crucial to properly regulate the amount of empathy and associated personal warmth. If the therapist is perceived as distant, cold, and unconcerned, the prospects for a good treatment outcome will be diminished. However, an overdone effort to be warm and empathic can also backfire. For example, a person with long-standing poor self-esteem or lack of basic trust could perceive an overzealous therapist's attempts to be understanding in a negative light (e.g., "Why should she care so much about a loser like me? The therapist must be lonely herself if she is trying so hard to get to know me. What is the therapist trying to get from me?").

Timing is also very important in making empathic comments. A common mistake is to weigh in heavily with attempts at empathy before patients sense that you adequately understand their plight. However, if you ignore a major display of emotional pain, even in the earliest phases of therapy, you may be seen as disconnected or unresponsive. Here are some good questions to ask yourself as you consider making empathic comments: How well do I understand this person's life circumstances and thinking style? Is this a good time to show empathy? How much empathy is needed now? Are there any risks to being empathic at this time with this patient?

Although well-placed empathic comments usually help strengthen the relationship and relieve emotional tension, there are instances in which attempts to be understanding can reinforce negatively distorted cognitions. For example, if you continually make assurances such as "I can understand the way you feel" to patients who believe that they have failed or their life is unmanageable, you may inadvertently validate their self-condemning and hopeless attitudes. If you are engaged in active listening and are repeatedly nodding your head "yes" while the patient expresses a litany of maladaptive cognitions, she may think that you agree with her conclusions. Or if you have a patient with agoraphobia and you feel so much empathy about the emotional pain of the disorder that you neglect using behavioral methods to break patterns of avoidance, the effectiveness of the therapy may be compromised.

One of the most important keys to showing accurate empathy is genuineness. Therapists who exhibit genuineness are able to communicate verbally and nonverbally in an honest, natural, and emotionally connected manner to show patients that they truly understand the situation. The genuine therapist is diplomatic in giving constructive feedback to patients but does not try to hide the truth. Actual negative events and outcomes are acknowledged as such, but the therapist is always trying to find strengths in patients that will help them cope better with the vicissitudes of life. Thus, one of the desirable personal characteristics of cognitive-behavior therapists is a genuine sense of optimism and a belief in the resilience and growth potential of patients.

Full expression of accurate empathy in CBT includes a vigorous search for solutions. It is not enough to show sensitive concern. The therapist needs to convert this concern into actions that reduce suffering and help the patient manage life problems. Therefore, the cognitive-behavior therapist blends appropriate empathic comments with Socratic questions and other CBT methods that encourage rational thinking and the development of healthy coping behaviors. Often the most effective empathic response involves asking questions that help the patient see new perspectives, instead of simply going along with the flow of a dysfunctional stream of thinking.

## Collaborative Empiricism

The term most often used to describe the therapeutic relationship in CBT is *collaborative empiricism*. These two words do a good job of capturing the essence of the treatment alliance. The therapist engages the patient in a highly collaborative process in which there is a shared responsibility for setting goals and agendas, giving and receiving feedback, and putting CBT methods into action in everyday life. Together the therapist and patient target problematic thoughts and behaviors, which are then scrutinized empirically for validity or utility. When actual flaws or deficits are detected, coping strategies for these difficulties are designed and practiced. However, the main job of the therapeutic relationship is to view cognitive distortions and unproductive behavioral patterns through an empirical lens that can reveal opportunities for increased rationality, symptom relief, and improved personal effectiveness.

The collaborative empirical style of the treatment relationship is illustrated throughout this book in a series of brief videos that demonstrate core CBT methods. We suggest you view two of these vignettes now from Dr. Wright's treatment of Kate, a woman with anxiety disorder. The first example is from an early session in which Dr. Wright is helping Kate understand how CBT can help her reverse a pattern of fearful thoughts, anxious emotions, and avoidance of the triggers for anxiety. Therapist and patient are building a solid relationship that will allow them to make progress toward reducing her symptoms. In the second example, Kate is being encouraged to take an empirical approach to modifying a set of maladaptive cognitions. A good treatment alliance is an essential requirement for doing this type of therapeutic work.

Before you watch the first video, we want to make a few suggestions on how to get the most out of viewing these demonstrations. As noted in the Preface, our goal in producing the video illustrations was to provide examples of how clinicians might implement CBT in actual sessions. The videos were not scripted tightly or designed to be perfect illustrations of the only possible way to treat each situation. Although we asked the clinicians to give the intervention their best effort, and we believe that the videos generally represent solid CBT interventions, you may think of alternative methods or variations in therapy style that might have worked better.

When we show videos in our classes, even when they are sessions conducted by masters such as Aaron T. Beck, we routinely find both strengths and opportunities for the therapist to do things differently. Therefore, we recommend that you ask yourself these types of questions when you view the video illustrations in this book: How did this vignette demonstrate the key principles of CBT? What did I like about the therapist's style? What, if anything, would I have done differently? It also may be useful to view the videos with a colleague or supervisor to compare notes and to generate additional ideas for therapy interventions. Finally, we want to remind you that the videos are designed to be watched in sequence at the point in the book where you are reading about the specific method illustrated in the vignette.

**Video 1.** Getting Started—CBT in Action: Dr. Wright and Kate (12:17)

**Video 2.** Modifying Automatic Thoughts: Dr. Wright and Kate (8:48)

## Therapist Activity Level in CBT

In addition to the nonspecific relationship qualities common to all effective therapists, cognitive-behavior therapists need to become proficient in demonstrating high levels of activity in treatment sessions. Cognitive-behavior therapists typically work intently at structuring therapy, pacing sessions to get the most out of the available time, developing an ever-evolving case formulation, and implementing CBT methods.

Therapists' activity levels are usually the highest in the early phases of treatment, when patients are more symptomatic and are being socialized to the cognitive-behavioral model. During this part of treatment, the therapist will typically shoulder most of the responsibility for directing the flow of sessions and will spend considerable time explaining and illustrating basic CBT concepts (see Chapter 4, "Structuring and Educating"). The therapist also may need to inject energy, animation, and a sense of hopefulness into the therapy, especially when the patient is severely depressed and is exhibiting pronounced anhedonia or psychomotor slowing. The following case example from the treatment of a depressed man demonstrates how the clinician may sometimes need to be quite active in helping the patient grasp and use CBT methods.

### Case Example

Matt was asked to do a thought record for homework after his second session but had trouble completing the assignment.

*Therapist:* We said that we would spend some time reviewing your homework from last week. How did it go?

*Matt:* I don't know. I gave it a try, but I was really tired after coming home every night. I never seemed to have enough time to work on it. *(Opens his therapy notebook and takes out the homework.)*

*Therapist:* Can we take a look at what you wrote on the sheet?

*Matt:* Sure, but I don't think I did a very good job with it.

The therapist and Matt look at Matt's thought record. The first column has an event ("Wife told me I wasn't fun anymore"); the second column (Thoughts) has no entries; and the third column includes a rating of his feelings ("Sad, 100%").

*Therapist:* Matt, I can tell that you are getting down on yourself about the homework. Sometimes when people are depressed, it's hard to do this sort of thing. But you did give it a good try, and you did identify a situation that stirred up lots of feelings. If it's all right with you, we can work on completing the other columns here.

*Matt (appearing relieved):* I was worried that I messed it up and that you would think I wasn't trying.

*Therapist:* No, I won't judge you. I just want to help you use these types of exercises to get better. Are you ready to talk about what happened when your wife made that remark?

*Matt:* Yes.

*Therapist:* I noticed that you wrote down the event and the sad feelings that occurred. But you didn't put anything down in the thoughts column. Can you think back to when your wife told you that you weren't any fun anymore and try to remember what might have been going through your mind when that happened?

*Matt:* It just blew me out of the water. It had been a hard day at work. So, after I came home, I sort of collapsed into my chair and started to read the paper. Then she really laid into me. I guess it upset me so much, I didn't want to write down what I was thinking.

*Therapist:* That's understandable. I can see that it really upset you. But if we can find out what you were thinking, we may be able to find some clues for ways to fight your depression.

*Matt:* I can tell you about it now.

*Therapist:* Let's use this thought record and write down some of the thoughts that you were having at the time. *(Takes thought record and is poised to write.)*

*Matt:* Well, I guess the first thought was "She's had it with me." Then I started seeing all the important things in my life slipping away.

*Therapist:* What were you thinking that you were going to lose?

*Matt:* I was thinking, "She's bound to leave me. I'll lose my family and my kids. My whole life will fall apart."

*Therapist:* Those are upsetting thoughts. Do you think they are completely accurate? I wonder if depression could be influencing your thinking?

The therapist then explained the nature of automatic thoughts and helped Matt examine the evidence for this stream of negative cognitions. As a result of the intervention, Matt concluded that it was highly likely that his wife was committed to keeping the relationship going but was

> growing frustrated with his depression. Matt's level of sadness and tension was reduced as the absolutistic nature of his cognitions faded and a behavioral plan was developed to respond to his wife's concerns. This example demonstrates how the therapist may need to take a very active role in explaining concepts, demonstrating central tenets of CBT, and assisting patients in becoming fully engaged in the treatment process.

You might have noted that the therapist talked more than Matt during much of this interchange. Although there is a great deal of variability from patient to patient and from session to session in how much the therapist will need to talk in CBT, early sessions may be marked by segments with a relatively high level of verbal activity by the therapist. Usually as therapy progresses and patients learn how to use CBT concepts, the therapist will be able to get points across, show empathic concern, and move therapy ahead with fewer words and less effort.

## The Therapist as a Teacher-Coach

Do you like to teach? Have you had experiences either being coached or coaching others? Because of the significant importance of learning in CBT, the treatment relationship has more of a teacher–student quality than in most other therapies. Good teacher-coaches in CBT transmit knowledge in a highly collaborative way, using the Socratic method to encourage the patient to be fully involved in the learning process. The following attributes of the therapeutic relationship can promote effective teaching and coaching:

- **Friendly.** Patients typically perceive good therapist-teachers as friendly and kind persons who do not intimidate, prod excessively, or admonish. They convey information in a positive and constructive manner.
- **Engaging.** To be especially effective in the teacher role in CBT, you will need to create a stimulating learning environment. Engage patients with Socratic questions and learning exercises that energize the therapy, but do not overwhelm them with more material or more complexity than they can handle. Emphasize teamwork and the collaborative process in learning.
- **Creative.** Because patients often come to therapy with a fixed, monocular style of thinking, clinicians may need to model more creative ways of viewing the situation and searching for solutions. Try to use learning methods that draw out the patient's own creativity and put these strengths to work in coping with problems.
- **Empowering.** Good teaching usually involves giving patients ideas or tools that allow them to make significant changes in their lives. The

empowering nature of CBT is heavily dependent on the educational nature of the therapeutic relationship.

- **Action oriented.** Learning in CBT is not a passive, armchair-style process. Therapist and patient work together to acquire knowledge that is put into action in real-life situations.

## Using Humor in CBT

Why should you consider using humor in CBT? After all, most of our patients are facing very serious problems such as the death of loved ones, the breakup of their marriages, medical illnesses, and the ravages of mental illnesses. Could attempts at humor be misconstrued as meaning that you are trying to trivialize, brush off, or ignore the gravity of the patient's problems? Could the patient see your effort to be humorous as a put-down? Is there a chance that the patient will think you are laughing *at* him instead of *with* him?

Of course there are risks in using humor in therapy. Clinicians need to be very careful to recognize potential pitfalls and to gauge the patient's ability to benefit from an injection of humor into the relationship. However, humor can have many positive effects on the patient's ability to recognize cognitive distortions, express healthy emotions, and experience pleasure. For many persons, humor is a highly adaptive coping strategy. It brings emotional release, laughter, and fun into their lives (Kuhn 2002). Yet when patients come to therapy, they often have lost or experienced a major decline in their sense of humor.

There are three main reasons to use humor in CBT. First, humor can normalize and humanize the treatment alliance. Because humor is such an important part of life and is often a component of good relationships, judicious and well-placed humorous comments can help promote the friendly, collaborative nature of CBT. The second reason to use humor is to assist patients with breaking out of rigid patterns of thinking and behaving. If the therapist and patient can gently laugh together about the foibles of extreme ways of viewing situations, the patient may be more likely to consider and adopt cognitive changes. The third reason for drawing on the potential of humor in CBT is the possibility that humor skills can be uncovered, strengthened, and enhanced as an important resource for fighting symptoms and coping with stress.

Humor in CBT rarely involves the therapist or the patient cracking jokes. A much more likely scenario involves the use of hyperbole in describing the impact of holding maladaptive beliefs or of persisting with a rigid, ineffective behavioral pattern. Key elements of this type of humor are that it be 1) spontaneous and genuine, 2) constructive, and 3) focused on an external problem or an incongruous way of thinking instead of a personal weakness. Humor that follows these guidelines can loosen the grip of a rigid, dysfunctional set of cognitions or behaviors. Video 2 includes several examples of the therapeutic use of humor in CBT. Dr. Wright and Kate were able to laugh together as they made progress in using the CBT model to attack Kate's anxiety symptoms.

Some therapists are naturally adept at using gentle humor in sessions, whereas others find this aspect of therapy awkward or difficult. Humor is by no means an essential part of CBT. So if you don't like to employ humor or don't have these skills, you can de-emphasize this aspect of therapy and focus on other elements of the collaborative empirical relationship. However, we still recommend that you ask patients if their sense of humor is one of their strengths and that you help them use their sense of humor as a positive coping strategy.

## Flexibility and Sensitivity

Because patients come to treatment with a wide variety of expectations, life experiences, symptoms, and personality traits, therapists need to be attuned to individual differences as they attempt to develop effective working relationships. A monolithic, one-size-fits-all type of therapeutic relationship should be avoided in favor of a flexible, individually tailored style that is sensitive to the unique characteristics of each patient. We suggest that you consider influences from three major domains of clinical interest when customizing treatment alliances: 1) situational issues, 2) sociocultural background, and 3) diagnosis and symptoms (Wright and Davis 1994).

### *Situational Issues*

Current life stresses such as bereavement after the death of a loved one, separation or divorce, job loss, financial problems, or medical illnesses may require adjustments in the therapeutic relationship. An example from our clinical practices is the treatment of a depressed woman who had recently experienced the death of her teenage son from suicide. Because of her profound grief, the therapist needed to make great efforts to be empathic, understanding, and supportive. Typical cognitive-behavioral interventions such as thought recording and examining the evidence were not used in the early part of this treatment because the therapist could better respond to the patient's gaping personal wounds by employing warm concern, active listening, and behavioral interventions to help her resume functioning in everyday life.

Environmental influences or stressors may at times lead patients to make special requests. A patient who is having a troubled marital relationship may ask that bills for therapy not be sent to his home, so that his wife will not know that he is seeing a therapist. A person who has had a surgical complication and is thinking of suing his doctor may stipulate that the surgeon not be contacted to provide medical records. A woman who is involved in a child custody battle may ask the therapist to be her advocate in court. Our general rule for responding to such requests early in therapy is to accept them at face value and to try to meet the patient's expectations unless there is an ethical conflict or professional boundary issue to consider. However, some patients may have expectations that are unrealistic or potentially damaging. Requests, either direct or implicit, for extensive friendship or physical intimacy need to be recognized and managed with firm, ethically responsible guidelines (Gutheil and Gabbard 1993; Wright and Davis 1994). Some other types of requests—such as for extending sessions beyond the normal time frame or for responding to a plethora of phone calls from the patient—may have a negative impact on the alliance. Even though patients can sometimes cite extraordinary situational issues to justify these demands, astute therapists will be aware of the dangers of going overboard in granting special favors.

### *Sociocultural Background*

Sensitivity to sociocultural issues is an essential component of forming authentic and highly functional working alliances. Among other personal variables, gender, race, ethnicity, age, socioeconomic status, religion, sexual orientation, physical disabilities, and educational level may influence both therapist and patient as they attempt to build a therapeutic relationship. Although clinicians typically seek to be unbiased and to be respectful of diverse backgrounds, beliefs, and behavior, we can have blind spots or lack of knowledge that can interfere with the treatment bond or completely derail our efforts to relate to the patient. Also, patients' biases can significantly impair their ability to benefit from working with therapists whose personal characteristics do not match the patients' expectations.

There are several useful strategies for becoming attuned to the impact of sociocultural influences on the treatment alliance. Our first recommendation is to be introspective in your work with patients from varied backgrounds. Don't assume that you are 100% sensitive to and tolerant of diversity in your patients. Watch closely for negative reactions to patients or evidence that sociocultural factors are limiting your therapeutic efforts. Are you having difficulty expressing empathy with a particular patient? Do you feel stiff or unnatural in treatment sessions? Are you dreading the appointment with this patient? Could any of these responses be due to your personal biases and attitudes? If you spot such reactions, then work out a plan to modify your negative perceptions in order to be more understanding and accepting of the patient.

The second strategy is to make a concerted effort to improve your knowledge of sociocultural differences that can influence the therapeutic relationship. For example, a heterosexual therapist who has limited training about the lesbian, gay, bisexual, or transgender (LGBT) culture and is noticing an aversion to working with patients who have an LGBT orientation might read literature about the LGBT experience, attend workshops designed to improve sensitivity, and view films intended to enhance understanding of issues related to sexual orientation (Austin and Craig 2015; Graham et al. 2013; Safren and Rogers 2001; Wright and Davis 1994). Also, clinicians may be able to form more effective alliances if they learn about a wide range of religious traditions and life philosophies. Although a limited amount of research has shown that patients with certain religious beliefs will have an affinity for therapists with similar spiritual backgrounds (Propst et al. 1992), our experiences in using CBT with patients from a variety of religions (or without any specific spiritual leaning) suggest that understanding, tolerance, and respect for different belief structures usually promote good therapeutic alliances.

Clinicians also need to be well versed in ethnic and gender issues that may influence the treatment process (Graham et al. 2013; Wright and Davis 1994). In addition to readings and sensitivity training, we suggest that you discuss such issues with experts in cultural diversity and with colleagues and friends to gain a full perspective on these potential influences on the therapeutic relationship. We have particularly valued input from coworkers and associates who have given us feedback about our attitudes. They have helped us deepen our awareness of how race, ethnicity, gender, and other sociocultural factors can affect the treatment process.

As you are learning more about sociocultural influences on the therapeutic relationship, we also recommend that you take time to examine your office setting for possible biases or slights that may make patients feel uncomfortable. Is the waiting room designed to accommodate persons with physical disabilities or who are grossly overweight? Does the literature in the waiting room convey any particular prejudice? Do office staff members treat all patients with equal respect and attention? Do the decorations of the office convey any unintended meaning that may be off-putting to persons from certain ethnic or cultural backgrounds? If you recognize any features of your office setting that could have a negative impact on therapeutic alliances, then work toward correcting and enhancing the treatment environment.

## *Diagnosis and Symptoms*

Each patient's illness, personality type, and cluster of symptoms can have a substantial influence on the therapeutic relationship. A manic patient may be intrusive and irritating, or he may be overly charming and seductive. Patients with substance use disorders often have cognitive and behavioral patterns that encourage them to deceive the therapist and themselves. A person with an eating disorder can work hard to convince the therapist of the validity of her maladaptive attitudes.

Personality disorders and traits also can have a highly significant effect on the therapist's efforts to establish an effective working alliance. The dependent patient may want to lean on the therapist. A person with obsessive-compulsive personality disorder may have difficulty expressing emotion in therapeutic interchanges. A schizoid patient may be very guarded and have problems trusting the therapist. And of course, a person with borderline personality disorder is likely to have had chaotic and unstable relationships, which can be carried over into the therapeutic arena.

Modifications in CBT methods for specific conditions, including personality disorders, are detailed in Chapter 10, "Treating Chronic, Severe, or Complex Disorders." Here we list three general strategies for managing the impact of the patient's illness and personality structure on the therapeutic alliance:

1. **Spot potential problems.** Be on the lookout for possible influences of symptoms and personality variables, and be ready to adjust your behavior to account for these differences. For example, you may need to pay special attention to developing trust with a person who has been traumatized and is experiencing posttraumatic stress disorder. Or you may want to loosen up, use humor, and try creative approaches to break through the rigidity of a person with obsessive-compulsive traits. If you are treating a woman with an eating disorder whom you suspect is not being fully honest with you about the extent of her unhealthy behavior (e.g., bingeing, purging, abusing laxatives, exercising excessively), open discussions about your concerns may be needed.
2. **Don't label the patient.** Labeling occurs when the clinician slips into using diagnostic terms such as *borderline, alcoholic,* or *dependent* in a pejorative manner. Negative attitudes about these types of behaviors may be subtle, under the surface, or overt. Once labeling occurs, the relationship becomes more distant or strained, the therapist may try less hard to work on symptoms, and the quality of the therapy is likely to deteriorate.

3. **Strive for equanimity.** Try to be like the calm in the eye of the storm. Be objective and steer a clear course for the therapy, even when you are responding to emotionally charged situations or are challenged by a demanding patient. Work on developing the capacity to deal with a wide range of clinical situations and personality types while avoiding overreactions, angry behavior, or defensive responses. Your temperament may already contain a healthy dose of equanimity. However, this attribute can be practiced and strengthened. One of the most valuable ways to increase your capacity for equanimity is to build skills in recognizing and managing transference and countertransference reactions, as discussed below.

## Transference in CBT

The concept of transference is derived from psychoanalysis and psychodynamic psychotherapy, but it is revised substantially in CBT to be consistent with cognitive-behavioral theories and methods (Beck et al. 1979; Sanders and Wills 1999; Wright and Davis 1994). As in other therapies, transference phenomena are viewed as a reenactment in the treatment relationship of key elements of previous important relationships (e.g., parents, grandparents, teachers, bosses, peers). However, in CBT the focus is not on unconscious components of the transference or on defense mechanisms but on habitual ways of thinking and acting that are recapitulated in the treatment setting. For example, if a man has a deeply held core belief (e.g., "I must be in control") and has long-standing behavioral patterns of controlling others, he may play out these same cognitions and behaviors in the therapeutic relationship.

Because CBT is typically a short-term treatment with a straightforward, highly collaborative therapist-patient alliance, the intensity of the transference is usually much lower than in longer-term, dynamically oriented psychotherapy. In addition, transference is not seen as a necessary or primary mechanism for learning or change. Nevertheless, an awareness of transference responses in patients and an ability to use this knowledge to improve treatment relationships and modify dysfunctional thought patterns are important parts of CBT.

In assessing transference in CBT, the therapist watches for schemas and associated behavioral patterns that are likely to have been developed within the context of significant past relationships. This evaluation serves two primary functions. First, the therapist is able to analyze the treatment relationship to learn about the patient's core beliefs and to examine in vivo the effects of these cognitions on the patient's behavior in important relationships. Second, the therapist can design interventions to curtail any negative effects of transference on the treatment bond or on the outcome of therapy.

If there is evidence that a core belief is influencing the therapist-patient relationship, the clinician needs to consider these questions:

1. **Is the transference a healthy or productive phenomenon?** If so, the therapist may elect to withhold any comments about the transference and allow it to continue as is.
2. **Do you think that there is potential for negative effects of the transference?** Perhaps the current state of the transference is neutral or benign, but there is a prospect for complications in the therapeutic relationship. When you spot transference reactions, try to think ahead to what may happen if the therapy keeps going and the relationship intensifies. Preventive actions (e.g., setting strict boundaries, detailing appropriate guidelines for the treatment alliance) may help avoid future problems.
3. **Is there a transference reaction that needs attention now?** When there is a transference reaction that is interfering with the collaboration, is blocking progress, or is having a destructive effect on the therapy, the therapist needs to take prompt action to address the problem. Interventions may include psychoeducation on the transference phenomenon, use of standard CBT techniques to modify automatic thoughts and schemas involved in the transference, behavioral rehearsal (practicing alternate, healthier behaviors in therapy sessions), and contracting to limit or stop certain behaviors.

### Case Example

The treatment of Carla, a 25-year-old woman with severe depression, by a middle-aged female therapist included work on bringing a transference reaction to light and using the transference to help the patient change. The patient's core beliefs (e.g., "I can never be a competent person"; "I'll never be able to satisfy my parents"; "I'm a failure") were negatively affecting the relationship because the patient was comparing herself to the therapist, a successful professional. Carla was also having automatic thoughts that the therapist was judging her and was thinking that she was lazy or dull because she was not always able to show success in implementing CBT self-help methods. As a result, Carla felt distant from the therapist and perceived her as a demanding person who didn't like her very much.

The therapist recognized that Carla's experiences of having hypercritical parents and always believing that she was inferior to others had set her up for having a strained therapeutic relationship. Therefore, the therapist openly discussed the transference reaction and then used CBT methods to correct distortions that were impairing the collaborative bond.

Some of the specific cognitions about the therapist that were targeted for change were the following: "She has everything going for her—I have nothing" (an automatic thought with a cognitive error: maximizing the positives of others and minimizing one's own strengths); "If she really got to know me, she would realize I'm a fraud" (a maladaptive schema that was driving a wedge between the patient and the therapist); and "I could never measure up to her standards" (a transference of beliefs about parents to the therapist).

After eliciting these cognitions, the therapist explained how automatic thoughts, core beliefs, and behaviors from other relationships can be reenacted in therapy and in other current interpersonal situations. Then she reassured Carla that she understood and respected her, but wanted to help build her self-esteem. They agreed that one way to improve Carla's self-image would be to talk regularly about the therapy alliance and to test out her assumptions about the therapist's attitudes and expectations. As treatment progressed, the therapeutic relationship became a healthy mechanism for Carla to see herself accurately and to develop more realistic, functional attitudes.

## Countertransference

Another responsibility of cognitive-behavior therapists is to look for possible countertransference reactions that may be interfering with the development of collaborative treatment relationships. Countertransference occurs in CBT when the relationship with the patient activates automatic thoughts and schemas in the clinician, and these cognitions have the potential for influencing the therapy process. Because automatic thoughts and schemas can operate outside your full awareness, a good way to spot possible countertransference reactions is to recognize emotions, physical sensations, or behavioral responses that may be stimulated by your cognitions. Common indicators that countertransference may be occurring are that you feel angry, tense, or frustrated with the patient; are becoming bored in the therapy; are relieved when the patient is late or cancels the appointment; have repeated difficulties working with a particular type of illness, symptom cluster, or personality dimension; or are finding yourself particularly attracted or drawn to a certain patient.

When you suspect that countertransference may be developing, you can apply the theories and methods of CBT described throughout this book to better understand and manage the reaction. Begin by trying to identify your automatic thoughts and schemas. Then, if it is clinically indicated and feasible, you can work on modifying the cognitions. For example, if you have automatic thoughts such as "This patient has no motivation…all he does is whine through the entire session…this therapy is going nowhere," you can try to spot your cognitive errors (e.g., all-

or-nothing thinking, ignoring the evidence, jumping to conclusions) and change your thinking to reflect a more balanced view of the patient's efforts and potential.

## Summary

An effective alliance between therapist and patient is an essential condition for implementation of the specific methods of CBT. As therapists engage patients in the process of CBT, they need to show understanding; appropriate empathy and personal warmth; and flexibility in responding to the unique features of each person's symptoms, beliefs, and sociocultural background. Good therapeutic relationships in CBT are characterized by a high degree of collaboration and an empirical style of questioning and learning. The collaborative empirical treatment alliance brings the therapist and patient together in a joint effort to define problems and search for solutions.

## References

Austin A, Craig SL: Transgender affirmative cognitive behavioral therapy: clinical considerations and applications. Prof Psychol Res Pr 46(1):21–29, 2015

Beck AT, Rush AJ, Shaw BF, et al: Cognitive Therapy of Depression. New York, Guilford, 1979

Beitman BD, Goldfried MR, Norcross JC: The movement toward integrating the psychotherapies: an overview. Am J Psychiatry 146(2):138–147, 1989 2643360

Graham JR, Sorenson S, Hayes-Skelton SA: Enhancing the Cultural Sensitivity of Cognitive Behavioral Interventions for Anxiety in Diverse Populations. Behav Ther (N Y N Y) 36(5):101–108, 2013 25392598

Gutheil TG, Gabbard GO: The concept of boundaries in clinical practice: theoretical and risk-management dimensions. Am J Psychiatry 150(2):188–196, 1993 8422069

Keijsers GP, Schaap CP, Hoogduin CAL: The impact of interpersonal patient and therapist behavior on outcome in cognitive-behavior therapy: a review of empirical studies. Behav Modif 24(2):264–297, 2000 10804683

Klein DN, Schwartz JE, Santiago NJ, et al: Therapeutic alliance in depression treatment: controlling for prior change and patient characteristics. J Consult Clin Psychol 71(6):997–1006, 2003 14622075

Kuhn C: The Fun Factor: Unleashing the Power of Humor at Home and on the Job. Louisville, KY, Minerva Books, 2002

Propst LR, Ostrom R, Watkins P, et al: Comparative efficacy of religious and nonreligious cognitive-behavioral therapy for the treatment of clinical depression in religious individuals. J Consult Clin Psychol 60(1):94–103, 1992 1556292

Rogers CR: The necessary and sufficient conditions of therapeutic personality change. J Consult Psychol 21(2):95–103, 1957 13416422

Safren SA, Rogers T: Cognitive-behavioral therapy with gay, lesbian, and bisexual clients. J Clin Psychol 57(5):629–643, 2001 11304703

Sanders D, Wills F: The therapeutic relationship in cognitive therapy, in Understanding the Counselling Relationship: Professional Skills for Counsellors. Edited by Feltham C. Thousand Oaks, CA, Sage, 1999, pp 120–138

Wright JH, Davis D: The therapeutic relationship in cognitive-behavioral therapy: patient perceptions and therapist responses. Cogn Behav Pract 1:25–45, 1994

# 3

# Assessment and Formulation

The process of evaluating patients for cognitive-behavior therapy (CBT) and performing case conceptualizations is based on a comprehensive treatment model. Although the cognitive and behavioral elements of understanding the patient's illness are given the greatest emphasis, biological and social influences are also considered to be essential features of the assessment and formulation. In this chapter, we discuss indications for CBT, patient characteristics that are associated with an affinity for this approach, and key dimensions of assessing suitability for therapy. We also introduce a pragmatic method for organizing case conceptualizations and developing treatment plans.

## Assessment

An assessment for CBT starts with the fundamental features of evaluation for any form of psychotherapy: a full history and mental status ex-

---

The case formulation worksheet mentioned in this chapter, located in Appendix 1, "Worksheets and Checklists," is also available as a free download in a larger format on the American Psychiatric Association Publishing Web site: https://www.appi.org/wright.

amination. Attention should be paid to the patient's current symptoms, interpersonal relationships, sociocultural background, and personal strengths, in addition to consideration of the impact of developmental history, genetics, biological factors, and medical illnesses. A detailed evaluation of influences from these multiple domains will allow you to produce a multifaceted case formulation, as detailed in the next section, "Case Conceptualization in CBT."

Completion of a standard interview and diagnosis will provide much of the information needed to assess the patient's suitability for CBT. Since the 1980s, CBT has been adapted for a large range of conditions, greatly broadening its scope beyond treatment of mild to moderate depressive and anxiety disorders (Wright et al. 2014). For example, in Chapter 10, "Treating Chronic, Severe, or Complex Disorders," we review modifications of CBT for bipolar disorder, schizophrenia, borderline personality disorder, and other conditions that are difficult to treat. We therefore suggest that most of the patients whom you evaluate for psychiatric treatment will be potential candidates for CBT, either alone or in combination with appropriate pharmacotherapy.

There are few absolute contraindications for use of CBT (e.g., advanced dementia, other severe amnestic disorders, and more transient states such as delirium or drug intoxication). Persons with severe antisocial personality disorder, malingering, or other conditions that markedly impair the development of a collaborative and trusting therapeutic relationship may be as likely to be poor candidates for CBT as they are for other forms of psychotherapy.

We discuss the use of longer-term methods of CBT in Chapter 10, "Treating Chronic, Severe, or Complex Disorders." Our focus in this chapter is on identifying the types of patients for whom CBT can be expected to work within a 2- to 4-month time frame. For this purpose, we have drawn from earlier contributions on brief psychodynamic psychotherapy (Davanloo 1978; Malan 1973; Sifneos 1972) and from the thoughtful work of Safran and Segal (1990). Safran and Segal developed a semistructured interview to assess patients' suitability for time-limited CBT. Although this interview has excellent psychometric characteristics, the Safran and Segal method is impractical for use outside of research settings because of the length of time to complete: 1–2 hours. The recommendations we make here are derived in part from Safran and Segal's contributions but are designed to be integrated into the initial evaluation as part of the standard psychiatric assessment.

Who are the ideal candidates for treatment with CBT alone? To some extent, time-limited CBT is best suited for people seeking therapy for a relatively acute, not overwhelming severe anxiety or depressive disorder.

**Table 3–1.** Dimensions to consider in evaluating patients for cognitive-behavior therapy

| |
|---|
| Chronicity and complexity |
| Optimism about the chances of success in therapy |
| Acceptance of responsibility for change |
| Compatibility with the cognitive-behavioral rationale |
| Ability to access automatic thoughts and identify accompanying emotions |
| Capacity to engage in a therapeutic alliance |
| Ability to maintain and work within a problem-oriented focus |

To these generic good-prognosis indicators we would add factors such as verbal skills, motivation to change, adequate financial resources, safe housing, and supportive family members or close friends. Fortunately, there is good evidence that the utility of CBT is *not* limited to individuals who would typically be considered easy-to-treat or ideal patients for this psychotherapy. Several additional dimensions of suitability for time-limited therapy are shown in Table 3–1 and discussed further below.

The first dimension noted in Table 3–1 is a general prognostic indicator: the *chronicity and complexity* of the patient's problems. You should adhere to the basic wisdom that long-standing problems typically warrant longer courses of therapy; the same can be said for treatment of depressive or anxiety disorders that are complicated by substance abuse, significant personality disorders, a history of early trauma or neglect, or other comorbid conditions. The patient's treatment history may provide important clues about the treatability of his condition. If you are the twelfth therapist in 25 years or are being asked to try a new approach after the failure of extensive courses of pharmacotherapy and psychotherapy, longer and more extensive treatment than a standard 12- or 16-week treatment program may be needed.

The second dimension, *optimism about the chances of success in therapy*, is also a global prognostic indicator across various forms of helping relationships (Frank 1973). High levels of pessimism can diminish a patient's ability to respond to therapy in several ways. Pessimism can reflect a patient's valid assessment that she has serious difficulties, particularly when there is a history of prior unsuccessful courses of treatment. Depression does tend to remove the so-called rose-colored glasses of well-being (i.e., the tendency of people to minimize their problems and overvalue their strengths). Nevertheless, demoralization can undercut the patient's capacity to engage in therapeutic exercises or, through a self-fulfilling prophecy, can discount evidence of progress. Because pessimism is associated with both hopelessness and suicidal ideation, you should be vigilant to the possibility that in some patients a marked level of pessimism may warrant alternate therapies or even hospitalization. In the most extreme sense, pessimism may conceal nihilistic delusions, which indicate the need for antipsychotic medication.

The third dimension, *acceptance of responsibility for change,* is linked to the model of motivation initially described by Prochaska and DiClemente (1992) and more fully elaborated as a central component of motivational interviewing (Miller et al. 2004). This approach encourages discussion about the treatment-seeking person's expectations about treatment and his apprehensions. The interview can elicit the person's general understanding about his illness and its treatment, as well as more specific knowledge and expectations about CBT. People who express strong preferences for a medical model of treatment may require more preparatory work before beginning psychotherapy than those who express genuine interest in CBT.

The fourth dimension, *compatibility with the cognitive-behavioral rationale,* concerns the specific impressions of both the patient and the therapist about the appropriateness of CBT. Just as in everyday life, first impressions are important, and people who give CBT high marks before beginning therapy tend to respond better than those who form more negative initial impressions. The willingness to perform self-help exercises or homework is another key aspect of compatibility. As we emphasize throughout this book, homework is a defining component of CBT. There is ample evidence that patients who do not regularly complete homework assignments are significantly less likely to respond to therapy than those who do (Thase and Callan 2006).

Although extreme pessimism may have potentially negative prognostic implications, the fifth dimension, *ability to access automatic thoughts and identify accompanying emotions,* reflects a real aptitude for CBT. Staying with the view that therapy builds on strengths, you will find that patients who are able to identify and speak aloud their negative automatic thoughts during periods of depressed or anxious mood typically can begin to use three- and five-column exercises earlier in the course of therapy. As a means to help uncover automatic negative thoughts, it can be useful in the initial evaluation to ask the patient about the thoughts and associated feelings she had while she was driving to the session or sitting in the waiting room. Questions to further probe the patient's ability to identify and express negative automatic thoughts (e.g., "What were you thinking during that situation?" or "What thoughts ran through your mind when you were feeling so blue?") are also typically used in assessing suitability for CBT. Difficulty with identifying fluctuations in emotional states is a disadvantage in CBT because patients will miss opportunities to identify *hot thoughts* (i.e., automatic negative thoughts experienced in concert with strong emotional states) and to practice ways of improving mood with cognitive restructuring methods.

The sixth relevant dimension in assessing suitability for short-term therapy deals with the patient's *capacity to engage in a therapeutic alliance.* Safran and Segal (1990) suggested that observations about behavior in sessions and questions about the patient's history of intimate relationships can provide important clues about his ability to form an effective treatment relationship. During the initial session, direct solicitation of feedback (e.g., "How do you feel about today's session?") and observations about the patient's ability to *connect* (e.g., eye contact, posture, and degree of comfort related to the therapist) are used to gauge capacity to engage in a helping alliance. Historical questions pertaining to the quality of relationships with parents, siblings, teachers, coaches, and romantic partners can provide useful information—particularly when repetitive patterns of disappointment, rejection, or exploitation are revealed. Likewise, if the patient has prior experiences with psychotherapy, his impressions about the quality of that dyad are likely to convey some information about what the future might hold in store.

The seventh and final dimension pertains to the patient's *ability to maintain and work within a problem-oriented focus.* From the perspective of Safran and Segal (1990), this dimension has two components: *security operations* and *focality.* The former refers to the patient's use of potentially therapy-disrupting behaviors to restore a sense of emotional security when psychologically threatened. *Focality,* by contrast, refers to the capacity to work within the structure of CBT sessions and to maintain attention on a relevant topic from start to finish.

In addition to completing a history, mental status exam, and evaluation of suitability for CBT, we recommend that you consider using standardized rating scales for measuring symptoms and tracking progress. Studies have shown solid benefits for "measurement-enhanced care," in which symptom severity is measured at each session (Forney et al. 2016; Guo et al. 2015). A number of self-rating scales can be used that require minimal effort and time from patients. We typically use the Patient Health Questionnaire-9 (PHQ-9; Kroenke et al. 2001; xxSpitzer et al. 1999) for measurement of depression and the Generalized Anxiety Disorder-7 (GAD-7; Spitzer et al. 2006) for measurement of anxiety. Both are free and available online (www.phqscreeners.com). Other options include the Beck Depression Inventory (Beck 1961), Center for Epidemiologic Studies Depression Rating Scale (CES-D; Radloff 1977), and the Penn State Worry Questionnaire (Meyer et al. 1990).

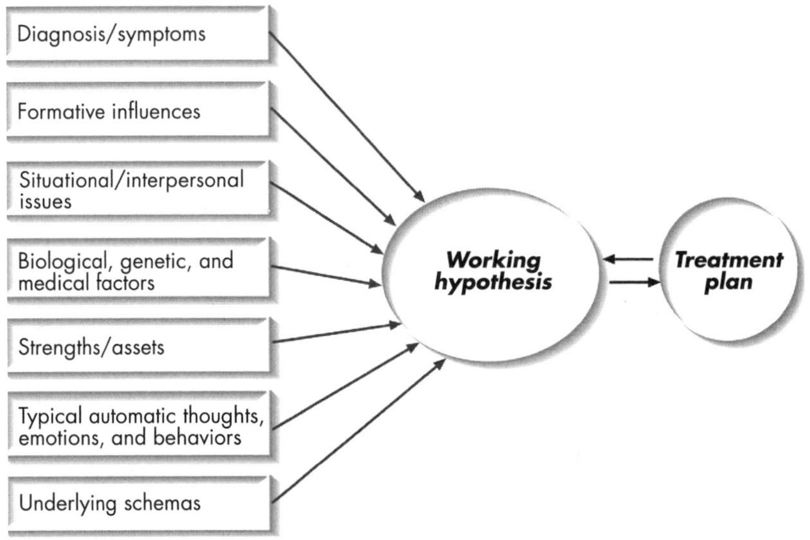


**Figure 3–1.** Case conceptualization flowchart.

## Case Conceptualization in CBT

The case conceptualization, or formulation, is a road map for your work with the patient. It brings together information from seven key domains: 1) diagnosis and symptoms; 2) contributions of childhood experiences and other formative influences; 3) situational and interpersonal issues; 4) biological, genetic, and medical factors; 5) strengths and assets; 6) typical patterns of automatic thoughts, emotions, and behaviors; and 7) underlying schemas (Figure 3–1). In short, all of the important findings from your assessment of the patient are considered in developing a case formulation.

At first glance, it may seem to be a daunting task to synthesize all this information in devising a specific plan for an individual patient. However, the system we describe in this chapter will give you a pragmatic and easy-to-use method for organizing case formulations. The pivotal step in conceptualizing a case is the formation of a working hypothesis (see Figure 3–1). The clinician uses cognitive-behavioral constructs to develop an individualized theoretical formulation relevant to the patient's particular blend of symptoms, problems, and resources. This working hypothesis is then used to direct treatment interventions.

Early in therapy, the case conceptualization may be just an outline or a sketch. You may be uncertain about the diagnosis or you may still be collecting critical parts of the data. You also might have just started to try some CBT interventions. However, it is vital to begin to think about the formulation from the very beginning of treatment. As you get to know the patient better, more observations and layers of complexity can be added to the formulation. You will be able to test your theories to see if they are accurate, and you will learn if your treatment methods are on target. If not, the formulation will need to be revised. For example, if you begin to recognize long-standing dependent features that are stalling progress, you will need to consider altering the treatment plan. If previously unrecognized strengths become apparent, the course of therapy can be changed to take advantage of these assets.

By the middle and late phases of CBT, the case conceptualization should mature to a well-orchestrated plan that provides a coherent and effective guide for each therapy intervention. If you reviewed a video- or audio-recorded session from this part of therapy and stopped the recording at any juncture, you should be able to explain your rationale for following the path you are taking at that moment and for the entire course of therapy. Ideally, you would also be able to describe the obstacles to be faced in achieving the best results and a plan for overcoming these obstacles.

The system that we recommend for developing case conceptualizations is based on guidelines established by the Academy of Cognitive Therapy. This organization's Web site (http://www.academyofct.org) contains detailed instructions for writing formulations that meet standards for certification in cognitive therapy. Case examples are also provided. We have distilled the main features of the Academy of Cognitive Therapy case conceptualization guidelines into a case formulation worksheet (Figure 3–2; see also Appendix 1, "Worksheets and Checklists," for blank copies of this form).

To complete the CBT case formulation worksheet, you will need to be able to perform a thorough assessment, as described in this chapter, and you will need to know the core theories and methods of CBT. Because you may not yet be armed with all the information and skills required for developing fully realized case conceptualizations, our goal at this point in the book is modest. We want to introduce formulation methods and to give some examples that will show how CBT constructs can be used in planning treatment. As you work your way through the rest of the book and gain additional experience in CBT, you can build expertise in performing case conceptualizations.

Figure 3–2 shows a case formulation worksheet that Dr. Wright developed for the treatment of Kate, the woman with anxiety disorder featured in Videos 1 and 2.

**Patient Name:** Kate

**Diagnoses/Symptoms:** Panic disorder with agoraphobia (fear of driving). Primary symptoms are panic attacks, hyperventilation, and avoidance. GAD-7 score=16 (moderate general anxiety)

**Formative Influences:** —

**Situational Issues:** New location for job requires driving across bridge over a large river and through heavy traffic; son has moved and now lives a 2-hour drive away; husband wants her to drive with him to Florida for a vacation.

**Biological, Genetic, and Medical Factors:** Mother has history of untreated anxiety. Father died suddenly of a heart attack when he was in his 50s. Kate has hypothyroidism and low vitamin D levels; both corrected with treatment.

**Strengths/Assets:** Intelligent, articulate, good sense of humor, support from family and coworkers.

**Treatment Goals:** 1) Reduce panic attacks to one a month or less, 2) learn skills for reducing anxiety and panic, 3) be able to drive self across bridge to work, and 4) drive to visit son and go on vacation with husband (do at least part of the driving by myself).

| Event 1 | Event 2 | Event 3 |
|---|---|---|
| Driving to pharmacy to pick up daughter's medicine. | Driving to get work supplies. | Thinking of driving across bridge with coworkers to new office. |
| **Automatic Thoughts** | **Automatic Thoughts** | **Automatic Thoughts** |
| "What if someone runs into me?"<br>"What if I get stranded?"<br>"I can't do it."<br>"What if I can't get back home?" | "I can't do it."<br>"Could I get somebody else to do it?"<br>"I'll pass out."<br>"Somebody's going to slam into my car." | "I might have a heart attack like my father did."<br>"I'll have to get out of the car."<br>"I can't do it." |
| **Emotions** | **Emotions** | **Emotions** |
| Anxiety, pounding heart, light-headedness, dizziness, difficulty breathing | Anxiety | Anxiety |

**Figure 3–2.** Case formulation worksheet for Kate.

| Behaviors | Behaviors | Behaviors |
|---|---|---|
| Drove to pharmacy because there were no other options. But gripped steering wheel so tightly it could have left "permanent marks." Typically avoids similar situations if possible. | Drove to get supplies but wanted to avoid the trip. Looked for escape options. | Planning ways to avoid going over the bridge. |
| **Schemas:** "I'm bound to be hurt"; "Always be on guard, the world is a very dangerous place"; "I'll die early like my father." **Working Hypothesis:** 1) Kate has unrealistic fears of driving, underestimates her ability to control or manage driving situations, and avoids the feared stimuli (especially bridges). 2) Her family background (e.g., father's sudden death, mother's tension and hypervigilance) contributed to the development of anxiety-ridden schemas and avoidance. 3) Death of classmate in car accident during high school primed her fear of driving. 5) Current situational factors (new location of work and pressure to drive) have played a role in triggering symptoms. **Treatment Plan:** 1) Cognitive restructuring (e.g., examining the evidence, spotting cognitive errors, using thought records, cognitive rehearsal) to teach Kate that her fears are unrealistic and that she can learn to cope with her anxieties; 2) breathing training, imagery, and deep muscle relaxation to provide tools for controlling anxiety; 3) graded exposure to driving situations; and 4) later in therapy, focus on revising maladaptive schemas. | | |

**Figure 3–2.** Case formulation worksheet for Kate. *(continued)*

## Case Example

Kate described a host of anxiety-related symptoms, including panic attacks, hyperventilation, physiological arousal, and avoidance of driving situations such as crossing bridges, congested highways, and long distances (beyond a restricted "safe zone"). She gave a history of a few panic attacks several years ago that led to emergency room visits on two occasions. All of her tests, including cardiograms, were normal. And a consultation with a cardiologist confirmed that she had no evidence of heart disease. Kate began to experience more frequent panic attacks (2–3 per week) when she was offered a promotion to an office manager position at a new location of the plate glass company where she has worked as an administrative assistant. The new facility, located across a large river, is scheduled to open in about 2 months. As the move has gotten closer, she has been thinking she may need to resign from a job that she has worked hard to acquire.

> Several formative influences from Kate's earlier years appear to have shaped her vulnerability to anxiety symptoms. Kate was the second of two children raised in a loving family environment with both parents present in the home. Although her mother never received treatment for anxiety, she is a tense woman, a worrier, who appears to be excessively concerned about danger and gave her children the message that the world is a very risky place.
>
> She was especially concerned about danger during the time when Kate was learning to drive. Like most parents she gave Kate repeated instructions to be careful because of the high risk of an accident among teenage drivers. When one of Kate's classmates was killed in a car wreck, her mother became so overwhelmed with anxiety and distress that she forbade Kate to drive for over 6 months.
>
> Another traumatic life experience contributed to Kate's panic attacks and avoidance of driving. During her mid-20s, her father died suddenly of a heart attack. The loss was devastating to her and triggered a fear that she would suffer the same fate at an early age.
>
> Fortunately, Kate had a number of strengths that could be tapped in the process of doing CBT. She was genuinely interested in learning about CBT and was willing to engage in exposure therapy—a key element of CBT for anxiety disorders. She was articulate and intelligent and had a good sense of humor. She was also free of personality disorders and had excellent support from her family members and coworkers. However, she had long-standing anxiety symptoms with well-entrenched patterns of avoidance of driving across bridges and traveling distances beyond a safe zone of familiar streets close to her home, frequently visited shops, and her old place of work. It also appeared that her family, friends, and coworkers were unknowingly reinforcing the anxiety by participating in her elaborate methods of avoidance (e.g., driving her across bridges or through heavy traffic, protecting her from going on trips that would require driving out of her safety zone, running errands for her).

As shown in Videos 1 and 2 (see Chapter 2, "The Therapeutic Relationship"), Kate was able to collaborate effectively in working toward reaching her goals (Figure 3–2): "1) reduce panic attacks to one a month or less, 2) learn skills for reducing anxiety and panic, 3) be able to drive self across bridge to work, and 4) drive to visit son and go on vacation with husband (do at least part of the driving by myself)."

In its case conceptualization guidelines, the Academy of Cognitive Therapy recommends that clinicians take both a *cross-sectional* and a *longitudinal* view of the cognitive and behavioral factors that may be influencing symptom expression. The cross-sectional part of the formulation involves looking at current patterns of how major precipitants (e.g., large-scale stressors such as a relationship breakup, job loss, new onset of a serious medical illness) and activating situations (commonly occurring events such as arguments with one's spouse, pressures at work, being exposed to a trigger for recurring anxiety symptoms) stimulate automatic thoughts, emotions, and behaviors. The longitudinal view takes developmental events and other formative influences into account, especially as they pertain to the shaping of core beliefs or schemas.

The case formulation worksheet shown in Figure 3–2 contains a cross-sectional analysis of three typical events in Kate's current environment that are associated with maladaptive cognitions, emotions, and behavior. In her response to the first event, driving to the pharmacy to pick up her daughter's antibiotics, she has automatic thoughts such as "What if someone runs into me?…What if I get stranded?… I can't do it.…What if I can't get back home?" The emotions and physical sensations associated with these cognitions are anxiety, increased heart rate, light-headedness, dizziness, and fast, irregular breathing. Although in this example Kate was able to drive to the pharmacy, she did so under considerable duress. And she clenched the steering wheel so hard that it could have left "permanent marks." Usually Kate avoided similar driving situations, thus contributing to a vicious cycle of chronic anxiety and escape behaviors. The second and third examples of situations that stir up automatic thoughts and anxiety (driving to get work supplies and thinking of driving across a bridge with coworkers to the new office) have similar outcomes. Kate has a flurry of intense automatic thoughts (e.g., "I'll pass out.… I can't do it.… I might have a heart attack like my father") and either avoids driving or tries to do so.

From the longitudinal perspective, Kate had formative experiences that appear to have contributed to the development of maladaptive core beliefs about the dangerousness of the world around her and her vulnerability to having a disaster befall her (e.g., "I'm bound to be hurt"; "Always be on guard, the world is a very dangerous place"; "I'll die early like my father").

Putting all of these observations together, Dr. Wright developed a working hypothesis that included these key features: 1) Kate was exhibiting the classic cognitive-behavioral features of anxiety disorders: unrealistic fears of situations, underestimates of her ability to control or manage these situations, intense emotional and autonomic arousal, and avoidance of the feared situation; 2) a developmental background of tension, wariness of danger, and sudden death of a loved one—and a family history of possible anxiety disorder in her mother—were likely contributors to the disorder; 3) the trauma of a classmate's fatal car accident added to her fears and focused them on risks of driving; and 4) current situational factors (a promotion to a job that required driving across a large river) likely played a role in triggering symptoms.

The treatment plan organized by Dr. Wright was directly linked to this working hypothesis. He decided to focus on modifying Kate's catastrophic automatic thoughts with Socratic questioning, examining the evidence, thought recording, and cognitive rehearsal. He also planned to give her training in breathing to reduce or resolve the hyperventilation she experienced in panic attacks. The most important part of the program was desensitization to the feared stimuli with a stepwise hierarchy for graded exposure. These methods are explained in detail and illustrated with videos in Chapter 5, "Working With Automatic Thoughts," and Chapter 7, "Behavioral Methods II: Reducing Anxiety and Breaking Patterns of Avoidance."

Although Dr. Wright believed that Kate's developmental experiences set her up for having anxiety-ridden core beliefs, he opted to target most of his treatment efforts on using cognitive techniques to identify and change automatic thoughts and to implement behavioral strategies to break her pattern of avoidance. These methods are consistent with the cognitive-behavioral model for treatment of anxiety. In an early session (shown in Video 2, "Modifying Automatic Thoughts"), he and Kate worked on a core belief about dying young. Later in therapy, he was able to help Kate understand and modify other schemas about vulnerability to danger.

Another case shown in the video illustrations that accompany this book demonstrates how to develop a conceptualization for a person with depression. Chapter 5, "Working With Automatic Thoughts," and Chapter 8, "Modifying Schemas," contain videos from the treatment of Brian, a young man who became depressed when he had problems making the transition to a move to a new city and a new job. We recommend that you wait until Chapters 5 and 8 to watch the videos from Dr. Sudak's treatment of Brian because they will give specific examples of how to perform the techniques described in these sections of the book. However, we briefly describe the case here as another example of a CBT case formulation. This conceptualization (Figure 3–3) should help you better understand the methods Dr. Sudak chose in this example of CBT for depression.

## Case Example

Brian is a 25-year-old man who recently moved to Philadelphia from his hometown after his employer, an information technology firm, was acquired by a larger company. Since the move he has become increasingly lonely and depressed. This is his first time away from home. Symptoms of depression include low mood, poor sleep, decreased appetite with a 10-pound weight loss, many self-condemning thoughts, and reduced interest and enjoyment in activities. Concentration has been good, and his work performance as a computer engineer hasn't appeared to suffer. He has not had suicidal thoughts or intent. His PHQ-9 score is 18.

Brian describes himself as "lost" since his move. Although he considered moving back home, there are no good jobs for him there. And he said he would be a "failure" if he returned to live with his mother. Before the move, he sang in a choir, was a runner, and enjoyed spending time with his male friends. However, all of these activities have stopped. For the last 3 months he has come back to his apartment after work to spend all of his time alone.

There is no previous history of treatment for depression. But Brian notes that he has always lacked confidence, and he remembers long periods of sadness as a child, especially after visits from his inconsistent father. Despite long absences, his father would show up without warning with offerings of gifts and apologies. In a few days, he would be "gone like the wind." A breakup with a long-term girlfriend from college was devastating to Brian. In retrospect, he says he should have gone for counseling then. He has never been suicidal. Brian has no history of medical problems.

An only child, Brian was raised in a semirural area in upstate New York. His parents separated when he was 18 months old. The family history is positive for alcohol abuse in his father. No family members have been treated for psychiatric illnesses, but Brian believes his mother has had chronic, low-grade depression. She started work as a housekeeper after her husband left her and is now the supervisor of housekeeping services for a small group of motels and restaurants in her town. Brian's relationship with his mother has been very strong. He describes her as "always in my corner."

Because of financial strains, Brian held part-time jobs as a high school and college student. He describes himself as "shy." Yet he developed close male friends and had a steady girlfriend from his junior year in high school until his sophomore year in college. She ended their relationship when Brian discovered she was seeing another man in secret. He hasn't dated anyone for more than a few times since then.

As shown in Figure 3–3, the case conceptualization brings together Dr. Sudak's major observations on Brian's history and cognitive-behavioral pathology to form a working hypothesis and a plan for implementing CBT. As you will note, Dr. Sudak decided to add an antidepressant to the treatment plan. With moderate to severe symptoms, Brian could have been treated with CBT alone. However, there was a possible history of depression earlier in his life, probable family history of depression, and enough symptoms to suggest a combined approach might offer advantages. The CBT elements of the plan were directed at reversing self-punishing automatic thoughts, helping Brian reengage in positive activities, break his pattern of social isolation, and revise long-standing maladaptive core beliefs.

The two examples of case formulations presented here demonstrate typical CBT conceptualizations for treatment of anxiety disorders and depression. In each example, the therapist brings together observations from the patient's current functioning, developmental history, and bio-

**Patient Name:** Brian

**Diagnoses/Symptoms:** Major depression. PHQ-9 score at beginning of treatment=18 (moderately high depression). Primary symptoms are deep sadness, low self-esteem with self-condemning thoughts, loss of energy and interest, and social isolation. No suicidal thoughts.

**Formative Influences:** Father is an alcoholic who left the family when Brian was 18 months old, but sporadically tried to make contact with Brian and his mother. There have been financial strains, and his mother has had to "work constantly" in a variety of housekeeping jobs to support them. She is very loving and a solid support for Brian, who lived with her until his recent move to Philadelphia. Brian was shy as a teenager and college student and dated infrequently. When his only steady girlfriend broke up with him, he was devastated. Since then he has had no dates and has been especially lonely since moving about 6 months ago.

**Situational Issues:** Move from his small hometown to take new job in large city, difficulty making new friends and developing relationships, breakup with girlfriend.

**Biological, Genetic, and Medical Factors:** Mother has probably been depressed chronically but has never been treated. Father is an alcoholic. No history of medical illnesses.

**Strengths/Assets:** College education; good job skills as computer engineer; support from mother and male friends in his hometown; loyal to his friends; previous interests in singing in choir, running, and hiking; no substance abuse.

**Treatment Goals:** 1) Reduce depressive symptoms (PHQ-9 less than 5); 2) build self-confidence in relationships so I feel like I "fit in;" 3) resume participation in positive activities and hobbies; 4) be able to date regularly (at least 2 times a month).

| Event 1 | Event 2 | Event 3 |
|---|---|---|
| Sitting in car. Not able to go into restaurant with people from work. | Alone at home after skipping the happy hour with coworkers. | I notice an attractive woman at work. |

**Figure 3–3.** Case formulation worksheet for Brian.

| Automatic Thoughts | Automatic Thoughts | Automatic Thoughts |
|---|---|---|
| "I'm never going to fit in with these people." "I'm never going to be one of them." "I don't understand why they would want me here." "I'm nobody to them." | "I'm so alone." "I'm never going to fit in." "I'll never be able to make a life here." "I'm not going to be able to do it." | "She would never want to go out with me." "She probably thinks I'm a loser." "I should have stayed in a place where I had a chance to find someone." |
| **Emotions** | **Emotions** | **Emotions** |
| Sad | Sad | Sad, anxious |
| **Behaviors** | **Behaviors** | **Behaviors** |
| Didn't attend the party. Went home and spent entire weekend in front of TV. | Stayed by self in apartment. | Turned the other way and acted like I didn't see her. |

**Schemas:** "People can't be counted upon"; "I must always being on guard or I will be hurt"; "I'm not good enough"; "I'll never find a woman who loves me."

**Working Hypothesis:** 1) Brian's life experiences with an unreliable father and rejection by his only close girlfriend shaped core beliefs such as "People can't be counted upon" and "I'm not good enough." 2) A recent move from his hometown to a much larger city has been a major precipitant for a depression in which he is riddled with automatic thoughts with themes of never fitting in and not being accepted. 3) These thoughts are associated with a deep sadness and avoidance of social contacts. 4) His social isolation and lack of pleasurable activities have become part of a vicious cycle of negative thinking and depressed behavior.

**Treatment Plan:** 1) Identify recurrent automatic thoughts related to depressed mood and social isolation; 2) teach skills to modify automatic thoughts (examining the evidence, recognizing cognitive errors, and thought recording); 3) use activity scheduling and other behavioral activation methods to increase involvement in pleasurable activities and build social contacts; 4) increase self-esteem and personal effectiveness by identifying and modifying schemas (examining the evidence, CBT rehearsal for modified schemas, behavioral experiments with social relationships); 5) pharmacotherapy with an antidepressant.

**Figure 3–3.** Case formulation worksheet for Brian. *(continued)*

medical background and articulates a hypothesis consistent with the cognitive-behavioral model. The treatment plans flow directly from the working hypothesis and are rooted in specific CBT constructs for the treatment of anxiety and depression. We recommend that you begin to use the CBT case formulation worksheet now by completing Learning Exercise 3–1 and that you continue to build skills in performing conceptualizations as you gain additional experience in CBT. Chapter 11, "Building Competence in Cognitive-Behavior Therapy," includes exercises in writing out full case conceptualizations and performing self-ratings on your ability to carry out this important function.

**Learning Exercise 3–1.** CBT Case Formulation Worksheet

1. Use the CBT case formulation worksheet (see Appendix 1, "Worksheets and Checklists") to develop a conceptualization for a patient you are treating.

2. Try to fill out as much of the form as possible. However, if you have not performed case conceptualizations before or are inexperienced with CBT, don't worry if all of the worksheet is not completed. If possible, identify at least one event that stimulates automatic thoughts, emotions, and a behavioral response. Also attempt to identify at least one underlying schema. If the patient hasn't reported any schemas yet, you can theorize about schemas that might be present.

3. Sketch out a preliminary working hypothesis and treatment plan based on your current knowledge of the patient and the basic CBT concepts you have already learned.

4. Continue to use the CBT case formulation worksheet as you treat additional patients with CBT.

## Summary

Assessment for CBT includes all the usual tasks of performing an initial evaluation, including taking a thorough history, evaluating the patient's strengths, and performing a mental status examination. However, special attention is devoted to eliciting typical patterns of automatic thoughts, schemas, and coping behaviors and to judging the patient's suitability for

CBT. Because CBT has been shown to be effective for a wide range of conditions—including major depression, anxiety disorders, and eating disorders—and can add to the effects of medication in the treatment of severe psychiatric disorders (e.g., schizophrenia and bipolar disorder), there are many indications for this treatment approach.

A broad, cognitive-behavioral-social-biological viewpoint is suggested for case formulation and treatment planning. To construct a refined and highly functional conceptualization, clinicians need to 1) perform a detailed assessment, 2) develop a cross-sectional analysis of the cognitive-behavioral elements of typical stressful situations in the patient's current life, 3) consider longitudinal (i.e., developmental) influences on the patient's core beliefs and habitual behavioral strategies, 4) formulate a working hypothesis, and 5) design a treatment plan that directs effective CBT techniques at the patient's key problems and strengths.

## References

Beck AT, Ward CH, Mendelson M, et al: An inventory for measuring depression. Arch Gen Psychiatry 4:561–571, 1961 13688369

Davanloo H: Evaluation and criteria for selection of patients for short-term dynamic psychotherapy. Psychother Psychosom 29(1–4):307–308, 1978 724948

Forney JC, Unützer J, Wrenn G, et al: A Tipping Point for Measurement-Based Care. Psychiatr Serv Sept 2016 27582237

Frank JD: Persuasion and Healing. Baltimore, MD, Johns Hopkins University Press, 1973

Guo T, Xiang Y-T, Xiao L, et al: Measurement-based care versus standard care for major depression: a randomized controlled trial with blind raters. Am J Psychiatry 172(10):1004–1013, 2015 26315978

Kroenke K, Spitzer RL, Williams JB: The PHQ-9: validity of a brief depression severity measure. J Gen Intern Med 16(9):606–613, 2001 11556941

Malan DJ: The Frontiers of Brief Psychotherapy. New York, Plenum, 1973

Meyer TJ, Miller ML, Metzger RL, Borkovec TD: Development and validation of the Penn State Worry Questionnaire. Behav Res Ther 28(6):487–495, 1990 2076086

Miller WR, Yahne CE, Moyers TB, et al: A randomized trial of methods to help clinicians learn motivational interviewing. J Consult Clin Psychol 72(6):1050–1062, 2004 15612851

Prochaska JO, DiClemente CC: The transtheoretical approach, in Handbook of Psychotherapy Integration. Edited by Norcross JC, Goldfried MR. New York, Basic Books, 1992, pp 301–334

Radloff LS: The Center for Epidemiologic Studies Depression (CES-D) Scale: a self-report depression scale for research in the general population. Appl Psychol Meas 1:385–401, 1977

Safran JD, Segal ZV: Interpersonal Process in Cognitive Therapy. New York, Basic Books, 1990

Sifneos PE: Short-Term Psychotherapy and Emotional Crisis. Cambridge, MA, Harvard University Press, 1972

Spitzer RL, Kroenke K, Williams JBW, Löwe B: A brief measure for assessing generalized anxiety disorder: the GAD-7. Arch Intern Med 166(10):1092–1097, 2006 16717171

Thase ME, Callan JA: The role of homework in cognitive behavior therapy of depression. J Psychother Integr 16(2):162–177, 2006

Wright JH, Thase ME, Beck AT: Cognitive-behavior therapy, in The American Psychiatric Publishing Textbook of Psychiatry, 6th Edition. Edited by Hales RE, Yudofsky SC, Roberts L. Washington, DC, American Psychiatric Publishing, 2014, pp 1119–1160

# 4 Structuring and Educating

To understand the value of structuring in cognitive-behavior therapy (CBT), place yourself for a moment in the position of a patient who is just starting treatment. Try to imagine what it would be like to be a person with deep depression who is overwhelmed by life stresses, who is having trouble concentrating, and who has little or no idea of how therapy will work. Add to this mix of confusion and symptomatic distress a sense of demoralization—a belief that you have expended most or all of your personal resources and have not been able to find a solution to your problems. You are feeling frightened and are not sure where to turn for help. If you were in this state of mind, what do you think you would be looking for in therapy?

Of course you would want a kind, empathic, wise, and highly skilled therapist, as we discuss in Chapter 2, "The Therapeutic Relationship: Collaborative Empiricism in Action." But you would probably also be looking for a clear direction—a hopeful and compelling path toward recovery from your symptoms. Structuring methods, beginning with goal formulation and agenda setting, can play a large role in providing a direction for change (Table 4–1). If the patient has been feeling defeated by a problem or is vexed by his inability to overcome a symptom, structuring methods can send a powerful message: *Stay focused on the key problems,*

**Table 4–1.** Structuring methods for cognitive-behavior therapy

| |
|---|
| Goal setting |
| Agenda setting |
| Performing symptom checks |
| Bridging sessions |
| Providing feedback |
| Pacing sessions |
| Assigning homework |
| Using therapy tools (recurrent) |

*and answers will follow.* Psychoeducation sends a related message of hope: *These methods can work for you.*

Structuring and educating go hand in hand in CBT because these therapy processes complement one another in promoting learning. Effective structuring techniques enhance learning by keeping treatment well organized, efficient, and on target. Good psychoeducational interventions, such as homework exercises and using a therapy notebook, contribute important elements to the structure of CBT. The overall goals of structuring and educating are to generate hope, boost the learning process, improve the efficiency of therapy, and help the patient build effective coping skills.

During the early part of treatment, the clinician may do a large part of the work in structuring and educating. However, as CBT proceeds to its conclusion, the patient takes increasing responsibility for defining and managing problems, staying on task in working toward change, and applying the core concepts of CBT in everyday life.

## Structuring CBT

### Goal Setting

The process of developing treatment goals provides a great opportunity to teach the patient the value of setting specific, measurable targets for change. Typically, the first goal-setting intervention is performed toward the end of the first session, when you have assessed the patient's main problems, strengths, and resources and have started to build a collaborative empirical relationship. If you take a few moments to educate the patient about effective goal setting, the process may go more smoothly, take less time, and lead to a better result. The following case example demonstrates how to introduce goal setting in the first session.

## Case Example

Janet, a 36-year-old woman, recently ended a long-term relationship with her boyfriend. She told the therapist that the relationship was "going nowhere." Janet decided to make the change because she believed she had "wasted enough time already." Despite believing that she had made the correct decision, Janet was very depressed. She blamed herself for being "stupid to stay with him for so long" and for "putting up with a loser." Janet's self-esteem was at rock bottom. She saw herself as a person who would not find happiness in life and was doomed to be "rejected by anybody I would really want." Since the breakup 6 weeks ago, Janet had stopped exercising and socializing with friends. She was sleeping, or trying to sleep, much of the time that she was not at work. Fortunately, Janet had not been thinking of suicide. During the earlier part of the session, she had told the therapist that she knew she had to get over the breakup and put her life back together.

*Therapist:* We've had a good talk so far, and I think we've learned a lot about your problems and your strengths. Could we try to set some goals for treatment?

*Janet:* Yes. I need to stop falling apart. I've been such a wimp about this whole thing.

*Therapist:* I think you're putting yourself down. But let's try to come up with some goals that will give you a sense of direction—that will point your way out of this depression.

*Janet:* I don't know…I guess I just want to be happy again. I don't like feeling this way.

*Therapist:* Getting better can be an ultimate goal of treatment. But what might help the most right now is to choose some specific objectives that will tell us what we want to focus on in our therapy sessions. You might try to pick some short-term goals that we could accomplish fairly soon and some longer-range goals that will stretch us to keep working on the things that are most important to you.

*Janet:* Well, I want to do something with my life now besides trying to sleep it away. One goal could be to get back into my exercise routine. And I need to find something to do with my time that takes my mind off the relationship with Randy.

*Therapist:* Those are two good short-term goals. Could we put down on our list that you will work toward resuming regular exercise and developing positive interests or activities to help you get over the relationship?

*Janet:* Sure. I'd like to do both of those things.

*Therapist:* It also would be good to state the goals in a way that we can tell when we are making progress. What kind of markers could we set that will let us know how we are coming along?

*Janet:* To be exercising at least three times a week.

*Therapist:* How about for the interests and activities?

*Janet:* Well, at least going out with friends once a week and not spending so much time in bed.

*Therapist:* Those goals will give us a good start. Could you try to write down some other short-term goals before our next session?

*Janet:* OK.

*Therapist:* Now let's try to set some longer-term goals for us to work on. We've talked about your low self-esteem. Do you want to do anything about that problem?

*Janet:* Yes, I'd like to feel good about myself again. I don't want to spend the rest of my life feeling like a failure.

*Therapist:* Can you put the goal into specific terms? What do you want to accomplish?

*Janet:* To see myself as a strong person who will be fine with or without a man in my life.

The therapeutic interchange continued with the therapist giving Janet positive feedback for articulating clear goals that could help her make productive changes. Then the therapist helped Janet articulate additional goals before closing the session with homework assignments related to the overall objectives of the therapy. [The strategy used here, behavioral activation, is covered in more detail in Chapter 6, "Behavioral Methods I: Improving Mood, Increasing Energy, Completing Tasks, and Solving Problems."]

*Therapist:* What steps could you take in this next week to make some progress toward meeting your goals? Can you pick one or two things that you could do that would make you feel better if you were able to accomplish them?

*Janet:* I'll go to my health club after work at least twice, and I'll call my friend Terry to see if she wants to go to a movie.

Goals should be reviewed and revised at regular intervals (at least every fourth session) throughout the treatment process. Sometimes goals set early in treatment become less important as issues or concerns are resolved or as you get to know the patient better. New goals may become apparent as therapy progresses, and adjustments in treatment methods may be needed to surmount barriers in reaching certain goals. It can be helpful to list the patient's goals in the health record in order to keep focused on working toward these objectives. You can also ask patients to list their treatment goals in a therapy notebook (see the "Psychoeducation" section later in this chapter). Some basic principles for effective goal setting in CBT are reviewed in Table 4–2.

## Agenda Setting

The agenda-setting process runs parallel to goal setting and uses many of the same principles and methods. In contrast to goal setting, which is di-

**Table 4–2.** Tips for goal setting in cognitive-behavior therapy (CBT)

| |
|---|
| Educate the patient on goal-setting techniques. |
| Try to avoid sweeping, overgeneralized goals that may be difficult to define or attain. Generating goals of this type may make the patient feel worse, at least temporarily, if they seem overwhelming or unreachable. |
| Be specific. |
| Guide patients to choose goals that address their most significant concerns or problems. |
| Choose some short-term goals that you believe could likely be attained in the near future. |
| Develop some long-term goals that will require more extensive work in CBT. |
| Try to use terms that make goals measurable and will help you gauge progress. |

rected at the entire course of therapy, agenda setting is used to structure individual sessions. As we noted in describing goal-setting methods, patients usually need to be educated on the benefits and methods of devising a productive agenda. During the first few sessions, the therapist may need to take the lead in shaping the agenda. However, most patients quickly learn the value of an agenda and come to subsequent sessions prepared to work on specific concerns.

Session agendas that are especially effective include some of the following features:

1. **Agenda items relate directly to the overall goals of therapy.** Session agendas should help you reach treatment goals. If you find that an agenda item is not linked to the overall goals of therapy, consider revising either the session agenda or the goal list. Perhaps the agenda item is superfluous or has limited relevance to the overall course of therapy. Alternatively, the suggested agenda item might point toward a new or reformulated goal.
2. **Agenda items are specific and measurable.** Well-defined agenda items might be, for example, "1) develop ways to cope with my boss's irritability, 2) reduce procrastination at work, and 3) check on progress with homework from last week." Vague or overly general agenda items that would require further definition or reformulation might be "1) my depression, 2) feeling tired all the time, and 3) my mother."
3. **Agenda items can be addressed during a single session, and there is a reasonable likelihood that some benefit will result.** Try to help the patient select items, or redefine items, so that progress is possible in a single session. If the item seems too large or overwhelming, take a

piece of it for work in the session or restate the item in terms that are more manageable. To illustrate, an unwieldy agenda item suggested by Janet ("I don't want to feel rejected all the time") was reformulated to make it a workable topic for a single session ("build ways to cope with feelings of rejection").

4. **Agenda items contain an achievable objective.** Instead of merely being a discussion topic (e.g., "problems with kids, my marriage, handling stress"), the agenda item includes some potential measure of change or leads the therapist and patient to work on a specific plan of action (e.g., "what to do about daughter's problems at school, argue less and have more shared activities with my husband, reduce tension at work").

Even though agendas are a mainstay of the structuring process, there can be liabilities to dogmatically following an agenda. Too much structure can be a bad thing if it stifles creativity, lends a mechanistic tone to therapy, or prevents you and the patient from following valuable leads. When agendas and other structuring tools are used to their best effect, they create conditions that allow spontaneity and creative learning to proliferate.

Achieving the right balance between structure and expressiveness has been a recurring theme in art, music, architecture, psychotherapy, and other major fields of human endeavor. For example, the success of one of the world's most famous gardens, Sissinghurst, is often attributed to the dynamic interplay between a finely wrought structure of hedges, trees, and statuary and the abundant and free-flowing plantings of colorful flowers within these borders (Brown 1990). We view the agendas and other structuring tools of CBT as promoters of the more creative aspects of therapy, in the same way that the structure of a symphony, a painting, or a garden allows the emotionally resonant part of the composition to have greater impact.

To apply this concept practically in CBT sessions, we suggest that you routinely set and follow agendas, but remember that these structures are not set in stone. Their only purpose is to help you and the patient concentrate your energies on gaining insights and learning new ways of thinking and behaving. If following an agenda item is not helpful and it is unlikely that further work with this issue on this day will bear fruit, then move on to another topic. If a new idea comes out during a session and you believe there would be significant potential in altering the agenda, then discuss your observations with the patient and collaboratively decide on whether to move in this direction. However, stick with agendas when they are working and use them to shape your efforts to help patients change.

Because agenda setting is such an important component of CBT, we have included two video illustrations of this procedure. In the first vignette, Dr. Wichmann, a psychiatry resident, demonstrates agenda setting during a second session. At this point in therapy, the patient, Meredith, is feeling somewhat overwhelmed by a number of problems. However, Dr. Wichmann is able to help her shape an agenda that identifies specific targets for change.

**Video 3.** Agenda Setting:
Dr. Wichmann and Meredith (3:16)

You may be wondering if agenda setting always goes as smoothly as it did in Dr. Wichmann's session with Meredith. Perhaps you are thinking, "My patient just wants to talk....It would be hard to set an agenda with her." Although we often find that patients respond well to requests for agenda setting, there can be challenges in implementing this core CBT method. So we have included another video illustration to demonstrate how to overcome obstacles in developing an effective agenda, and we have provided Troubleshooting Guide 1 to help you gain skills in managing problems with agenda setting.

As you watch this next video, think about how you might overcome similar problems in agenda setting with your patients. Dr. Brown realized that allowing Eric to ventilate about his father for most of the session (a nondirective approach) would be unlikely to help Eric gain needed CBT skills. So Dr. Brown politely interrupted him, reinforced the value of agenda setting, and showed him how to define an agenda that would yield positive results.

**Video 4.** Difficulty Setting an Agenda:
Dr. Brown and Eric (2:50)

## Symptom Checks

The basic structure of CBT sessions includes several standard procedures that are performed each time the patient comes to therapy. In addition to agenda setting, most cognitive-behavior therapists include a brief symptom check or rating at the beginning of the session (Beck 2011). A simple, quick method is to ask patients to rate their level of depression, anxiety, or other symptoms on a scale of 0–10 points, where 10 equals the highest level of distress and 0 equals no distress. Even better, you can administer short, self-report questionnaires at each session. We especially recommend the Patient Health Questionnaire–9 (PHQ-9; Kroenke et al.

## Troubleshooting Guide 1
### Challenges in Working With an Agenda

1. **The patient launches into detailed or rambling accounts from the beginning of the session despite your request to set an agenda.** This challenge in implementing CBT may be especially common in individuals who have had previous experiences with nondirective therapy and have been encouraged to talk freely in an unstructured way. Other patients may have a natural inclination to be very talkative or have problems focusing on problem solving. During early sessions, explain the collaborative nature of CBT. If applicable, ask the patient about prior therapy experiences and discuss how the problem-oriented approach of CBT might differ. Ask permission to interrupt occasionally to help the patient stay on track to reach treatment goals. As done by Dr. Brown in Video 4, demonstrate that following an agenda leads to productive outcomes.

2. **The patient suggests too many agenda items or identifies a number of problems that seem overwhelming.** Step back to assess how the proposed agenda items fit with the overall goals of therapy, and work with the patient to plan an overall strategy that deals with concerns in a sequential fashion. Explain that progress is most likely if a smaller number of agenda items (usually two or three) are targeted in each session and these items are discussed in enough depth to develop action plans and effective coping skills.

3. **The patient suggests too few agenda items.** If the patient draws a blank when asked to set an agenda or lists only one or two items that don't appear to offer much opportunity for gain, the therapist can ask questions to stimulate ideas. "Could we take a look at our notes from the last session to see if there are topics we can work on today?" "How about reviewing your treatment goals so we're not missing something?" "Any stressful events that have triggered automatic thoughts?" Alternatively, the therapist can take the lead in generating agenda items. Perhaps the patient is ignoring or downplaying issues that need attention. Examples might include alcohol overuse, procrastinating on overdue projects from work, or avoiding social contacts.

## Troubleshooting Guide 1 *(continued)*
## Challenges in Working With an Agenda

4. **The patient typically neglects to place homework on the agenda.** As noted in the section "Homework" later in this chapter, routine inclusion of homework on session agendas increases the chances that exercises will be completed and be effective. If the patient doesn't add homework to the agenda, you can do so. In a kind manner, point out the importance of consistent follow-up on the self-help activities done outside sessions.

5. **The patient frequently veers off the agenda or spends much of the session ventilating about stressful events without learning CBT methods for coping with these events.** If the patient is a natural storyteller and feels frustrated by the structured nature of CBT, budget a modest amount of time for open discussions. In these cases, it is best if the majority of the effort is devoted to working on specific agenda items, while some time is set aside for the patient to report on what has happened since the last visit. To enlist the patient's cooperation in such structuring of sessions, you might say something like the following: "You are wonderful at telling about your experiences. I appreciate learning about the people in your life and the problems you face. But I've found that I can get caught up in the details of the story and do not make enough time to teach you something new. The session ends before we have a chance to practice ways to deal with your problems. What I would like to suggest is that we both do a better job at setting aside enough time for the work of CBT. What do you think?"

6. **You are uncomfortable with structuring therapy.** Previous training in supportive or psychodynamically oriented therapy may make it difficult for some therapists to take an active role in setting agendas, interrupting patients, and redirecting the flow of conversation. In addition, some therapists may have personality traits or background experiences that make them hesitant to interrupt others. If you have difficulty asking patients to be more focused in their conversations, review this issue with a supervisor and practice polite ways to interrupt. For example, you might say, "Do you mind if we pause for a moment to decide how to best use our time today? I can tell that the argument with your sister upset you. But we haven't set our agenda yet. I want to be sure we get the most out of our session."

2001) and the Generalized Anxiety Disorder 7-Item Scale (GAD-7; Spitzer et al. 2006). The PHQ-9 covers the nine core symptoms of major depressive disorder, including a question on suicidal ideation, and the GAD-7 targets seven common symptoms of anxiety. Both scales are in the public domain, so they can be administered without charge. And they are used widely in clinical practice and research. Table 4–3 lists several valuable self-report rating scales and their sources.

The symptom check provides a valuable estimate of progress and adds a consistent structuring item to the therapy session. Another reason to routinely perform a symptom check is the possibility that it will improve treatment outcome. As noted in Chapter 3, "Assessment and Formulation," routine use of self-rating scales has been found to improve treatment outcome and is a cornerstone of measurement-enhanced care.

To save time for therapeutic work in sessions, some clinicians ask patients to come early for appointments and to complete self-report questionnaires in the waiting room, either on paper or on a computer or electronic notepad. Integration of these ratings with the electronic health record can allow clinicians and patients to see graphic displays of treatment outcomes and to direct their attention toward achieving maximum gains.

In addition to the symptom check, we also perform a brief update with enough questions to obtain an accurate picture of how the patient is doing, assess progress, and learn about new developments. This symptom-check and brief-update segment of the session usually takes only a few minutes.

Some cognitive-behavior therapists routinely set the agenda before doing the symptom check/brief update and thus include symptom assessment as a standard agenda item. Others perform the symptom check in the very beginning portion of the session as a prelude to the agenda-setting process. In the templates for session structures provided later in this chapter (see "Structuring Sessions Throughout the Course of CBT"), we use the strategy of performing a symptom check/brief update as the first element of the session.

## Bridging Between Sessions

Although most of the structuring effort is directed at managing the flow within a single session, it is usually helpful to ask a few questions that will help the patient follow through on issues or themes from the previous meeting. Homework, one of the standard structuring elements, ties sessions together and keeps therapy focused on key issues or interventions that stream through multiple visits. However, we recommend that you go beyond checking the homework, to be sure that important directions from

**Table 4–3.** Brief self-report rating scales

| Rating scale | Application | Source | Reference |
|---|---|---|---|
| Patient Health Questionnaire–9 (PHQ-9) | Depression | www.phqscreeners.com | Kroenke et al. 2001 |
| Quick Inventory of Depressive Symptomatology (QIDS-16) | Depression | www.ids-qids.org | Rush et al. 2003 |
| Beck Depression Inventory (BDI) | Depression | www.pearsonclinical.com | Beck et al. 1961 |
| Generalized Anxiety Disorder 7-Item Scale (GAD-7) | Anxiety | www.phqscreeners.com | Spitzer et al. 2006 |
| Penn State Worry Questionnaire (PSWQ) | Anxiety | at-ease.dva.gov.au/professionals/files/2012/11/PSWQ.pdf | Meyer et al. 1990 |
| Beck Anxiety Inventory | Anxiety | www.pearsonclinical.com | Beck et al. 1988 |

*Note.* All scales in this table can be used clinically for not-for-profit use without royalty payment, with the exception of the Beck Depression and Beck Anxiety Inventories. Check rights information on the Web site for each scale before use.

earlier meetings are not set aside or forgotten with the press of newer initiatives. One useful way to bridge sessions is to take a few moments early in the visit to review your therapy notes and to ask the patient to review her notebook to look for follow-up items for the day's agenda.

## Feedback

In some forms of psychotherapy, limited emphasis is given to providing feedback to the patient. However, cognitive-behavior therapists go out of their way to provide and request feedback to help keep the session structured, build the therapeutic relationship, give appropriate encouragement, and correct distortions in information processing. It is usually recommended that cognitive-behavior therapists stop at several points in each session to elicit feedback and check for understanding. The patient is asked questions such as the following: "How do you think the session is going so far?" "Before we go on, I want to pause a moment to see if we are both on the same track.... Can you summarize what you've learned so far?" "What do you like about the therapy?" "What suggestions do you have for things you would like for me to do differently?" or "What are your take-home points from today's session?"

Constructive and supportive feedback is also given to the patient at frequent intervals (Table 4–4). Many times the feedback is just a phrase or two that provides direction for the session. For example, the therapist might say, "We're making good progress today, but I think we'd get the most out of the session if we put off discussing your job until next week and focused our attention on the problem with your daughter." A statement like this would be best followed by a request for feedback from the patient: "How does this idea sound to you?" In giving feedback, there can be a fine line between providing accurate information that gives the patient appropriate encouragement and making statements that could be perceived as being either overly positive or critical. The suggestions in Table 4–4 may help you give your patients feedback that is well received and moves the therapy ahead.

Some of the impetus for attention to the feedback process in CBT has come from the extensive studies of information processing in depression (Clark et al. 1999). The weight of evidence from these investigations suggests that persons with depression hear less positive feedback than nondepressed control subjects and that this bias in information processing may play a role in the persistence of depressogenic cognitions (Clark et al. 1999). In addition, studies of persons with anxiety disorders have found that these conditions are associated with a maladaptive information processing style (see Chapter 1, "Basic Principles of Cognitive-Behavior Ther-

**Table 4–4.** Tips for giving feedback in cognitive-behavior therapy

| |
|---|
| Provide feedback that helps patients stick to the agenda. You can make comments such as "You've started to talk about a new problem; before we go in that direction, let's stop to think about how we want to use the rest of our time today." |
| Provide feedback that enhances the organization, productivity, and creativity of the therapy session. Spot digressions, but also take note if an unexpected breakthrough or unplanned revelation appears to hold considerable promise. |
| Be genuine. Offer encouragement, but don't go overboard in praising the patient. |
| Try to make constructive comments that identify strengths or gains and also may suggest further opportunities for change. Be careful to avoid giving feedback that may make patients think you are judging them negatively or are unhappy with their efforts in therapy. |
| You can summarize main points of therapy as a way of giving feedback. However, it can become tedious if you are continually summarizing the content of therapy. Giving a capsule summary once or twice a session will usually suffice. Asking the patient to give the capsule summary can enhance collaboration and learning. |
| Use feedback as a teaching tool. Be a good coach, and let patients know when they are picking up valuable insights or skills. You can use comments such as "Now we're getting somewhere" or "You really made that homework assignment pay off" to highlight areas of progress or lessons you hope they will retain. |

apy"). For example, a person with agoraphobia may have been told many times by family members and friends that her fears are unfounded, but the message does not get through.

We suggest that you keep these research findings in mind when you are giving feedback to your patients. You might need to help them understand that depression or anxiety can place a filter on their perceptions and that things you or others say to them may not be heard as intended. You may also want to help your patients work on skills of giving and receiving accurate feedback. An especially useful way of doing this is by modeling effective ways of processing feedback in the therapeutic relationship.

## Pacing

How can you make best use of the time in therapy sessions? When should you switch to a new agenda item? How long should you continue to work on a topic when you seem to be stalled or are having trouble making progress? How directive should you be in helping the patient stay focused on the current issue? Are you moving so fast that the patient is having trouble grasping and remembering key concepts? Would it help to go back over a topic to review what has been learned? These are the types of questions that you will need to answer to pace sessions at a high level of productivity while maintaining an excellent therapeutic relationship.

In our experience with supervising CBT trainees, we have found that pacing skills are hard to learn from reading about therapy. The nuances of timing therapy interventions and asking questions that effectively shape the structure of sessions are best learned through repeated practice, role-playing, receiving supervision on recorded therapy sessions, and watching videos of experienced therapists.

The main strategy to keep in mind as you work on pacing CBT sessions is the effective use of a problem-oriented or goal-oriented questioning style. Nondirective or supportive therapists may simply follow the patient's lead in carrying on a therapeutic dialogue. However, if you are doing CBT, you will need to actively plan and focus the line of questioning. Based on the case formulation, you will guide the patient toward productive discussion of specific topics and will usually stick with a theme until an intervention yields results, an action plan can be developed, or a follow-up homework assignment can be arranged. Because artful pacing is one of the more difficult CBT skills to acquire, we offer Troubleshooting Guide 2; it provides possible solutions for common problems in gaining maximum benefit from therapy time.

There are a number of video illustrations in this book that demonstrate pacing techniques in CBT. We suggest that you keep pacing and timing issues in mind as you view the brief vignettes that are included in later chapters. Sources for additional videos of CBT, including our other illustrated guides for CBT (*Cognitive-Behavior Therapy for Severe Mental Illness*; Wright et al. 2009, and *High-Yield Cognitive-Behavior Therapy for Brief Sessions*; Wright et al. 2010) and sessions conducted by master therapists such as Aaron T. Beck, Judith Beck, Christine Padesky, are provided in Appendix 2, "Cognitive-Behavior Therapy Resources."

## Homework

Homework serves many purposes in CBT. The most important function of homework is building CBT skills for managing problems in real-life situations. But homework also is used to add structure to therapy by providing a routine agenda item for each therapy visit and by serving as a bridge between individual sessions. For example, if homework to complete a thought record for an anticipated stressful event (e.g., meeting with a boss, attempting to face a feared social situation, or trying to resolve a conflict with a friend) was suggested at the previous visit, this assignment would

**Troubleshooting Guide 2**
**Difficulty Pacing Sessions**

1. **Therapy time is used inefficiently.** You note that there are many digressions and sessions lack clarity or sharp focus. Possible solutions include 1) increasing your attention to setting a well-tuned agenda, 2) asking for and giving more feedback, 3) checking overall therapy goals to see if you are staying on target to reach those goals, and 4) reviewing a recorded session with a supervisor to spot and correct inefficiencies.

2. **Only one agenda item is covered when two or three other important items are neglected or given only cursory attention.** There are some occasions when a decision to spend the entire session on one agenda item is the best course to take. In this situation, other agenda items can be delayed until the next visit. However, a general pattern of not covering listed agenda items suggests that you are not thinking ahead and making strategic decisions about how to use therapy time. Try having a discussion with the patient at the beginning of the session about allocating therapy time for each agenda item. You don't have to nail the timing down to the minute, but you can try to prioritize the items and get a general idea of how much time each item should take.

3. **You have difficulty making collaborative decisions on the direction of therapy.** Pacing and timing decisions are being made only by you. The patient either has not been asked to give feedback or passively accepts all your decisions and is content to let you always be in the driver's seat. Or the patient is controlling much of the direction of the session without getting or accepting feedback from you. In these types of situations, there is a problem with balance in the therapeutic relationship. Try to improve the flow and pace of sessions by emphasizing joint decision-making on a) choice of topics, b) how much time and effort are spent on a topic, and c) when to move ahead to another topic.

### Troubleshooting Guide 2 *(continued)*
### Difficulty Pacing Sessions

4. **The session ends without any sense of movement or action that could lead to progress.** Well-paced sessions are typically directed toward a change that the patient can make that will help relieve symptoms, manage a problem, or prepare him to manage a future situation. If you find that your sessions are ending without any sense of resolution or forward movement, review the case formulation, devise some strategies for change, and plan ahead to the next visit. Are you suggesting homework assignments that help the patient follow through with lessons learned in therapy sessions? If not, refine homework assignments to include an action plan for change. Also ask the patient to summarize the main "take away" points from the session. If she has difficulty doing so, or there are no specific takeaways that can be identified, focus more effort on developing them.

5. **You give up prematurely on a topic that shows promise.** This pacing problem is commonly observed in sessions conducted by CBT trainees. Generally, the yield from a therapy session is greater when a small number of topics are discussed in depth than when a large amount of ground is covered superficially.

6. **Your skills in phrasing questions and managing therapy transitions need further development.** Although some clinicians seem to have an abundance of native talent for asking just the right questions to make sessions flow smoothly and efficiently, most of us need to practice, watch ourselves on video, and get good supervision before we can master interviewing techniques in CBT. Viewing recorded sessions (or listening to audio recordings) is a particularly important method of gaining skills in pacing and timing. When you observe recorded sessions, try to spot areas where you could have sharpened the focus of the questioning. Stop the playback and brainstorm several different options for questions you might have asked. Also watch sessions conducted by experienced cognitive-behavior therapists to get ideas on how to ask the most effective questions and make excellent therapy transitions.

be placed on the agenda for the current session. Even if the patient does not complete the assignment or has difficulty carrying it out, there are usually benefits to discussing the homework.

When assignments work out well, review points can be made so that learning is reinforced during the session. Tie-ins to the agenda for the current visit, or ideas or issues that have been stimulated by the homework, may suggest new agenda items. When problems are encountered in completing homework, it often helps to explore the reasons why the assignment was not done or why it didn't work out as planned. Perhaps you did not explain the assignment clearly. Is it possible that you suggested homework that was seen as too difficult, too easy, or not relevant to the patient's challenges?

A strategy that usually works well is to explore any barriers that the patient experienced in carrying out the assignment. Was he feeling so overwhelmed with work that he didn't think he could take the time to do the homework? Was he afraid that coworkers, children, or others would see his homework? Was he feeling so exhausted that he couldn't get organized to start the exercise? Has there been a long pattern of procrastination? Did the word *homework* set off some negative associations from experiences in school? There can be numerous reasons why patients do not follow through with homework assignments. If you can discern the reasons why this happened, you will be in a better position to make future homework assignments a more successful experience.

We discuss homework at a number of places in this book because it is one of the most useful tools in CBT (e.g., Troubleshooting Guide 3 addresses problems in completing homework in Chapter 6, "Behavioral Methods I: Improving Mood, Increasing Energy, Completing Tasks, and Solving Problems"). As you will see, the wide variety of interventions for changing maladaptive cognitions and behavior (e.g., thought records, examining the evidence, activity scheduling, and exposure and response prevention) described in later chapters are used extensively as homework assignments. Although your main focus in suggesting homework will be to put a CBT method into action or to help the patient cope with a troubling situation, try to keep in mind the importance of structure in CBT and the central role of homework in providing this structure.

## Structuring Sessions Throughout the Course of CBT

Some elements of session structure are maintained during all phases of CBT. However, early sessions are typically characterized by more structure than later sessions. In the beginning of therapy, patients are usually more symptomatic, may have more difficulty concentrating and remembering, are more likely to be feeling hopeless, and have not yet gained CBT skills for organizing efforts to cope with problems. By the later parts of therapy, less structure should be required because patients have made progress in resolving symptoms, have acquired expertise in using CBT self-help methods, and can take increased responsibility for managing their own therapy. As we have noted before, one of the goals of CBT is to help patients become their own therapists by the end of treatment.

In Tables 4–5, 4–6, and 4–7, we provide templates for session structures for the early, middle, and late phases of CBT. Each session includes the common features of agenda setting, a symptom check, homework review, CBT work on problems or issues, a new homework assignment, and feedback. The amount of structure and the content of the session vary as the therapy matures to its conclusion. These templates are provided for general guidance only and are not meant to be used as a one-size-fits-all system for structuring therapy. However, we have found that these basic outlines can be customized to fit the needs and attributes of most patients and provide structures that help reach treatment goals.

**Table 4–5.** Session structure outline: early phase of treatment

1. Greet patient.
2. Perform a symptom check.
3. Set agenda.[a]
4. Review homework from previous session.[b]
5. Conduct cognitive-behavior therapy (CBT) work on issues from agenda.
6. Socialize to cognitive model. Teach basic CBT concepts and methods.
7. Develop new homework assignment.
8. Review key points, give and elicit feedback, and close session.

*Note.* Examples of CBT work in the early part of therapy include identifying mood shifts, spotting automatic thoughts, making two- or three-column thought records, identifying cognitive errors, scheduling activities, and conducting behavioral activation. There is an emphasis in the beginning phases of CBT on demonstrating and teaching the basic cognitive model. Feedback is typically given and requested several times during the visit and at the end of the session.
[a]Some therapists prefer to set the agenda before performing a symptom check.
[b]Homework may be reviewed and/or assigned at multiple points in the session.

**Learning Exercise 4–1.** Structuring CBT

1. Enlist a fellow trainee, colleague, or supervisor to help you practice structuring methods for CBT. Use role-

**Table 4–6.** Session structure outline: middle phase of treatment

1. Greet patient.
2. Perform a symptom check.
3. Set agenda.
4. Review homework from previous session.
5. Conduct cognitive-behavior therapy (CBT) work on issues from agenda.
6. Develop new homework assignment.
7. Review key points, give and elicit feedback, and close session.

*Note.* Examples of CBT work in the middle part of therapy include identifying automatic thoughts and schemas, making five-column thought records, providing graded exposure to feared stimuli, and conducting beginning-level or midlevel work on changing schemas. Therapy goals should be reviewed periodically throughout the middle phase of therapy, but a review is usually not placed on the agenda for every session. The amount of structure may begin to decline gradually in the middle phase of CBT if the patient is demonstrating increased skill in organizing efforts to tackle problems.

**Table 4–7.** Session structure outline: late phase of treatment

1. Greet patient.
2. Perform a symptom check.
3. Set agenda.
4. Review homework from previous session.
5. Conduct cognitive-behavior therapy (CBT) work on issues from agenda.
6. Work on relapse prevention; prepare for termination of therapy.
7. Develop new homework assignment.
8. Review key points, give and elicit feedback, and close session.

*Note.* Examples of CBT work in the late phase of therapy include identifying and modifying schemas, making five-column thought records, developing action plans to manage problems and/or practice revised schemas, and completing exposure protocols. Therapy goals are reviewed periodically throughout the late phase of CBT, and goals for work beyond therapy are formulated. There is a focus on identifying potential triggers for relapse and using procedures such as cognitive-behavioral rehearsal to help the patient stay well after therapy ends. The amount of structure is reduced in the late phase of CBT as the patient takes progressively more responsibility for implementing CBT methods in daily life.

playing to practice setting goals and agendas at different phases of therapy.

2. Ask the helper to role-play a patient who has difficulty setting agendas. Discuss options you may have for helping the patient define productive agenda items. Then try to implement these strategies.

3. Use the role-playing exercise to practice giving and receiving feedback. Ask the helper to give you constructive criticism. Are you perceived as giving supportive, helpful, and clear feedback?

4. Rehearse giving homework assignments. Again, ask the helper to give you an honest appraisal of your skills. Does she have any suggestions for how you might improve the homework assignment?

5. Implement the structuring methods described in this chapter in work with your patients. Discuss your experiences with a supervisor or colleague.

## Psychoeducation

There are three principal reasons why honing your teaching skills can help you maximize your effectiveness as a cognitive-behavior therapist. First, CBT is based on the idea that patients can learn skills for modifying cognitions, controlling moods, and making productive changes in their behavior. Your success as a therapist will rest in part on how well you teach these skills. Second, effective psychoeducation throughout the therapy process should arm patients with knowledge that will help them reduce the risk of relapse. Finally, CBT is geared toward helping patients become their own therapists. You will need to educate your patients on how to continue to use cognitive and behavioral self-help methods after the conclusion of therapy. Some methods for providing this education are outlined in Table 4–8 and are described in the subsections below.

### Mini-Lessons

There are occasions in therapy sessions when short explanations or illustrations of CBT theories or interventions may be used to help the patient understand concepts. A lecturing style is avoided in these mini-lessons in favor of a friendly, engaging, and interactive educational style. Socratic questions can be used to stimulate the patient to get involved in the learning process. Written diagrams or other learning aids can also enhance the educational experience. We often use a circular diagram that shows the linkage between events, thoughts, emotions, and behavior when we first explain the basic cognitive-behavioral model. This technique works best if you can diagram an example from the patient's life.

A demonstration of psychoeducation on the CBT model is provided in Video 1. In this video, Dr. Wright helps Kate understand the relationship

**Table 4–8.** Psychoeducational methods

| |
|---|
| Providing mini-lessons |
| Writing out an exercise in session |
| Using a therapy notebook |
| Recommending readings |
| Using computer-assisted cognitive-behavior therapy |

between environmental triggers, automatic thoughts, emotions, and behaviors. Using an emotionally charged example from her recent experiences, he generates an engaging learning experience that is likely to be remembered and used. The diagram shown in Figure 4–1 was a major feature of the educational work done in this therapy session.

**Video 1.** Getting Started—CBT in Action: Dr. Wright and Kate (12:17)

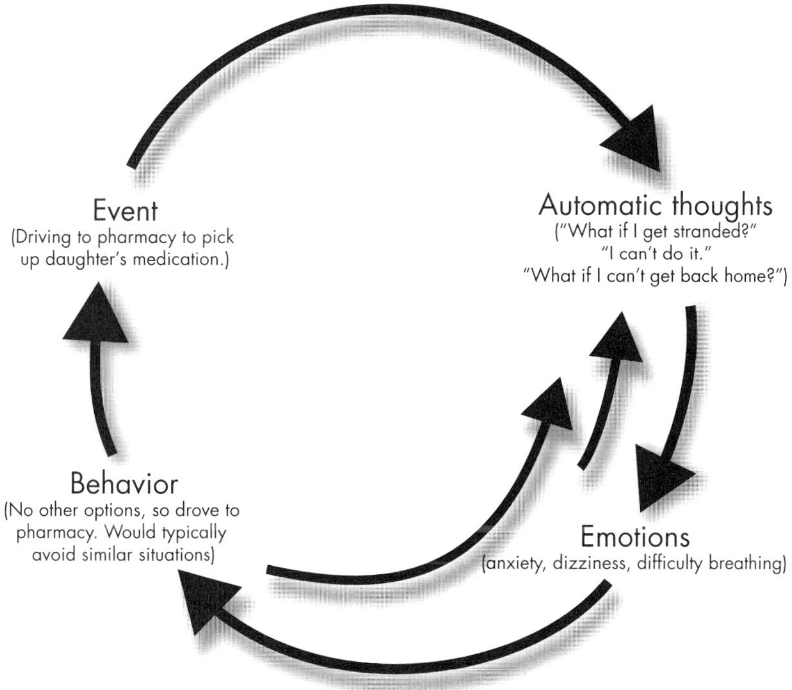


**Figure 4–1.** Kate's diagram of the cognitive-behavior therapy model.

## Exercise Template

A good way to educate patients on CBT methods is to write out an example of an exercise in a therapy session while explaining how the procedure works. Then the written exercise can be given to the patient as a template for future work, and a copy can be made for the chart. Seeing the method in writing can help patients learn the concept quickly and retain it. Some possible applications of this technique include drawing a diagram of the CBT model, as shown in Video 1; writing out a thought record (see Figure 5–1 in Chapter 5, "Working With Automatic Thoughts"); completing an exercise in examining the evidence (see Figure 5–2 in Chapter 5); and filling out a coping card (see Table 5–5 and Figures 5–6 and 5–7 in Chapter 5).

## Therapy Notebook

Exercises from therapy sessions, homework assignments, handouts, rating scales, notes on key insights, and other printed or electronically produced materials can be organized in a therapy notebook (in paper and/or digital format). We are strong proponents of the use of therapy notebooks because they promote learning, can enhance follow-through with homework assignments, and can help patients remember and use CBT concepts for many years after therapy ends. For example, a man whom one of us had treated in the past called to schedule a session after a divorce. He had not been seen in the past 10 years, but he reported that he had routinely consulted his therapy notebook for assistance in using CBT to manage the stresses in his life. Although he had been troubled by the divorce, he had successfully used CBT methods to avoid slipping back into depression. After one booster session, he decided that he could continue to use self-help CBT techniques and would not need ongoing therapy.

We typically introduce the idea of a therapy notebook during the first or second session and then reinforce the value of this method throughout the course of treatment. A bonus of therapy notebooks is that they can help structure CBT if they are consulted or augmented as a routine part of each session. Therapy notebooks are also extremely valuable for inpatient CBT applications, in which the efforts of individual therapy, group treatments, homework review sessions, and other activities can be organized and enhanced with this recording method (Wright et al. 1993).

## Readings

Self-help books, handouts, or other materials available in print or on the Internet are often used in CBT to educate patients and to get them involved in learning exercises outside treatment sessions. We typically recommend at least one self-help book to our patients and give them guidance on what chapters they might find helpful at different points in the therapy. For example, *Breaking Free From Depression: Pathways to Wellness* (Wright and McCray 2011) has two introductory chapters that help people assess symptoms and set useful goals. These chapters offer a good starting point for a person who is in the earliest stage of therapy. Chapters on automatic thoughts, core beliefs, and behavioral exercises are then recommended as therapy turns to these topics. Readings from this book about medications can be suggested when patients are receiving pharmacotherapy or are interested in learning about biological treatments for depression.

When you assign readings, try to choose materials that are appropriate for the stage of therapy; the patient's education level, cognitive capacity, and psychological sophistication; and the type of symptoms that are being experienced. In addition, materials should be selected to meet the special needs of patients. Large print may be required if patients have visual acuity problems, or audio recordings or video recordings may be needed for persons who cannot read. We keep a wide range of choices in mind when we use readings to augment CBT.

A list of recommended readings and Web sites for patients is included in Appendix 2, "Cognitive-Behavior Therapy Resources." Popular CBT self-help books include *Feeling Good: The New Mood Therapy* (Burns 2008), *Breaking Free From Depression: Pathways to Wellness* (Wright and McCray 2011), and *Mind Over Mood: Change How You Feel by Changing the Way You Think* (Greenberger and Padesky 2015). Useful books for persons with anxiety disorders include *Mastery of Your Anxiety and Panic* (Craske and Barlow 2006) and *The Anti-Anxiety Workbook* (Antony and Norton 2009). *Stop Obsessing! How to Overcome Your Obsessions and Compulsions* (Foa and Wilson 2001) is a widely used self-help resource for obsessive-compulsive disorder. And useful CBT methods for bipolar disorder are provided in *The Bipolar Workbook: Tools for Controlling Your Mood Swings* (Basco 2015).

We suggest that you read several of the self-help books and review some of the other resources listed in Appendix 2, "Cognitive-Behavior Therapy Resources," so that you will be prepared to discuss specific educational materials with your patients. The Web sites identified in Appendix 2 can also provide valuable information on CBT. The Academy of Cognitive Therapy has an excellent Web site (http://www.academyofct.org) that has educational materials for both clinicians and patients. The Web site of the Beck Institute (http://www.beckinstitute.org) offers suggested readings and has a CBT bookstore.

Becoming an expert in providing psychoeducation requires both knowledge and practice. The next learning exercise can help you gain valuable experience in learning how to be a good teacher and coach for your patients.

**Learning Exercise 4–2.** Psychoeducation in CBT

1. Make a list of at least five main components of CBT for which you believe psychoeducation should be routinely provided (e.g., basic cognitive-behavioral model, the nature of automatic thoughts). What are the essential lessons you want to get across?

2. Add to this list

   a. Specific ideas for educating patients in each of the areas you have identified.

   b. Suggested readings or other educational resources for each topic.

3. Ask a colleague, fellow trainee, or supervisor to help you role-play methods for providing psychoeducation. Pay special attention to maintaining the collaborative empirical relationship and avoiding an overly didactic teaching style.

## Computer Technology in the Delivery of CBT

Have you thought about how computer programs or apps might help you perform CBT? Traditional psychotherapy relies completely on the therapist to coach the patient on therapy principles, provide insights, measure progress, give feedback, and build CBT skills. However, there has been escalating interest in ideas for integrating computer technology into the treatment process. A number of studies have demonstrated effectiveness of computer-assisted CBT (CCBT), in which a computer program is used to significantly reduce the amount of therapist time required for successful treatment (Adelman et al. 2014; Andersson and Cuijpers 2009; Davies et al. 2014; Newman et al. 2014; Richards and Richardson 2012; Thase et al. 2017; Wright 2004, 2016; Wright et al. 2005). For example, CCBT with a multimedia program (*Good Days Ahead*; Wright 2004; Wright et al. 2005) has been shown to be as effective as standard CBT in treating depressive symptoms in drug-free patients, despite lowering the total amount of therapist time by about one-half in one study and two-thirds in another (Thase et al. 2017; Wright 2016; Wright et al. 2005). The computer-assisted approach was more effective than standard CBT in helping patients acquire knowledge about CBT (Thase et al. 2017; Wright 2016; Wright et al. 2005).

Fully developed computer programs for CBT may go beyond the provision of psychoeducation to include a broad array of therapeutic experiences (Andersson and Cuijpers 2009; Marks et al. 2009; Thase et al. 2017; Wright 2004, 2016). *Good Days Ahead* provides an online experience that utilizes video, audio, and a variety of interactive exercises to help patients apply CBT principles in fighting depression and anxiety. This program also tracks the user's responses (including mood graphs, comprehension scores, lists of automatic thoughts and schemas, action plans to cope with problems, and other data) to assist the clinician in monitoring progress and guiding the patient in use of the computer software.

Examples of other multimedia programs for CBT that have been studied in controlled trials and are being used in clinical practice include *FearFighter* (Kenwright et al. 2001; Marks et al. 2009), a program from the United Kingdom that is directed primarily at using behavioral methods for anxiety disorders, and *Beating the Blues* (Proudfoot et al. 2003), another program from the United Kingdom. *Beating the Blues* was shown to have an additive effect to pharmacotherapy in primary care patients with depression in an initial study (Proudfoot et al. 2003). In contrast to the generally favorable results of studies of CCBT for depression and anxiety (Adelman et al. 2014; Richards and Richardson 2012; Thase et al. 2017; Wright 2016), a larger trial involving the addition of *Beating the Blues* or another widely used program, *Mood Gym* (Gilbody et al. 2015), to treatment as usual for depression in primary care patients failed to show any additional benefit.

Findings of this latter study underscore the importance of providing adequate human support for patients participating in computer-assisted therapy for depression. A mean of less than 7 minutes of technical support and no clinician time was given (Gilbody et al. 2015). Completion rates were very low—only 18% for *Beating the Blues* and 16% for *Mood Gym* (Gilbody et al. 2015). However, studies of CCBT with *Good Days Ahead* coupled with modest amounts of clinician support observed completion rates of about 85% (Thase et al. 2017; Wright 2016; Wright et al. 2005).

One of the most interesting applications of computer technology in CBT has been the use of virtual reality to assist in exposure therapies for anxiety disorders and related diagnoses. Programs have been developed and tested for height phobia, fear of flying, agoraphobia, and posttraumatic stress disorder, among other disorders (Morina et al. 2015; Rothbaum et al. 1995, 2000, 2001; Turner and Casey 2014; Valmaggia et al. 2016). Virtual reality is used to simulate feared situations so that the therapist can conduct in vivo exposure therapy in the office for situations such as riding in a glass elevator, flying in an airplane, or traumatic experiences.

A variety of apps are available for mobile deployment of commonly used CBT exercises, including pleasant events scheduling, breathing training, relaxation, and thought logging (Aguilera and Muench 2012; Dagöö et al. 2014; Possemato et al. 2016; Van Singer et al. 2015; Watts et al. 2013). However, a comprehensive review of 52 CBT apps for panic disorder found that most were insufficiently evidence based and had low content quality (Van Singer et al. 2015). Typically apps are used for a circumscribed CBT activity and do not provide comprehensive CCBT experiences such as those developed for *Good Days Ahead, FearFighter, Beating the Blues*, or other multimedia CBT programs. Yet, Watts et al. (2013) have described successful adaptation of a program for depression using text and cartoons for mobile delivery. We anticipate that the content and breadth of mobile apps will be enhanced with further development.

In evaluating computer technology for use in CBT, clinicians should be aware of confidentiality issues, Health Insurance Portability and Accountability Act (HIPAA) regulations, and need for secure encryption (APA Council on Psychiatry & Law 2014). Commercially available programs for CCBT should meet established requirements for security of data if any personal health information is collected and/or stored.

The use of computer technology to help therapists educate and treat patients is one of the newer developments in CBT. Although some clinicians have questioned whether CCBT might impair the therapeutic relationship or be perceived by the patient in a negative way, there is a long track record of studies showing excellent acceptance by patients (Andersson and Cuijpers 2009; Colby et al. 1989; Johnston et al. 2014; Kim et al. 2014; Thase et al. 2017; Wright 2016; Wright et al. 2002). As with any other therapy tool, you will be able to make the best use of computer programs if you make an effort to familiarize yourself with the materials and then gain experience with using them in clinical practice. Web sites that give information on computer programs for CBT are listed in Appendix 2, "Cognitive-Behavior Therapy Resources." We think that the pervasive use of computers in society, lack of access to empirically tested psychotherapies, evidence for the efficiency and effectiveness of CCBT, and increased sophistication and appeal of CBT programs and apps will lead to a merging of human effort and technology in the practice of CBT.

## Summary

Structuring and educating are complementary processes in CBT. Structuring can generate hope, organize the direction of therapy, keep sessions on target to meet goals, and promote learning of CBT skills. Psychoeducation is primarily directed at teaching the core concepts of CBT, but it also adds to the structure of therapy by using recurring educational methods such as therapy notebooks in each session.

Cognitive-behavior therapists add structure to treatment by setting goals and agendas, performing symptom checks, providing and receiving feedback, assigning and checking homework, and pacing sessions effectively. Another part of the therapist's role is to be a good teacher or coach. Within the framework of the Socratic method, clinicians give mini-lessons, suggest readings, and may utilize innovative methods such as CCBT. Structuring and educating methods work best when they are integrated smoothly into the therapy session and are used to support and facilitate the more expressive, emotionally charged components of therapy.

## References

Adelman CB, Panza KE, Bartley CA, et al: A meta-analysis of computerized cognitive-behavioral therapy for the treatment of DSM-5 anxiety disorders. J Clin Psychiatry 75(7):e695–e704, 2014 25093485

Aguilera A, Muench F: There's an app for that: information technology applications for cognitive behavioral practitioners. Behav Ther (N Y N Y) 35(4):65–73, 2012 25530659

Andersson G, Cuijpers P: Internet-based and other computerized psychological treatments for adult depression: a meta-analysis. Cogn Behav Ther 38(4):196–205, 2009 20183695

Antony MM, Norton PJ: The Anti-Anxiety Workbook: Proven Strategies to Overcome Worry, Phobias, Panic, and Obsessions. New York, Guilford, 2009

APA Council on Psychiatry & Law: Resource Document on Telepsychiatry and Related Technologies in Clinical Psychiatry. Approved by the Joint Reference Committee. Arlington, VA, American Psychiatric Association, January 2014

Basco MR: The Bipolar Workbook, Second Edition: Tools for Controlling Your Mood Swings. New York, Guilford, 2015

Beck AT, Ward CH, Mendelson M, et al: An inventory for measuring depression. Arch Gen Psychiatry 4:561–571, 1961 13688369

Beck AT, Epstein N, Brown G, Steer RA: An inventory for measuring clinical anxiety: psychometric properties. J Consult Clin Psychol 56(6):893–897, 1988 3204199

Beck JS: Cognitive Behavior Therapy: Basics and Beyond, 2nd Edition. New York, Guilford, 2011

Brown J: Sissinghurst: Portrait of a Garden. New York, HN Abrams, 1990

Burns DD: Feeling Good: The New Mood Therapy, Revised. New York, HarperCollins, 2008

Clark DA, Beck AT, Alford BA: Scientific Foundations of Cognitive Theory and Therapy of Depression. New York, Wiley, 1999

Colby KM, Gould RL, Aronson G: Some pros and cons of computer-assisted psychotherapy. J Nerv Ment Dis 177(2):105–108, 1989 2915214

Craske MG, Barlow DH: Mastery of Your Anxiety and Panic, 4th Edition. Oxford, UK, Oxford University Press, 2006

Dagöö J, Asplund RP, Bsenko HA, et al: Cognitive behavior therapy versus interpersonal psychotherapy for social anxiety disorder delivered via smartphone and computer: a randomized controlled trial. J Anxiety Disord 28(4):410–417, 2014 24731441

Davies EB, Morriss R, Glazebrook C: Computer-delivered and web-based interventions to improve depression, anxiety, and psychological well-being of university students: a systematic review and meta-analysis. J Med Internet Res 16(5):e130, 2014 24836465

Foa EB, Wilson R: Stop Obsessing! How to Overcome Your Obsessions and Compulsions. New York, Bantam Books, 2001

Gilbody S, Littlewood E, Hewitt C, et al; REEACT Team: Computerised cognitive behaviour therapy (cCBT) as treatment for depression in primary care (REEACT trial): large scale pragmatic randomised controlled trial. BMJ 351:h5627, 2015 DOI: 10.1136/bmj.h5627 26559241

Greenberger D, Padesky CA: Mind Over Mood: Change How You Feel by Changing the Way You Think, 2nd Edition. New York, Guilford, 2015

Johnston L, Dear BF, Gandy M, et al: Exploring the efficacy and acceptability of Internet-delivered cognitive behavioural therapy for young adults with anxiety and depression: an open trial. Aust N Z J Psychiatry 48(9):819–827, 2014 24622977

Kenwright M, Liness S, Marks I: Reducing demands on clinicians by offering computer-aided self-help for phobia/panic: feasibility study. Br J Psychiatry 179:456–459, 2001 11689405

Kim DR, Hantsoo L, Thase ME, et al: Computer-assisted cognitive behavioral therapy for pregnant women with major depressive disorder. J Womens Health (Larchmt) 23(10):842–848, 2014 25268672

Kroenke K, Spitzer RL, Williams JB: The PHQ-9: validity of a brief depression severity measure. J Gen Intern Med 16(9):606–613, 2001 11556941

Marks IM, Cuijpers P, Cavanagh K, et al: Meta-analysis of computer-aided psychotherapy: problems and partial solutions. Cogn Behav Ther 38(2):83–90, 2009 20183689

Meyer TJ, Miller ML, Metzger RL, Borkovec TD: Development and validation of the Penn State Worry Questionnaire. Behav Res Ther 28(6):487–495, 1990 2076086

Morina N, Ijntema H, Meyerbröker K, Emmelkamp PMG: Can virtual reality exposure therapy gains be generalized to real-life? A meta-analysis of studies applying behavioral assessments. Behav Res Ther 74:18–24, 2015 26355646

Newman MG, Przeworski A, Consoli AJ, Taylor CB: A randomized controlled trial of ecological momentary intervention plus brief group therapy for generalized anxiety disorder. Psychotherapy (Chic) 51(2):198–206, 2014 24059730

Possemato K, Kuhn E, Johnson E, et al: Using PTSD Coach in primary care with and without clinician support: a pilot randomized controlled trial. Gen Hosp Psychiatry 38:94–98, 2016 26589765

Proudfoot J, Goldberg D, Mann A, et al: Computerized, interactive, multimedia cognitive-behavioural program for anxiety and depression in general practice. Psychol Med 33(2):217–227, 2003 12622301

Richards D, Richardson T: Computer-based psychological treatments for depression: a systematic review and meta-analysis. Clin Psychol Rev 32(4):329–342, 2012 22466510

Rothbaum BO, Hodges LF, Kooper R, et al: Effectiveness of computer-generated (virtual reality) graded exposure in the treatment of acrophobia. Am J Psychiatry 152(4):626–628, 1995 7694917

Rothbaum BO, Hodges L, Smith S, et al: A controlled study of virtual reality exposure therapy for the fear of flying. J Consult Clin Psychol 68(6):1020–1026, 2000 11142535

Rothbaum BO, Hodges LF, Ready D, et al: Virtual reality exposure therapy for Vietnam veterans with posttraumatic stress disorder. J Clin Psychiatry 62(8):617–622, 2001 11561934

Rush AJ, Trivedi MH, Ibrahim HM, et al: The 16-Item Quick Inventory of Depressive Symptomatology (QIDS), clinician rating (QIDS-C), and self-report (QIDS-SR): a psychometric evaluation in patients with chronic major depression. Biol Psychiatry 54(5):573–583, 2003 12946886

Spitzer RL, Kroenke K, Williams JB, Löwe B: A brief measure for assessing generalized anxiety disorder: the GAD-7. Arch Intern Med 166(10):1092–1097, 2006 16717171

Thase ME, Wright JH, Eells TD, et al: Improving efficiency and reducing cost of psychotherapy for depression: computer-assisted cognitive-behavior therapy versus standard cognitive-behavior therapy. Unpublished paper submitted for publication; data available on request from authors. Philadelphia, PA, January 2017

Turner WA, Casey LM: Outcomes associated with virtual reality in psychological interventions: where are we now? Clin Psychol Rev 34(8):634–644, 2014 25455627

Valmaggia LR, Latif L, Kempton MJ, Rus-Calafell M: Virtual reality in the psychological treatment for mental health problems: An systematic review of recent evidence. Psychiatry Res 236:189–195, 2016 26795129

Van Singer M, Chatton A, Khazaal Y: Quality of smartphone apps related to panic disorder. Front Psychiatry 6:96, 2015 26236242

Watts S, Mackenzie A, Thomas C, et al: CBT for depression: a pilot RCT comparing mobile phone vs. computer. BMC Psychiatry 13:49, 2013 DOI: 10.1186/1471-244X-13-49 23391304

Wright JH: Computer-assisted cognitive-behavior therapy, in Cognitive-Behavior Therapy. Edited by Wright JH (Review of Psychiatry Series, Vol 23; Oldham JM and Riba MB, series eds). Washington, DC, American Psychiatric Publishing, 2004, pp 55–82

Wright JH: Computer-assisted cognitive-behavior therapy for depression: progress and opportunities. Presented at National Network of Depression Centers Annual Conference, Denver, Colorado, September, 2016

Wright JH, McCray LW: Breaking Free From Depression: Pathways to Wellness. New York, Guilford, 2011

Wright JH, Thase ME, Beck AT, et al (eds): Cognitive Therapy With Inpatients: Developing a Cognitive Milieu. New York, Guilford, 1993

Wright JH, Wright AS, Salmon P, et al: Development and initial testing of a multimedia program for computer-assisted cognitive therapy. Am J Psychother 56(1):76–86, 2002 11977785

Wright JH, Wright AS, Albano AM, et al: Computer-assisted cognitive therapy for depression: maintaining efficacy while reducing therapist time. Am J Psychiatry 162(6):1158–1164, 2005 15930065

Wright JH, Turkington D, Kingdon D, Basco MR: Cognitive-Behavior Therapy for Severe Mental Illness. Washington, DC, American Psychiatric Publishing, 2009

Wright JH, Sudak DM, Turkington D, Thase ME: High-Yield Cognitive-Behavior Therapy for Brief Sessions: An Illustrated Guide. Washington, DC, American Psychiatric Publishing, 2010

Wright JH, Wright AS, Beck AT: Good Days Ahead. Moraga, CA, Empower Interactive, 2016

# 5

# Working With Automatic Thoughts

Methods designed to reveal and change maladaptive automatic thoughts lie at the heart of the cognitive-behavioral approach to psychotherapy. One of the most important basic constructs of cognitive-behavior therapy (CBT) is that there are distinctive patterns of automatic thoughts in psychiatric disorders and efforts to revise these styles of thinking can significantly reduce symptoms. Therefore, cognitive-behavior therapists often devote large portions of treatment sessions to the task of working with automatic thoughts.

There are two overlapping phases in the CBT approach to automatic thoughts. First the therapist helps the patient *identify* automatic thoughts. Then the focus shifts to learning methods to *modify* negative automatic thoughts and turn the patient's thinking in a more adaptive direction. In clinical practice, there is rarely a sharp division between these phases. Identification and change occur together as part of a progressive process of developing a rational thinking style. Commonly used methods for identifying and changing automatic thoughts are listed in Tables 5–1 and 5–2.

---

Items mentioned in this chapter that are available in Appendix 1, "Worksheets and Checklists," are also available as a free download in larger format on the American Psychiatric Association Publishing Web site: https://www.appi.org/wright.

**Table 5–1.** Methods for identifying automatic thoughts

| |
|---|
| Recognizing mood shifts |
| Psychoeducation |
| Guided discovery |
| Thought recording |
| Imagery exercises |
| Role-play exercises |
| Checklists |

**Table 5–2.** Methods for modifying automatic thoughts

| |
|---|
| Socratic questioning |
| Examining the evidence |
| Identifying cognitive errors |
| Thought change records |
| Generating rational alternatives |
| Decatastrophizing |
| Reattribution |
| Cognitive rehearsal |
| Coping cards |

## Identifying Automatic Thoughts

### Recognizing Mood Shifts

In the early stages of CBT, clinicians need to help patients understand the concept of automatic thoughts and assist them with recognizing some of these cognitions. We typically introduce this topic in the first session or another early session, when the patient displays a burst of automatic thoughts that drives an intense emotional response. A good rule of thumb is to regard any display of emotion as a sign that significant automatic thoughts have just occurred. Astute therapists will take advantage of these mood shifts to help uncover salient automatic thoughts and to teach patients about the basic cognitive-behavioral model.

Mood shifts are especially useful in uncovering automatic thoughts because they typically generate cognitions that are emotionally charged, immediate, and of high personal relevance. Beck (1989) noted that "emotion is the royal road to cognition" because thought patterns that are linked to significant emotional expression offer rich opportunities for drawing out some of the patient's most important automatic thoughts and schemas. Another reason for focusing on mood shifts is the impact of emotion on memory. Because emotional charging tends to increase a person's memory for events (Wright and Salmon 1990), therapy interventions that stimulate emotion may enhance recall and thus make it more likely that the patient will grasp and utilize the concept of automatic thoughts.

## Psychoeducation

The educational methods described in Chapter 4, "Structuring and Educating," can be an important part of helping patients learn to identify automatic thoughts. We usually devote time in the beginning of therapy to brief explanations of the nature of automatic thoughts and how they influence emotion and behavior. These explanations may work best if they follow the identification of a mood shift or relate to a specific stream of thoughts that have been uncovered during a therapy session. Video 1, introduced in Chapter 4, demonstrates psychoeducation about automatic thoughts. If you haven't seen this video yet, we suggest that you view it now.

## Guided Discovery

Guided discovery is the most frequently used technique for identifying automatic thoughts during therapy sessions. A brief sample illustrates questioning with simple guided-discovery methods.

### Case Example

Anna, a 60-year-old woman with depression, described herself as feeling disconnected from both her daughter and her husband. She was sad, lonely, and defeated. After retiring from a job as a teacher, she had hoped to have good times with her family. But now she was thinking, "No one needs me any longer.... I don't know what I'll do with the rest of my life."

*Therapist:* You've been talking about how the problem with your daughter has been upsetting you. Can you remember an example of something that happened recently?

*Anna:* Yes, I tried to call her three times yesterday. I didn't hear back till 10 o'clock at night, and she seemed irritated that I had been calling her all day.

*Therapist:* What did she say?

*Anna:* Something like "Don't you know I'm busy all day with my job and the kids? I can't drop everything to call you back right away."

*Therapist:* And what went through your mind when you heard her say that?

*Anna:* "She doesn't need me anymore.... She doesn't care.... I'm just a pest."

*Therapist:* And did you have any more thoughts—ideas that were popping through your mind at the time?

*Anna:* I guess I really got down on myself. I was thinking that I was pretty worthless—that no one needs me anymore. I don't know what I'll do with the rest of my life.

Some additional strategies for working with automatic thoughts are provided here. These guidelines are not absolute rules but are offered as tips for detecting automatic thoughts through guided discovery.

### *Guided Discovery for Automatic Thoughts: High-Yield Strategies*

1. **Pursue lines of questioning that stimulate emotion.** Remember that emotions such as sadness, anxiety, or anger are signs that the topic is important to the patient. Affectively laden cognitions can serve as beacons that you are on the right track.
2. **Be specific.** Questioning for automatic thoughts almost always goes better if it is targeted on a situation that is clearly defined and memorable. Discussion of general topics often leads to reports of broadly sketched or diffuse cognitions that do not give the degree of detail needed for fully effective interventions. Examples of specific situations that might lead to discovery of important automatic thoughts are 1) "I had a job interview last Monday"; 2) "I tried to go to a party in the neighborhood, but I got so nervous that I couldn't do it"; and 3) "My girlfriend dumped me, and I'm totally miserable."
3. **Focus on recent events instead of the distant past.** Sometimes it is important to lead the questioning process toward remote happenings, especially if the patient has posttraumatic stress disorder related to long-standing issues, a personality disorder, or a chronic condition. However, questioning about recent events usually offers the advantage of accessing automatic thoughts that actually occurred in the situation and that may be more amenable to change.
4. **Stick with one line of questioning and one topic.** Try to avoid jumping around among different topics. It is more important to do a thorough job of bringing out a series of automatic thoughts in a single situation than to explore an array of cognitions about multiple situations. If patients can learn to fully identify their automatic thoughts for one problematic concern, they are more likely to be able to do this on their own for other significant issues in their lives.
5. **Dig deeper.** Patients commonly report just a few automatic thoughts or seem to get in touch with only superficial cognitions. When this

happens, the therapist can ask additional questions that help the patient tell the full story. Further inquiry should be done in a sensitive manner so that the patient does not feel pushed. Questions such as the following might be used: "What other thoughts did you have in the situation?" "Let's try to stay with this a little bit longer, OK?" "Can you remember any other thoughts that might have been going through your mind?"

If these types of simple questions don't yield results, the therapist can try to move the process along by using Socratic questions that stimulate a sense of inquiry:

*Patient:* When I heard that Georgette was moving to Chicago, I was crushed. She is my only real friend.
*Therapist:* Did you have any more thoughts about her moving?
*Patient:* Not really—I just know that I'll really miss her.

The therapist notes that the patient is very sad and suspects that more intense automatic thoughts are below the surface.

*Therapist:* I have a hunch that you might have had some other thoughts. When you heard that she was leaving, what thoughts popped into your mind about yourself? How did you see yourself right after you learned the bad news?
*Patient (after a pause):* That I'm not any good at making friends.…I'll never have another friend like her.…My life is going nowhere.
*Therapist:* If those types of thoughts are true, how do you see yourself ending up?
*Patient:* Alone.…I think it's hopeless; nothing will ever change.

6. **Use your empathy skills.** Try to imagine yourself in the same situation as the patient. Get inside this person's head and think as he might think. By doing this with many patients, you can build your skills in understanding the cognitions that are common to a wide variety of conditions, and you will become more adept at sensing patients' key automatic thoughts.
7. **Ask for uncensored automatic thoughts.** To uncover immediate and intense automatic thoughts, it may help to discuss the natural tendency to cover over or edit raw thoughts that patients might think would be offensive or make the therapist think poorly of them. During such discussions, therapists can normalize the common urge to not report thoughts that may be laced with profanity or other incendiary words. And they can give reassurance that patients will not be judged on the content of their thoughts. Instead the therapist wants to hear the true, first-order automatic thoughts to give the most assistance. Patients who have problems

with anger at themselves or others are especially prone to censor their reports of automatic thoughts. For example, think of a patient with road rage. Helping a person with this difficulty may hinge on eliciting the inflammatory thoughts that fuel sudden bursts of extreme anger.

8. **Rely on the case formulation for direction.** The case formulation, even if it is in an early stage of development, can provide invaluable help in deciding on lines of inquiry. Knowledge of precipitants and stressors will suggest important topics for discussion. Assessment of the patient's symptoms, strengths, vulnerabilities, and background history will allow the therapist to customize questions for the individual patient. One of the most useful aspects of the formulation is the differential diagnosis. If panic disorder is suspected, questions can be directed at uncovering automatic thoughts about catastrophic predictions of bodily harm or loss of control. If the patient appears to be depressed, the questioning will typically lead to themes of low self-esteem, negative views of the environment, and hopelessness. When mania or hypomania is present, the therapist will need to adjust questioning techniques to account for a tendency to externalize blame, deny personal responsibility, and have grandiose automatic thoughts. We strongly recommend that clinicians who are learning CBT acquire a good understanding of the cognitive-behavioral model for each of the major psychiatric disorders (see Chapter 3, "Assessment and Formulation," and Chapter 10, "Treating Chronic, Severe, or Complex Disorders"). This information can provide an excellent road map for using guided discovery to identify automatic thoughts.

Video 5, drawn from Dr. Donna Sudak's treatment of Brian, demonstrates several of the guided-discovery methods noted above. Brian's history and case conceptualization are featured in Chapter 3, "Assessment and Formulation," and a series of other vignettes from his treatment will appear later in this chapter and in Chapter 8, "Modifying Schemas." As you view Video 5, try to spot the methods Dr. Sudak uses to uncover Brian's automatic thoughts and think of how you might use similar methods with your patients.

In this first video from Brian's treatment, Dr. Sudak asks questions that help him see the link between triggering events (e.g., sitting alone in his car after avoiding a social occasion), automatic thoughts (e.g., "I'm never going to fit in with these people....I'm never going to be one of them"), and his intense sadness. They agree that his negative automatic thoughts should be a prime target for therapy.

**Video 5.** Eliciting Automatic Thoughts:
Dr. Sudak and Brian (9:09)

## Thought Recording

Writing automatic thoughts down on paper (or using a computer or smartphone) is one of the most helpful and frequently used CBT techniques. The recording process draws the patient's attention to important cognitions, provides a systematic method to practice identifying automatic thoughts, and often stimulates a sense of inquiry about the validity of the thought patterns. Just seeing thoughts written down on paper often sets off a spontaneous effort to revise or correct maladaptive cognitions. Furthermore, thought recording can be a powerful springboard for the therapist's specific interventions to modify automatic thoughts (see the section "Thought Change Records" later in this chapter).

Thought recording is typically introduced in the early phase of therapy in a simplified manner that helps patients learn about automatic thoughts without overloading them with too much detail. More elaborate thought recording with features such as labeling cognitive errors, examining the evidence, and generating rational alternatives (see the section "Thought Change Records" later in this chapter) is usually delayed until the patient gains experience and confidence in identifying automatic thoughts. One method commonly used in the opening part of therapy is to ask patients to use two or three columns to record their thinking, first in a therapy session and then as a homework assignment. A two-column thought record might include listings of events and automatic thoughts (or automatic thoughts and emotions). A three-column record could contain spaces for noting events, automatic thoughts, and emotions. Figure 5–1 shows a thought recording exercise from the treatment of Anna, the 60-year-old woman with depression described earlier this chapter, in the section "Guided Discovery."

Efforts to teach patients thought recording methods and have them begin to log automatic thoughts often go smoothly. However, sometimes there can be challenges in using this valuable method. Patients may have adherence problems in doing thought records for homework, not understand the process, or get discouraged with automatic thoughts that seem impossible to change. So we've included a video to give you an example of how a therapist can overcame difficulties in implementing thought recording.

In this illustration, Dr. Brown finds that Eric did not do a homework assignment to log automatic thoughts. Using a nonjudgmental questioning style, he asks Eric to tell him what happened. After Eric explains that he didn't see the point in writing down how bad he was feeling and that he wanted to get away from the thoughts that were upsetting him, Dr. Brown admits that he may have not adequately prepared him for the as-

| Event | Automatic thoughts | Emotions |
|---|---|---|
| My husband decided to play poker on Friday night instead of going to the movies with me. | "I'm boring. It's no wonder he wants to spend so much time with his friends. It's a wonder he hasn't left me." | Sadness, loneliness |
| It's Monday morning and I have nothing to do, nowhere to go. | "I'm ready to scream. I can't stand my life. I was stupid to retire." | Sadness, tension, anger |
| A woman at church said I was lucky to be retired and not have to deal with the students every day. | "If only she knew how miserable I am. I don't have any friends. My family doesn't care how I feel. I'm a total mess." | Anger, sadness |

**Figure 5–1.** Anna's three-column thought record.

signment. The next step, discussing the rationale for thought recording, sets the stage for doing a thought record in the session. As you will see, the technique of performing a missed homework assignment in session—one of the best methods of responding to homework nonadherence—is successful in revealing important automatic thoughts and helping Eric understand the value of thought recording. Further tips for addressing homework adherence problems are detailed in Chapter 6, "Behavioral Methods I: Improving Mood, Increasing Energy, Completing Tasks, and Solving Problems."

**Video 6.** Difficulty With Thought Recording: Dr. Brown and Eric (6:31)

## Imagery

When patients have difficulty elaborating their automatic thoughts, an imagery exercise often can yield excellent results. This technique involves helping patients relive important events in their imagination to get in touch with the thoughts and feelings they had when the events occurred. Sometimes all that is needed is to ask patients to go back in time and to imagine themselves in the situation. However, it often helps to set the stage by using prompts or questions to rekindle their memories of events.

Methods of using imagery to identify automatic thoughts are demonstrated by Dr. Brown in his therapy with Eric. In this vignette, Eric has difficulty describing any of the automatic thoughts he had when his father came into his room and questioned him about finding a job. Noting that Eric appeared to be very upset about the interchange, Dr. Brown sus-

**Table 5–3.** How to help patients use imagery

1. Explain the method and its rationale.
2. Use a supportive and encouraging vocal tone. The quality of your voice and your questioning style should convey a message that the experience is safe and will be helpful.
3. Suggest that the patient try to remember what she was thinking in advance of the incident. "What led up to the event?" "What was going on in your mind as you approached the situation?" "How did you feel before the interaction began?"
4. Ask questions that promote recollection of the occurrence, such as "Who was there?" "How did the other people appear?" "What were the physical surroundings?" "Were there any sounds or smells that you can recall?" "What were you wearing?" or "What else can you picture about the scene before anything was said?"
5. As the scene is described, use stimulating questions that intensify the image and help the patient go deeper to remember automatic thoughts.
6. Use imagery exercises to underscore the importance of recognizing mood shifts as avenues to automatic thoughts.

pected there were important automatic thoughts that might be accessed with imagery techniques. After asking Eric to revisit the scene to immerse himself in the experience via imagery, intense automatic thoughts were revealed (e.g., "There's nothing I can do about it.... I'm not good enough.... I'm going to feel like this forever").

**Video 7.** Using Imagery to Uncover Automatic Thoughts: Dr. Brown and Eric (6:44)

The clinician's skill in explaining and facilitating imagery can make a big difference in how fully patients engage in this experience. Contrast, for example, an intervention that includes little or no preparation for imagery, followed by a rather mechanical statement (e.g., "Think back to the time your father came into the room, and describe what was going through your mind"), with the evocative coaching and questioning techniques used by Dr. Brown in the video illustration. Strategies for enhancing the effectiveness of imagery are listed in Table 5–3.

## Role-Play

Role-playing involves the therapist taking the role of a person in the patient's life—such as a boss, a spouse, a parent, or a child—and then trying to simulate an interchange that might stimulate automatic thoughts.

Roles also can be reversed by having the patient play the other person while the therapist plays the patient. Role-playing is used less frequently than other techniques such as guided discovery and imagery because it requires a special effort to set up and implement. Also, implications for the therapeutic relationship and boundaries between patient and therapist need to be considered when deciding to use this approach. Some questions that you might ask yourself before embarking on a role-play exercise are the following:

1. **How would role-playing this particular scene with this important figure in the patient's life affect the therapeutic relationship?** For example, would the advantages of my role-playing this patient's abusive father outweigh any disadvantages of me being seen in a negative light or possibly being identified with the father? Could the role-play have a favorable influence on the therapy relationship? Will the patient be able to perceive that I am being supportive and helpful by playing this role?
2. **Is the patient's reality testing strong enough to see this experience as a role-play and to return to an effective working relationship after the role-play is completed?** Caution should be exercised if the patient has significant characterological problems such as borderline personality disorder, has experienced severe abuse, or has psychotic features. However, experienced cognitive therapists have learned how to use role-play effectively under these conditions. We recommend that beginning cognitive therapists use role-play primarily with persons who have problems such as acute depression or anxiety disorders; for such patients, the role-playing experience usually will be seen as a straightforward attempt to help them understand their thinking.
3. **Would this role-play tap into long-standing relationship issues, or would it be focused on a more circumscribed event?** As a general rule, it is best to orchestrate role-plays early in therapy that deal with here-and-now concerns. After the patient and therapist gain experience in doing targeted role-plays for specific current situations, they can use this method to explore automatic thoughts associated with emotionally loaded topics such as feeling rejected or unloved by a parent.

Despite these notes of caution, role-play can be an especially useful method of revealing automatic thoughts and is typically viewed by patients as a positive demonstration of the therapist's interest and concern. Later in this chapter, we will discuss how role-play can be used to modify automatic thoughts (see the section "Generating Rational Alternatives" later in this chapter). You will also have the opportunity to use role-play as a method for learning CBT. Role-play can be an excellent way for trainees to practice CBT techniques. A wide variety of therapy interactions can be simulated, stopped and started, tried in a different manner, discussed, and rehearsed. In addition, taking the patient role in training applications of this method can help clinicians get a sense of what patients might experience in the CBT process. We suggest that you work on building your skills in role-playing and other CBT techniques for identifying cognitions by doing the following learning exercise:

**Learning Exercise 5–1.** Identifying Automatic Thoughts

1. Ask another trainee in CBT, a supervisor, or a colleague to help you practice identifying automatic thoughts. Do a series of role-play exercises in which you have the opportunity to be the therapist and your helper plays a patient. Then reverse roles to expand your experiences in using the techniques.

2. Use a mood shift to draw out automatic thoughts.

3. Implement the principles of guided discovery described earlier in this chapter. For example, focus on a specific situation, develop a formulation to direct the questioning, and try to dig deeper to bring out additional automatic thoughts.

4. Practice using imagery for a situation in which the "patient" is having trouble recognizing automatic thoughts. Ask a series of questions that set the scene and help evoke memories of the event.

5. Do a role-play within a role-play. For this part of the exercise, you will ask your helper to construct a scenario in which you will educate the "patient" on the role-play method and then use role-play methods to elicit automatic thoughts.

6. After practicing these methods with a helper, implement them with your patients.

## Checklists for Automatic Thoughts

The most extensively researched checklist for automatic thoughts is Hollon and Kendall's (1980) Automatic Thoughts Questionnaire (ATQ). Although this questionnaire has been used primarily in empirical studies to measure changes in automatic thoughts associated with treatment, it also can be used in clinical settings when patients have difficulty detecting their cognitions. The ATQ has 30 items (e.g., "I'm no good"; "I can't stand this anymore"; "I can't finish anything"), which are rated for frequency of occurrence on a five-point scale from 0 ("Not at all") to 4 ("All of the time").

The computer program *Good Days Ahead* (Wright et al. 2016) contains an extensive module on automatic thoughts that teaches patients how to recognize and change these cognitions. One component of the *Good Days Ahead* program is the development of customized lists of negative automatic thoughts and counterbalancing positive thoughts. Users of this program can draw cognitions from an inventory of common automatic thoughts and can also type in any other thoughts they can identify. An automatic thoughts checklist from *Good Days Ahead* is presented in Table 5–4 and is also available at: https://www.appi.org/wright.

## Modifying Automatic Thoughts

### Socratic Questioning

When learning to become a cognitive-behavior therapist, it is easy to fall into the trap of bypassing Socratic questioning in favor of thought recording, examining the evidence, coping cards, or other CBT methods with specific forms or procedures. However, we place Socratic questioning first on our list of methods for changing automatic thoughts because the questioning process is the backbone of cognitive interventions to change dysfunctional thinking. Although Socratic questioning is somewhat harder to learn and to implement with skill than more structured interventions, it can pay great dividends in your effort to modify automatic thoughts. Some of the benefits of Socratic questioning are enhancement of the therapeutic relationship, stimulation of a sense of inquiry, improved understanding of important cognitions and behaviors, and promotion of the patient's active engagement in therapy.

Methods for Socratic questioning are explained in Chapter 1, "Basic Principles of Cognitive-Behavior Therapy," and Chapter 2, "The Therapeutic Relationship: Collaborative Empiricism in Action." Listed below are some key features of Socratic questioning to keep in mind as you use this method to modify automatic thoughts:

1. **Ask questions that reveal opportunities for change.** Good Socratic questions often open up possibilities for patients. Using the basic CBT model as a guide (thoughts influence emotions and behavior), try to

**Table 5–4.** Automatic thoughts checklist

**Instructions:** Place a check mark beside each negative automatic thought that you have had in the past 2 weeks.

____I should be doing better in life.
____He/she doesn't understand me.
____I've let him/her down.
____I just can't enjoy things anymore.
____Why am I so weak?
____I always keep messing things up.
____My life's going nowhere.
____I can't handle it.
____I'm failing.
____It's too much for me.
____I don't have much of a future.
____Things are out of control.
____I feel like giving up.
____Something bad is sure to happen.
____There must be something wrong with me.

*Source.* Adapted with permission from Wright JH, Wright AS, Beck AT: *Good Days Ahead*. Moraga, CA, Empower Interactive, 2016. Copyright © Empower Interactive, Inc. All rights reserved. Available at: https://www.appi.org/wright.

ask questions that help patients see how changing their thinking can reduce painful emotions or improve their ability to cope.

2. **Ask questions that get results.** Socratic questions work best when they break through a rigid, maladaptive thought pattern to show patients reasonable and productive alternatives. New insights are developed, and the change in thinking is associated with a positive emotional shift (e.g., anxious or depressed mood is improved). If your Socratic questions don't seem to produce any emotional or behavioral results, then step back, review the case formulation, and revise your strategy.
3. **Ask questions that get patients involved in the learning process.** One of the goals of Socratic questioning is to help patients become skilled in "thinking about thinking." Your questions should stimulate your patients' curiosity and encourage them to look at new perspectives. Socratic questions should serve as a model for questions that patients can start asking themselves.
4. **Pitch questions at a level that will be productive for the patient.** Considering the patient's level of cognitive functioning, symptomatic distress, and ability to concentrate, ask questions that will offer enough

challenge to make patients think but will not overwhelm or intimidate them. Effective Socratic questions should make patients feel better about their cognitive abilities, not stupid or dense. Ask Socratic questions that you believe patients have a good chance of being able to answer.

5. **Avoid asking leading questions.** Socratic questions should not be used to establish the therapist as an expert (i.e., the therapist knows all the answers and leads the patient to these same conclusions) but should be a method for enhancing the patient's ability to think flexibly and creatively. Of course, you will have some idea of where Socratic questions might lead and what results you hope to achieve, but ask questions in a manner that respects patients' ability to think for themselves. Let patients do the work in answering questions whenever possible.
6. **Use multiple-choice questions sparingly.** Typically, good Socratic questions are open-ended. A large number of answers or permutations of answers are possible. Although yes-or-no questions or multiple-choice questions may be effective on some occasions, the majority of Socratic questions should leave room for a variety of responses.

## Examining the Evidence

The strategy of examining the evidence can be a powerful method for helping patients modify automatic thoughts. This technique involves listing evidence for and against the validity of an automatic thought or other cognition, evaluating this evidence, and then working on changing the thought to be consistent with the newfound evidence. There are two video illustrations of using examining the evidence to change automatic thoughts.

The first video illustration is from Dr. Sudak's treatment of Brian. They work on modifying one of his most troubling automatic thoughts, "I'll never fit in." A two-column worksheet was used to record evidence for this thought and to note the alternatives they generated (Figure 5–2). In this session from early in therapy, Dr. Sudak asks open-ended questions to find evidence, both pro and con. Then she takes the lead to help him understand that he hasn't had much experience in adapting to a move to a new city. She also normalizes his loneliness. In later sessions, she will put more emphasis on Brian taking the lead in generating alternative thoughts.

**Video 8.** Examining the Evidence: Dr. Sudak and Brian (11:58)

Automatic thought: I'll never fit in.

| Evidence for automatic thought: | Evidence against automatic thought: |
|---|---|
| 1. I'm so different from everybody. | 1. I've worked together with Jack on several projects. We work well together. We have some things in common. |
| 2. It's been 3 months since I've been here, and nothing is changing. | 2. I say hi to some people at my apartment building. |
| 3. It's getting worse. | 3. Before I came to Philadelphia, I had friends from running cross-country and singing in a choir. |
| | 4. I keep in touch with friends from my hometown. |

Cognitive errors: Overgeneralizing[a]

Alternative thoughts: I haven't had much experience with moving away and establishing a life for myself. It is normal to be lonely in these types of situations. Maybe my friends who have moved have had similar problems.

**Figure 5–2.** Examining-the-evidence worksheet.

[a]Additional cognitive errors are reflected in the automatic thought and in some of the evidence for the automatic thought. For example, Brian is using all-or-nothing thinking when he says the word "never," is ignoring the evidence that he is fitting in to some extent now and has done so in the past, and is magnifying how different he is from others. Although only one cognitive error is recorded here, Dr. Sudak will help him learn more about recognizing cognitive errors in future sessions.

The second video illustration shows Dr. Wright working with Kate to check the validity of her automatic thought "I'm going to pass out." This vignette was shown earlier in Chapter 2, "The Therapeutic Relationship: Collaborative Empiricism in Action," as an example of a collaborative empirical therapeutic relationship. We suggest that you view this video again, with your attention focused now on learning ways to implement the technique of examining the evidence. Dr. Wright demonstrates an intervention in examining the evidence that does not include a written worksheet. Examining the evidence can be performed quickly as part of a series of therapy interventions as in this example, or can be done in a more detailed manner with worksheets as shown in Dr. Sudak's treatment of Brian (see Figure 5–2). Generally, we recommend that examining the evidence be implemented in its full version with listing of written evidence at least once in the early part of therapy to teach patients how to use this valuable method. Exercises in examining the evidence also make excellent homework assignments. A copy of the blank worksheet is provided in Appendix 1, "Worksheets and Checklists."

**Video 2.** Modifying Automatic Thoughts: Dr. Wright and Kate (8:48)

**Learning Exercise 5–2.** Examining the Evidence

1. Ask a colleague to help you build your skills in examining the evidence by doing a role-play exercise.

2. When you examine the evidence, use a worksheet (see Appendix 1, "Worksheets and Checklists") and write out evidence for and against the automatic thought.

3. Next implement the examining-the-evidence method with one of your patients and discuss your efforts with a supervisor.

## Identifying Cognitive Errors

Definitions and examples of commonly encountered cognitive errors are given in Chapter 1, "Basic Principles of Cognitive-Behavior Therapy." To help patients spot their cognitive errors, you will first have to educate them on the nature and types of these problems in reasoning. We have found that having the patient read about cognitive errors in a book written for the general public—such as *Breaking Free From Depression: Pathways to Wellness* (Wright and McCray 2011), *Feeling Good* (Burns 2008), or *Mind Over Mood* (Greenberger and Padesky 2015)—and using a cognitive therapy computer program such as *Good Days Ahead* (Wright et al. 2016) are usually effective ways to get these concepts across. You can try to explain cognitive errors in therapy sessions, but patients usually require other learning experiences, such as those noted above, before they can fully grasp these ideas. Also, providing explanations of cognitive errors in therapy sessions can be time-consuming and may divert your efforts from other important topics or agendas. Therefore, we usually briefly explain cognitive errors in a treatment session when there is an obvious example of one of these distortions in logic. Then we suggest a homework assignment to further the learning process. You can make copies of the definitions of cognitive errors from Chapter 1, "Basic Principles of Cognitive-Behavior Therapy," to use as a handout for your patients. An effort to teach a patient to spot cognitive errors is illustrated in the following case.

### Case Example

Max, a 30-year-old man with bipolar disorder, reported a flare of intense irritability and anger during an argument with his girlfriend, Rita. She had called Max to tell him she was held up at work and would be about an hour late for a date to go out for dinner. They had a reservation for 7 P.M., but Rita didn't arrive at his house until almost 9 P.M. By that time Max was in quite a fury. He reported that he "screamed at her for 30 minutes" and then went to a bar without her.

In the therapy session, the clinician noted that Max had a number of maladaptive automatic thoughts that were laced with cognitive errors.

*Therapist:* Can you think back over the situation to tell me the automatic thoughts that were going through your mind? Try to speak the thoughts out loud now so that we can understand why you got so upset.

*Max:* She only cares about herself and her big-time job. She doesn't think about me at all. This relationship is going nowhere. She makes me look like a jerk!

*Therapist:* You told me that you felt guilty this morning and believe that you overreacted to her being late. You also said that you love her and want to make the relationship work. I think it might help to look at what you were thinking in the situation. It sounds like you took an extreme view of her behavior.

*Max:* Yes, I guess I was really wound up tight. Sometimes I get that way and go way overboard.

*Therapist:* One of the things that seemed to be happening was that you were thinking in extremes. Sometimes we call this "all-or-nothing" or "absolute" thinking. For example, your automatic thought "She doesn't care about me at all" is very absolute and gives no room for you to consider any other information about how she treats you. How did thinking like this make you feel and act?

*Max:* I got into a rage and said some really hurtful things to her. If I keep doing this, I'll ruin the relationship.

The therapist then explained the concept of cognitive errors and how spotting these distortions could help Max better manage his emotions and behavior.

*Therapist:* So, I've told you about these things we call cognitive errors. Would you be willing to read something about them before the next session? You could also try to identify some of these cognitive errors on your thought records.

*Max:* Sure. I think that's a good idea.

There can be multiple opportunities for helping patients learn how to spot cognitive errors and reduce the frequency and intensity of these distortions in logic. A thought change record (described in the next section and illustrated there in Figure 5–3) can be used to identify cognitive errors in specific automatic thoughts. Cognitive errors also can be recognized in other interventions such as examining the evidence and decatastrophizing (a method detailed later in this chapter). For many patients, spotting and labeling cognitive errors is one of the more challenging parts of building cognitive therapy skills. These thinking errors have been repeated over and over for many years and have become an automatic part of information processing. Therefore, the therapist may need to repetitively draw the patient's attention to this phenomenon and suggest multiple ways to practice thinking in a more balanced and logical manner.

Sometimes patients can get confused in their effort to identify cognitive errors. The definitions of the various errors can be difficult to understand, and there can be considerable overlap between the different types of errors in reasoning. It is a good idea to explain in advance that it might take some time to gain experience in spotting cognitive errors. We tell patients that it's not important to label the errors exactly each time (e.g., to discriminate between ignoring the evidence and overgeneralizing) or to recognize all of the cognitive errors that might be involved in an automatic thought (many automatic thoughts include more than one type of cognitive error). We try to convey the message that they shouldn't worry about getting this part of CBT exactly right. Recognizing any cognitive errors can help them think more logically and cope better with their problems.

## Thought Change Records

Self-monitoring, a key element of CBT, is fully realized through five-column thought records and similar thought recording methods designed to help patients change automatic thoughts. The thought change record (TCR), a five-column thought record, was recommended as a high-impact procedure by Beck and colleagues (1979) in their classic book, *Cognitive Therapy of Depression*, and continues to be used heavily in CBT applications. The TCR encourages patients to 1) recognize their automatic thoughts, 2) apply many of the other methods described in this chapter (e.g., examining the evidence, identifying cognitive errors, generating rational alternatives), and 3) observe positive outcomes in their efforts to modify their thinking. We typically suggest that patients complete TCRs on a regular basis for homework and that they bring these records to therapy sessions. Sometimes patients are able to use the TCR on their own to make substantive changes in thinking. On other occasions, they may get stuck and not be able to generate rational alternatives. Regardless of the level of success in using this tool outside therapy sessions, the TCR often provides rich material for discussions in therapy and serves as a springboard for further interventions to modify automatic thoughts.

In the TCR method, two columns, "Rational response" and "Outcome," are added to the three-column record typically used for identifying automatic thoughts. Patients are instructed to use the first column to write down an event or a memory of an event that stimulated automatic thoughts. The second column is used to record the automatic thoughts and the degree of belief in the thoughts at the time they occurred. Emotions are recorded in the third column.

Ratings of how much patients believe their automatic thoughts to be true (on a scale of 0%–100%) and of the degree of emotion associated with the automatic thoughts (on a scale of 1%–100%) are a vital part of the thought change process. Often in the early parts of therapy, patients will rate their automatic thoughts as 100%—or close to 100%—believable. After completing the rest of the TCR and exploring ways of changing their thinking, they are usually able to produce dramatic reductions in the degree of belief in their automatic thoughts and substantial improvement in the emotional distress associated with the thoughts. Observing these changes on the TCR can be a powerful reinforcer for practicing CBT methods and using them in daily life.

Ratings of the degree of belief in automatic thoughts also can give the therapist significant leads about the malleability or resistance to change of these cognitions. Clusters of automatic thoughts that remain quite believable in the face of contradictory evidence may suggest that a deeply held schema or an ingrained behavioral pattern will need to be addressed or that more vigorous efforts to use methods such as reattribution, role-play, or cognitive rehearsal will be required. Also, thoughts that persistently generate unpleasant emotions or physical tension can be targeted for more intensive CBT interventions.

The fourth column, "Rational response," is the centerpiece of the TCR. This column is used to record rational alternatives to maladaptive automatic thoughts and to rate the modified thoughts for degree of belief. Rational alternatives can be developed using a number of methods discussed in this chapter. However, the TCR alone often stimulates patients to consider alternatives and to develop a more rational thinking style. Some cognitive-behavior therapists suggest that the fourth column of the TCR be used to note cognitive errors identified in the automatic thoughts, thus promoting analysis of logical errors as a way of building rational thinking. However, you can recommend that patients avoid or delay labeling cognitive errors on the TCR if you think this process would overload them or would not be beneficial at the present time.

The fifth and last column of the TCR is used to document the outcome of the patient's effort to change automatic thinking. We generally ask patients to write down the emotions from column 3 and to again rate the intensity of their feelings using a scale of 0%–100%. The last column also can be used to observe any changes in behavior or to record plans that have been developed for coping with the situation. In most cases, there will be positive changes noted in the outcome column. In situations where there is little or no improvement recorded in the outcome column, the therapist can use this information to identify roadblocks and to devise methods of surmounting these obstacles.

A completed TCR from the treatment of Richard, a man with social phobia described in Chapter 1, "Basic Principles of Cognitive-Behavior Therapy," is illustrated in Figure 5–3. In this example, Richard had a flood of negative automatic thoughts as he was preparing to attend a neighborhood party. Although Richard typically avoided going to social events by either declining invitations outright or making a last-minute excuse, he was now trying to apply CBT principles to conquer his fear. Note that Richard was able to generate some rational alternatives to his automatic thoughts and that he has started to build skills for coping with anxiety (see Chapter 7, "Behavioral Methods II: Reducing Anxiety and Breaking Patterns of Avoidance," for behavioral techniques for anxiety disorders). A blank TCR is included in Appendix 1, "Worksheets and Checklists," so that you can make copies of the TCR to use in your clinical practice.

**Learning Exercise 5–3.** Using the Thought Change Record

1. Make copies of the blank TCR in Appendix 1, "Worksheets and Checklists."
2. Identify an event or situation from your own life that stimulated anxiety, sadness, anger, or some other unpleasant emotion.
3. Complete the TCR, identifying automatic thoughts, emotions, rational responses, and the outcome of using the thought record.
4. Introduce the TCR method to at least one of your patients in a therapy session. Ask this person (or persons) to complete a TCR for a homework assignment, and review the TCR in subsequent sessions.
5. If the patient(s) has problems implementing the TCR or is not making as much progress with this method as hoped, troubleshoot solutions for these difficulties.

| Situation | Automatic thought(s) | Emotion(s) | Rational response | Outcome |
|---|---|---|---|---|
| a. *Describe* event leading to emotion *or*<br>b. Stream of thoughts leading to emotion *or*<br>c. Physiological sensations. | a. *Write* automatic thought(s) that preceded emotion(s).<br>b. *Rate* belief in automatic thought(s), 0%–100%. | a. *Specify* sad, anxious, angry, etc.<br>b. *Rate* degree of emotion, 1%–100%. | a. *Identify* cognitive errors.<br>b. *Write* rational response to automatic thought(s).<br>c. *Rate* belief in rational response, 0%–100%. | a. *Specify and rate* subsequent emotion(s), 0%–100%.<br>b. *Describe* changes in behavior. |
| Preparing to attend a neighborhood party | 1. I won't know what to say. (90%) | Anxious (80%)<br>Tense (70%) | 1. *Ignoring the evidence, magnifying.* I read a lot and listen to the news on public radio. I've been practicing how to make small talk. I do have something to say. I just need to start saying it. (90%) | Anxious (40%)<br>Tense (40%)<br>I went to the party and stayed for over an hour. I was nervous, but I did OK. |

**Figure 5–3.** Richard's thought change record.

| Situation | Automatic thought(s) | Emotion(s) | Rational response | Outcome |
|---|---|---|---|---|
| | 2. I'll look like a misfit. (75%) | | 2. *Magnifying, overgeneralizing, personalizing.* I'm really exaggerating here. I might look a bit nervous, but people will be more interested in their own lives than in judging how I look. I'm a competent person. (90%) | |
| | 3. I'll clutch and want to leave right away. | | 3. *Jumping to conclusions, catastrophizing.* I will be nervous, but I need to stick it out and face my fear. I've rehearsed how to act at the party. So I don't need to leave right away or make an excuse to not attend. (80%) | |

**Figure 5–3.** Richard's thought change record. *(continued)*

*Source.* Adapted from Beck AT, Rush AJ, Shaw BF, et al.: *Cognitive Therapy of Depression*. New York, Guilford, 1979, pp. 164–165. Reprinted with permission of Guilford Press. Available at: https://www.appi.org/wright.

## Generating Rational Alternatives

In teaching patients how to develop logical thoughts, it is important to emphasize that CBT is not "the power of positive thinking." Attempts to replace negative thoughts with unrealistic positive thoughts are usually doomed to failure, especially if the patient has suffered real losses or traumas or is facing problems with a high likelihood of adverse outcomes. It may be that the patient has lost a job because of declining performance, has experienced the breakup of an important relationship, or is trying to cope with a significant physical illness. In such situations, it is unrealistic to try to gloss over the problems, ignore possible personal flaws, or minimize genuine risks. Instead, the therapist should try to help the patient to view the circumstances in the most rational way possible and then work out adaptive ways to cope.

You might consider these options when you coach your patients on how to develop logical thoughts:

1. **Explore different perspectives.** Depression and other mental disorders often narrow the focus of thinking to self-condemning and anxiety-generating cognitions while blocking out more adaptive, reasonable alternatives. To help patients overcome this tendency, you can ask them to imagine seeing themselves from a different perspective. They could try to think like a scientist or a detective—someone who avoids jumping to conclusions and searches for all of the evidence. Another strategy is to suggest they put themselves in the place of a trusted friend or family member. What might this person say about them? Also, patients can be asked to imagine giving advice to another person who is in a similar situation—a technique used to good effect by Dr. Sudak in her treatment of Brian (see Video 9). Or they might visualize an affirming and effective coach who is building their personal strengths by helping them see positive, but accurate, alternatives. Each of these related strategies encourages patients to step outside their current framework of thinking to consider other viewpoints that may be more rational, adaptive, and constructive.
2. **Brainstorm.** Explain that brainstorming involves letting your creativity run free to come up with a wide range of possibilities. To get the most from this technique, patients should be encouraged to suspend any "yes, but" from their thinking process. Suggest they list as many ideas as possible without considering whether they are practical or on target. Then they can sort through the possibilities to see which ones may be logical alternatives. Brainstorming can help patients break out of their tunnel vision to see options that otherwise would have gone unrecognized.

3. **Move out of the current time frame.** Try to help patients get in touch with the ways that they saw themselves before they became depressed or anxious or how they might see themselves if their symptoms were resolved. If patients can recall scenes in which they had considerable success or had a wellspring of positive feelings (e.g., graduating from school, being in a loving relationship, having a child, receiving an award, being hired for a new job), they may be able to recall adaptive thoughts that are being forgotten in the crush of their current problems. Ask questions such as "What alternatives would your old self see that your depressed self has ignored?" "What advice would your old self give you?" or "How would you see the situation if you weren't depressed any longer?"
4. **Ask others for their opinion.** People with depression, anxiety, and other conditions turn inward and draw conclusions without the benefit of feedback or suggestions from others. Although there are risks in asking others for their opinions, judicious discussions with trusted friends, family, or coworkers can help patients gain accurate perspectives. To facilitate productive discussions, you can coach patients on ways to check out their thinking with others that will limit risks and increase the chances of success. Ask questions such as "How much can you trust this person to tell you the truth and still be supportive?" "What are the risks in asking this person for feedback?" and "How could you cope if you get a disappointing response?" You can also role-play possible scenarios in advance to prepare the patient to ask effective questions. Teach the patient how to frame questions that will protect her interests while still getting at the truth.

There are two video illustrations that demonstrate methods of generating rationale alternatives. The first of these videos shows Dr. Sudak helping Brian build skills for generating rational alternatives. They are working on one of Brian's recurrent and especially troubling automatic thoughts—"I'll never fit in." Dr. Sudak begins by asking Brian to identify cognitive errors in his automatic thoughts. After Brian notes that he has been using all-or-nothing thinking and overgeneralization, Dr. Sudak suggests he try to generate an alternative thought. His first attempt at a revision ("I might be able to fit in") is greeted by positive feedback by Dr. Sudak. However, she thinks this modification is unlikely to "fortify" him enough to lead to substantive change. So Dr. Sudak asks him to view the situation of "fitting in" through the lens of a friend who has had a similar challenge of moving to a new city. As you view this video, you'll be able to see how this strategy unlocked Brian's potential to generate a number of realistic, alternative thoughts.

▶ **Video 9.** Developing Rational Alternatives: Dr. Sudak and Brian (8:50)

The second demonstration of finding rational alternatives comes from Dr. Brown's treatment of Eric. In Video 10, Eric shows Dr. Brown a TCR (first three columns of event, automatic thoughts, and emotions) that was completed for a homework assignment. Eric was sitting in his car outside a noodle shop while he was considering going to a job interview for a line cook position. From a host of negative automatic thoughts on the TCR, Eric chose "What's the point of trying?" for them to target during the session. As you view the video, try to spot the methods Dr. Brown uses to help Eric move toward finding alternatives to his automatic thought. Note how Dr. Brown asks artful questions to overcome the barrier of Eric's inability to generate any evidence against his self-defeating cognitions. Dr. Brown has more difficulty in helping Eric develop rational alternatives than Dr. Sudak had with Brian. However, it is likely that Dr. Brown's persistence and patience will pay off in articulating specific alternatives to Eric's maladaptive automatic thoughts.

▶ **Video 10.** Difficulty Finding Rational Alternatives: Dr. Brown and Eric (10:37)

**Learning Exercise 5–4.** Generating Rational Alternatives

1. Practice the use of Socratic questioning, examining the evidence, and generating rational alternatives in a role-play exercise with a colleague. Try to be creative in thinking of ways to open up the "patient's" mind.

2. Next, work with one of your patients to generate rational alternatives. Focus on asking good Socratic questions. Encourage the patient to think like a scientist or a detective in looking for different ways of seeing the situation. Or instruct the patient on the brainstorming technique. Your goal is to help the patient learn methods for breaking out of tunnel vision.

3. If possible, record a video or audio of these interviews and review them with a supervisor. One of the best ways of becoming an expert in using CBT to generate rational alternatives is to see yourself in action, get feedback on your interview style, and hear suggestions on how to ask effective Socratic questions.

## Decatastrophizing

Catastrophic predictions about the future are very common in persons with depression and anxiety. These predictions are frequently influenced by the cognitive distortions observed in these disorders, but sometimes the fears are on target. Thus the decatastrophizing procedure does not always attempt to negate the catastrophic fear. Instead, the therapist may elect to help the patient work on ways to cope with a feared situation in case it does come true.

### Case Example

Terry, a 52-year-old depressed man who was in his second marriage, expressed great anxiety about the possibility that his wife would leave him. Because the relationship did appear shaky, his therapist decided to use the *worst-case scenario* technique to help him decatastrophize and better manage the situation.

*Terry:* I think she is at the end of her rope with me. I couldn't survive another rejection.

*Therapist:* I can tell that you are very worried and upset. What do you think the chances are of your staying together?

*Terry:* About 50–50.

*Therapist:* Because you are predicting a high likelihood of a breakup, it might help to think ahead to what would happen if she did file for divorce. What is the worst outcome that you could imagine?

*Terry:* I'd be destroyed…a two-time loser with no future. She's everything to me.

*Therapist:* I know that it would be very tough if your marriage did end in divorce, but let's take a look at how you could cope. We can start with checking out your predictions. You said that you would be destroyed. Can we look at the evidence to see if that would be true?

*Terry:* I suppose I wouldn't be totally destroyed.

*Therapist:* What parts of you or your life wouldn't be destroyed?

*Terry:* My kids would still love me. And my brothers and sisters wouldn't give up on me. In fact, some of them think that I'd be better off ending the marriage.

*Therapist:* Any other parts of your life that would still be OK?

*Terry:* My job, as long as I don't get too depressed to do it. I can keep playing tennis with my friends. You know that tennis is a big outlet for me.

The therapist proceeded with questions to help Terry modify his absolutistic, catastrophic thoughts. By the end of this interchange, Terry had developed a different view of his reactions to a possible divorce.

*Therapist:* Before we go on, can you sum up what we've learned about how you might react if you did have to face a divorce?

*Terry:* It would be a big blow, and I don't want it to happen. But I'd try to look at all of the things I do have instead of thinking only about what I'm losing. I still have my health and the rest of my family. I have a good job and some close friends. She's been a big part of my life, but she isn't everything. Life would go on. Maybe I'd be better off in the long run, like my brother tells me.

The therapist then suggested that they work on a coping plan to be used in case a divorce should actually occur. [See the "Coping Cards" section later in this chapter for more information.]

Decatastrophizing also is a valuable technique for helping individuals with anxiety disorders. For example, persons with social phobia commonly have fears that they will be exposed as anxious or socially incompetent and that this revelation will be too painful to bear. You can try the following types of questions to reduce catastrophic predictions in social phobia: "What is the worst thing that could happen if you went to the party?" "What would be terrible about not having much to say?" "Could you tolerate this for at least 15 minutes?" "How does feeling anxious at a party compare with other terrible things, like having a serious illness or losing a job?" The thrust of such questions is to help patients see that their predictions of dire consequences and inability to cope are inaccurate.

## Reattribution

In Chapter 1, "Basic Principles of Cognitive-Behavior Therapy," we describe the findings of studies on attributional biases in depression. Attributions are the meanings people assign to events in their lives. To refresh your memory, we briefly summarize the three dimensions of distorted attributions:

1. **Internal versus external.** Depressed persons tend to internalize blame or responsibility for negative outcomes, whereas nondepressed persons make balanced or external attributions.
2. **General versus specific.** In depression, attributions are more likely to be sweeping and global than isolated to a specific flaw, insult, or problem. An example of a generalized attribution is "That fender bender was the last straw; everything in my life is going downhill."
3. **Invariant versus variable.** Depressed persons make attributions that are invariant and predict little or no chance of change—for example,

"I will never find love again." In contrast, nondepressed persons are more likely to think "This too will pass."

A variety of different methods can help patients make healthier attributions to significant events in their lives. Any of the other techniques described in this chapter can be employed, such as Socratic questioning, TCRs, or examining the evidence. However, we typically initiate reattribution by briefly explaining the concept and then drawing a graphic on a piece of paper to demonstrate the dimensions of attributions (Figure 5–4). Then we ask questions that prompt the patient to explore and possibly change her attributional style.

### Case Example

Sandy, a 54-year-old woman, was having trouble coping with the revelation that her married daughter, Maryruth, was having an affair. She blamed herself excessively, believed that her daughter was ruining her entire life, and thought that Maryruth's future was very dim. The therapist began with questions targeted at correcting Sandy's internalized attributions. [The diagram in Figure 5–4 was used to record Sandy's answers.]

*Therapist:* How much do you blame yourself for your daughter's problems now?

*Sandy:* A lot—probably about 80%. I should never have gone along with her idea to go to that college. She went wild up there, and she hasn't been herself since. I knew it was a bad idea for her to marry Jim. I should have told her what I thought about him. They don't have anything in common.

*Therapist:* We'll check out all of this blame you are putting on yourself later. But for now, can you just make a mark on the graph to show how much you think you are responsible for the problem?

*(Sandy places a mark at about the 90% level.)*

*Therapist:* OK, now let's try to think about what a healthy level of blame would be. Where would you like to be on the graph?

*Sandy:* I know I get down on myself too much. But I think I should still try to help and should take *some* of the responsibility. Probably 25% is about right.

*(Sandy places a mark at about the 25% level.)*

Although the therapist believed that Sandy was still taking too much blame for the situation, she didn't press the issue at that time. They proceeded to make graphs for the other dimensions of attributions [see Figure 5–4] and then began to discuss ways to move attributions in the desired direction.

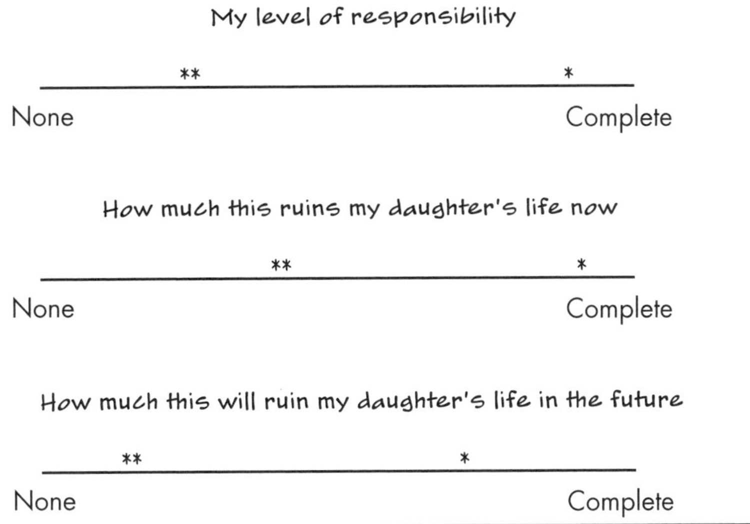


**Figure 5–4.** Sandy's attribution scales.
*What I think today.
**A healthy view of the situation.

One of the techniques that can be used to modify attributions is to ask the patient to brainstorm about a variety of possible contributors to negative outcomes. Because patients often have tunnel vision that is focused on their own faults, it can help to ask questions that prompt them to think of different perspectives—for example, "How about other people who could have influenced the situation: the in-laws? his buddies?" "What about the role of luck or fate?" "Could genetics be involved?" After going through a series of these types of questions, we sometimes use a pie graph to help patients take a multidimensional view of the situation. Figure 5–5 shows a pie graph that Sandy constructed for her attributions about blame for her daughter's problems.

**Learning Exercise 5–5.** Decatastrophizing and Reattribution

1. Again, ask a colleague to help you learn CBT procedures by doing role-play exercises. Ask your helper to role-play a situation in which decatastrophizing and reattribution for changing automatic thoughts might be used.

2. Then try out each of the techniques.

3. When you practice decatastrophizing, focus on correcting distorted predictions. But also work on

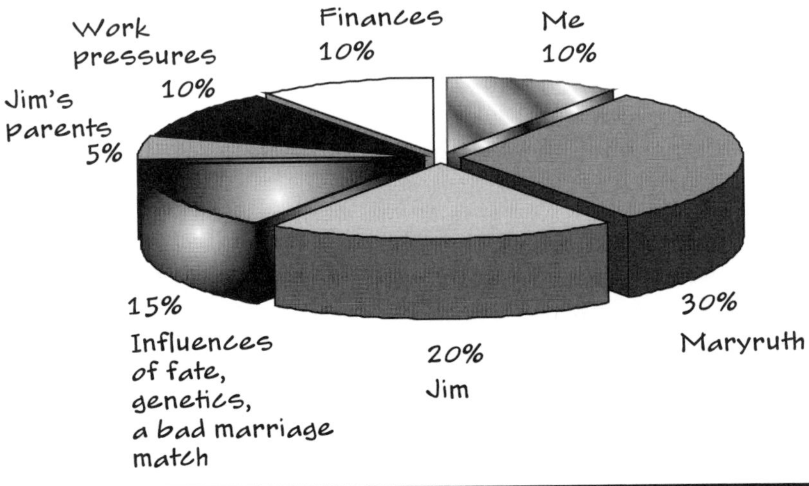


**Figure 5–5.** Sandy's pie graph: the positive effects of reattribution.

preparing the "patient" to cope with possible adverse outcomes.

4. Next, choose an automatic thought that might respond to a reattribution intervention. Explain attributional biases, and then use a graphic (as in Figure 5–4) and/or a pie graph (as in Figure 5–5) to help the "patient" make healthier attributions.

5. The last step in this learning exercise is to implement both procedures with actual patients and to discuss your efforts with a supervisor.

## Cognitive Rehearsal

When you are facing an important meeting or task, do you ever think through in advance what you are going to say? Do you rehearse your thoughts and behaviors so that you will have a greater chance of success? We use this strategy in our own lives, and we have found that it can help patients take the lessons of therapy into real-world situations.

When we explain this technique to patients, we often use the example of top athletes such as downhill skiers, who can visualize the challenges of a competitive situation and prepare their minds for the course ahead. A skier might use imagery to think about how she would react in a variety of situations. How would she compensate if she hit a patch of ice or a strong wind began to blow? The skier would also probably coach herself on keeping a positive mind-set to calm her anxieties and focus on competing in the race.

Cognitive rehearsal is usually introduced in a therapy session after the patient has already done some groundwork with other methods to change automatic thoughts. These earlier experiences prepare the patient to "put it all together" in orchestrating an adaptive response to a potentially stressful situation. One way of doing cognitive rehearsal is to ask the patient to take these steps: 1) think through a situation in advance, 2) identify possible automatic thoughts and behavior, 3) modify the automatic thoughts by writing out a TCR or doing another CBT intervention, 4) rehearse the more adaptive way of thinking and behaving in your mind, and then 5) implement the new strategy.

Of course, it often helps to coach patients on methods that will help them increase the chances of achieving their goals. They can be asked Socratic questions to help them see different options, mini-didactic interventions can be used to teach them skills, and experiments can be tried to test out possible solutions. However, often the most useful technique is rehearsing in a therapy session before trying out the new plan in vivo. Dr. Wright used this method with Kate to help her prepare for a drive with her coworkers to visit their new offices.

**Video 11.** Cognitive Rehearsal: Dr. Wright and Kate (9:31)

## Coping Cards

Coping cards can be a productive way to help patients practice key CBT interventions learned in therapy sessions. Either index cards (3×5 inches) or smaller cards (business-card size) can be used to write down instructions that patients would like to give themselves to help them cope with significant issues or situations. Or patients can use a smartphone or other device to record coping strategies. When used to best effect, coping cards identify a specific situation or problem and then succinctly detail a coping strategy with a few bullet points that capture the fundamentals of the plan. Table 5–5 presents some tips for helping patients write coping cards that work.

In Video 11, Dr. Wright helps Kate record the ideas from a cognitive rehearsal exercise on a coping card. Kate wrote down these adaptive cognitions on a coping card and planned to keep the card in her purse so she could review it frequently before riding with her coworkers over the big bridge to check out their new office (Figure 5–6).

**Table 5–5.** Tips for developing coping cards

1. Choose a situation that is important to the patient.
2. Plan therapy interventions with the goal of producing coping cards.
3. Assess the patient's readiness to implement strategies with a coping card. Don't try to do too much too soon. Start with a manageable task. Delay tackling overwhelming concerns or issues until the patient is prepared to meet these challenges.
4. Be specific in defining the situation and the steps to be taken to manage the problem.
5. Boil the instructions down to their essence. Highly memorable instructions are more likely to stick.
6. Be practical. Suggest strategies that have a high likelihood of success.
7. Advocate frequent use of the coping card in real-life situations.

**Situation:** Driving across bridge with coworkers to new office.

**Coping strategies:**

I'm different from my dad. He was a smoker and diabetic.

My cardiologist says I have a zero percent chance of having a heart attack.

I can do this even if it is hard.

I can practice doing some skills to help me.

**Figure 5–6.** Kate's coping card.

Another example of a coping card comes from the treatment of Max, the man with bipolar disorder who reported intense anger in his relationship with his girlfriend (Figure 5–7). Additional interventions described in the chapters on behavioral methods might be added later to help him deal more effectively with his anger, but Max has made a good start.

**Learning Exercise 5–6.** Cognitive Rehearsal and Coping Cards

1. Identify a situation in your own life for which advance rehearsal might help you be more effective or assured. Now go through the situation in your mind, identifying possible automatic thoughts, emotions, rational responses, and adaptive behaviors. Next, practice thinking and acting in the most adaptive way you can imagine.

**Situation:** My girlfriend comes in late or does something else that makes me think she doesn't care.

**Coping strategies:**

Spot my extreme thinking, especially when I use absolute words like never or always.

Stand back from the situation and check my thinking before I start yelling or screaming.

Think of the positive parts of our relationship—I think she does love me. We've been together for 4 years, and I want to make it work.

Take a "time-out" if I start getting into a rage. Tell her that I need to take a break to calm down. Take a brief walk or go to another room.

**Figure 5–7.** Max's coping card.

2. Distill the efforts of your cognitive rehearsal exercise into a coping card. Follow the tips for writing coping cards in Table 5–5. Write out specific bullet points that will coach you on the best way to handle the situation.

3. Practice cognitive rehearsal with at least one of your patients. Choose a situation that you believe the patient could manage better if it were thought through in advance. Also, try to pick rehearsal opportunities that might reduce the risk for symptom worsening or relapse. Examples might include going back to work, getting bad news about the health of a relative, and being criticized by a significant other.

4. Write out a least three coping cards with your patients. Promote use of the cards by asking patients to implement the coping strategies as homework assignments.

## Summary

CBT focuses on identifying and changing automatic thoughts because these cognitions have a strong influence on emotions and behavior. During the early phase of working with automatic thoughts, therapists teach patients about this stream of private, often unchecked cognitions and help them tune in to this internal dialogue. Guided discovery is the most important method used to uncover automatic thoughts, but many other techniques are available. Recognizing a mood shift is a powerful way of showing patients the impact of automatic thinking on their feelings.

Other valuable methods for eliciting automatic thoughts include thought recording, imagery, role-play, and the use of checklists.

After the patient learns to identify automatic thoughts, therapeutic efforts can shift to the use of interventions for modifying these cognitions. Effective Socratic questioning is the cornerstone of the change process. TCRs also are used extensively in CBT to help patients develop a more logical and adaptive thinking style. Therapists can draw from a variety of other useful techniques—such as examining the evidence, decatastrophizing, reattribution, cognitive rehearsal, and coping cards—to revise automatic thoughts. As CBT moves from early to later phases, patients gain skills in modifying automatic thoughts that they can use on their own to reduce symptoms, cope better with life stresses, and decrease the chance of relapse.

## References

Beck AT: Cognitive therapy and research: a 25-year retrospective. Paper presented at the World Congress of Cognitive Therapy, Oxford, UK, June 28–July 2, 1989

Beck AT, Rush AJ, Shaw BF, et al: Cognitive Therapy of Depression. New York, Guilford, 1979

Burns DD: Feeling Good: The New Mood Therapy, Revised. New York, HarperCollins, 2008

Greenberger D, Padesky CA: Mind Over Mood: Change How You Feel by Changing the Way You Think, 2nd Edition. New York, Guilford, 2015

Hollon SD, Kendall PC: Cognitive self-statements in depression: development of an automatic thoughts questionnaire. Cognit Ther Res 4:383–395, 1980

Wright JH, McCray LW: Breaking Free From Depression: Pathways to Wellness. New York, Guilford, 2011

Wright JH, Salmon P: Learning and memory in depression, in Depression: New Directions in Research, Theory, and Practice. Edited by McCann D, Endler NS. Toronto, ON, Wall & Thompson, 1990, pp 211–236

Wright JH, Wright AS, Beck AT: Good Days Ahead. Moraga, CA, Empower Interactive, 2016

# Behavioral Methods I 6

## Improving Mood, Increasing Energy, Completing Tasks, and Solving Problems

Low energy, decreased interest in or enjoyment of activities, and difficulty completing tasks or solving problems are common complaints of people with depression. Not engaging in potentially pleasurable or rewarding activities often results in an aggravation of symptoms. A vicious cycle can ensue in which an individual's reduced involvement in pleasurable or productive activities is followed by a further lack of interest or enjoyment, low mood (feelings of sadness and despair), increased helplessness, or worthlessness. This reaction, in turn, may lead to the individual's further disengagement in pleasurable or rewarding activities and a subsequent worsening of depressive symptoms. Eventually, a downward spiral may continue to occur until the individual may assume that he is incapable of experiencing pleasure, completing tasks, or solving problems. Patients with the deepest levels of depression may become abjectly hopeless and give up on any attempts to change.

Cognitive-behavioral methods for treating depression and other psychiatric disorders include specific interventions designed to reverse patterns of diminishing activity levels, energy depletion, worsening anhedonia, and reduced abilities to complete tasks. In this chapter, we discuss and illustrate some of the most useful behavioral interventions for helping people with these types of difficulties. Although the techniques described here are most often used in treatment of depression, they also can be applied successfully in cognitive-behavior therapy (CBT) for other conditions, such as anxiety disorders, eating disorders, and personality disorders (see Chapter 10, "Treating Chronic, Severe, or Complex Disorders").

When implementing behavioral procedures, it is important to remember the principle that engaging in pleasurable or rewarding activities is likely to be associated with improved mood and sense of accomplishment. Likewise, modifications in negative automatic thoughts or schemas can help promote adaptive behavior. Thus, behavioral methods are used in concert with cognitive techniques as an overall strategy for reaching treatment goals. The examples in this chapter illustrate how behavioral and cognitive interventions often augment each other and how therapists can blend these techniques in clinical practice.

The term *behavioral activation* can be used to describe any method designed to reenergize patients and help them make positive changes. These methods can range from simple one- or two-step *behavioral action plans,* to *activity scheduling,* to fully developed *graded-task procedures*.

## Behavioral Action Plans

A practical and doable *behavioral action plan* can engage the patient in a process of positive change and instill a sense of hope. The therapist helps the patient to choose one or two specific activities that could lead to an improvement in mood and then assists with working out a realistic plan to carry out this activity. Behavioral activation is often used in the first few sessions before more detailed cognitive-behavioral analysis or more complex interventions can be performed (e.g., activity schedules, cognitive restructuring). However, we also have found that this technique can be applied at other stages of therapy when a simple, targeted behavioral action plan can be used with significant benefit. The following example shows how this method can be used to rapidly engage patients in productive activities very early in therapy.

1. Go to grocery store to buy healthy food for week.
2. Schedule a specific time, Sunday morning at 10 A.M., when I am more likely to go.
3. Reward myself by stopping at my favorite bakery on the way home.

**Figure 6–1.** Meredith's behavioral action plan.

## Case Example

Meredith is a 30-year-old woman, in her sixth month of pregnancy, who is experiencing depression. Her symptoms have been at a moderate level of severity since the second month of pregnancy, when she began to experience depression. Her first and only previous depressive episode occurred when she was in school at a community college. She took sertraline and received some supportive counseling at that time. The medication seemed to help, but she doesn't want to take medication now because of her pregnancy.

She is a server in an upscale restaurant and hopes to keep working as long as possible. Her associate degree is in information technology, but she hasn't been able to find employment in that field. She currently lives alone, and her family lives near her home. Although she has not received much support from her mother, who is also depressed, her older brother, who is married and has two children, is very supportive. She also has two close friends—one friend from her childhood and another from work. Her pregnancy was unplanned, but she always wanted to have a family. She has positive feelings about the baby, but she is often self-critical because she does not expect that she will be a good mother. She also criticizes herself for eating "junk food" and not maintaining a healthy diet. Meredith wants to stay friends with her baby's father, for the sake of the child, but doesn't want to rekindle a romantic relationship.

Meredith reports no other psychiatric history except as previously noted. She has had no suicidal ideation or suicidal behavior. There are no physical illnesses, and her pregnancy has gone well other than her experience of some back pain, heartburn, and decreased energy.

In Video 12, Meredith and Dr. Wichmann, a psychiatry resident, focus on some ways to help Meredith become more active again. Near the end of this second session, they develop a promising behavioral action plan (Figure 6–1). The small section of dialogue shown below will give you an idea of how Dr. Wichmann shaped this intervention. We suggest you take time now to view the video so you can see how to build a specific plan that has a good chance of success.

**Video 12.** Behavioral Action Plan: Dr. Wichmann and Meredith (3:34)

*Dr. Wichmann:* If you could do one thing this week that could help make you feel better, what do you think that might be?

*Meredith:* I think I want to eat healthy.

*Dr. Wichmann:* When you say that you want to eat healthy, can you tell me what you mean by that?

*Meredith:* I want to completely cut out fast food. I want to have more set meals, and I just want to eat healthy food.

*Dr. Wichmann:* All of those ideas you named are very important.... I just wonder if all of those things that you named can be a lot to take on at once. Do you think there are some smaller, more specific goals that you could work on...toward that?

*Meredith:* I think I at least need to go to the grocery.

*Dr. Wichmann:* OK. Has that been something you haven't been doing?

*Meredith:* No, not lately. I've been just grabbing food at work or going for fast food on the way home.

*Dr. Wichmann:* Well, going to the grocery, I think, is a more doable goal and something that you can hopefully work toward more easily than just eating healthy all at once. What are some possible barriers or obstacles that could make it difficult for you to get to the grocery?

Because Meredith was moderately depressed and was having difficulty engaging in any activities that gave her a sense of well-being or pleasure, Dr. Wichmann was careful to avoid a behavioral action plan that would be too challenging or would be unlikely to be accomplished. In this case, Meredith chose some actions that she thought would be helpful, but Dr. Wichmann suggested she plan a less ambitious activity. There were several other strategies used to increase the likelihood that Meredith would be able to complete the action plan. These included asking her about potential obstacles or barriers to completing the plan and then engaging her in problem solving to address these obstacles. Also, Dr. Wichmann urged the patient to identify a specific day and time to complete the activity. Finally, Dr. Wichmann wrote the behavioral action plan on a card to serve as a reminder to carry out the plan. Dr. Wichmann and Meredith collaborated well in developing the behavioral action plan. Note that Dr. Wichmann asked Meredith for suggestions based on her previous experiences, rather than simply telling Meredith what to do.

When patients seek treatment, they are usually interested in making changes. They want to start moving in a positive direction, and they are looking for guidance for steps that they can begin to take. Therefore, when the therapist suggests taking an immediate behavioral action (even if it is rudimentary) during the initial sessions, this request is usually greeted by patients as a sign that they will be able to work together with the therapist on making bigger gains and on solving larger problems. Behavioral action plans don't use fancy or complicated techniques, but they can help patients start to break out of patterns of withdrawal or inactivity

**Table 6–1.** Tips for using behavioral action plans

1. **Develop a collaborative relationship before trying behavioral activation.** Don't put the cart before the horse. Without good collaboration between patient and therapist, attempts to implement behavioral action plans may fail. Part of the reason the patient may carry out the task is that he wants to work with you and can understand the reasons for making changes.
2. **Let the patient decide.** Although you can help guide the patient to actions that may be helpful, whenever possible, ask him to make suggestions to develop an action plan and then offer the patient some choices for implementing the plan.
3. **Judge the patient's readiness to change.** Before suggesting behavioral action plans, gauge the patient's motivation and openness for taking this step. If the patient is not interested in doing things differently right now or is not ready to take action, defer the intervention. On the other hand, if the patient is open to start moving in a positive direction, capitalize on the moment.
4. **Prepare the patient for behavioral activation.** Lead up to the assignment with Socratic questions or other cognitive-behavior therapy interventions that pave the way for change. Try to ask questions that educate the patient about the benefits of taking action or that tap into motivations for doing things differently. One of the best questions is "How would this change make you feel?" If the answer is positive and the action stands a reasonable chance of being effective, the patient will be more likely to follow through.
5. **Design assignments that are manageable.** Choose behavioral activation exercises that match the patient's energy level and capacity to change. Check out the details of the behavioral plan to be sure that it offers enough challenge but doesn't overload the patient. If needed, do brief coaching on ways to make the plan work out well.
6. **Facilitate the implementation of the action plan.** Ask the patient to identify a specific date and time to complete the activity. Identify and address any barriers to doing the activity and, if any are present, assist the patient in addressing these obstacles. Always write the assignment down as a reminder to do the assignment.

and show them that progress can be made. This type of intervention may also be used to good effect in later stages of therapy or in the maintenance phase of treatment of chronic conditions. The suggestions listed in Table 6–1 may help you implement effective behavioral action plans.

## Activity Scheduling

When fatigue and anhedonia progress to the point that patients feel exhausted and believe that they can experience little or no pleasure, they may benefit from activity scheduling. This systematic behavioral method is frequently used in CBT to reactivate people and help them find ways to improve their interest in life. Activity scheduling is most often used with patients who have moderate to severe depression. However, it can also have a place in the treatment of other patients who have difficulty organizing their days or engaging in productive activities. Activity scheduling focuses on activity assessment and increasing mastery and pleasurable activities. These methods, introduced in Juliana's case below, are described further following the case example.

### Case Example

Juliana had severe depression and was a good candidate for activity scheduling. She was a 22-year-old, single Puerto Rican woman who had suffered the loss of her brother in a car accident a year before she started treatment with CBT. After her brother's death, Juliana dropped out of college to return home to comfort her parents. However, her own grief was intense and unrelenting. She was unable to make herself go back to school the following semester. Her parents understood Juliana's grief and did not force her to resume college or get a job. Juliana's friends tried to be supportive for many months after her brother's death. But when she consistently rejected offers to go out to dinner and stopped returning phone calls, her friends eventually began to drift away.

Juliana was well cared for by her family. There was no real need for her to work, so no demands were placed on her. After about a year, her parents thought that Juliana had overcome much of the sadness from the loss of her brother. Yet there had been a distinct change in her behavior. She had developed a more serious demeanor, a preference for solitude, and a greater tendency toward introspection. Juliana's parents felt comfortable leaving her at home when they were at work or traveling out of town, because she appeared to be better. However, one evening her mother came home early from work and found Juliana preparing to hang herself in her closet.

After a brief hospitalization and initiation of pharmacotherapy, Juliana improved to the point that she could be referred to a cognitive-behavior therapist for outpatient treatment. Given the severity of her symptoms, one of the first treatment initiatives was to increase Juliana's activities so that she could benefit from the support of friends, feel better about her personal appearance, practice her social skills, and in general feel more like her old self. The intervention began with an assessment of her current level of activity, experiences that gave her pleasure, and the amount of mastery she felt over her world.

## Activity Assessment

Because depressed patients tend to underreport positive experiences, emphasize negative perceptions, and focus more on failures than on successes, self-reports may not be as accurate as a log of activities kept for a day or a week between therapy sessions. The activity assessment, or activity monitoring, also may be used for noting patterns in engaging in pleasurable or rewarding activities and corresponding changes in mood. Patients who recognize the association between specific types of activities and their mood may be more likely to engage in additional activities to improve their mood and decrease the severity of their depression.

The activity schedule form presented in Figure 6–2 can be assigned as homework but should be started during the session to ensure that the patient understands the rationale for activity scheduling and to practice how to use the form. Beginning with the day of the therapy session, ask the patient to fill in her activities for each time block before the treatment session. Encourage her to write in the activities that actually occurred, no matter how mundane. For example, activities might include bathing, dressing, eating, traveling, talking with others on the phone or in person, watching television, and sleeping. If the patient has pronounced loss of energy or significant problems concentrating, it may be best to ask her to complete the schedule for only 1 day, or a part of a day. Inpatient applications of activity scheduling often employ a daily activity schedule instead of a weekly activity schedule (Wright et al. 1993).

To determine the impact of activities listed on a weekly or daily schedule, ask the patient to rate the degree of enjoyment experienced for each, as well as the sense of mastery or accomplishment that was associated with the activity. A scale of either 0–5 or 0–10 can be used (Beck et al. 1979, 1995; Wright et al. 2014). On a 0–10 scale, a rating of 0 on mastery suggests that the activity provided no experience of accomplishment, whereas a rating of 10 indicates a great sense of accomplishment. When coaching patients to use both of these rating scales, it is often helpful to ask them for specific examples of activities that correspond to no pleasure/accomplishment, moderate pleasure/ accomplishment, and a great deal of pleasure/accomplishment. Some patients will give a low rating to simple tasks such as washing dishes or making themselves a cup of coffee because they do not consider those activities to be meaningful. When this underestimation occurs, help them try to recognize the value of participating in everyday activities. Another strategy that is often used when rating specific activities is to have patients rate their mood level, using a 0–10 scale, while engaging in each activity or at the end of each day. This mood rating helps patients to become more aware of how specific activities are associated with changes in their mood.

Patients should try to give themselves credit for small accomplishments, because progress is generally made in small, incremental steps. Some simple tasks might receive high ratings for mastery. For example, after a patient has been immobilized by depression for some time, mak-

**Weekly Activity Schedule**

**Instructions:** Write down your activities for each hour and then rate them on a scale of 0–10 for mastery **(m)**, or degree of accomplishment, and for pleasure **(p)**, or amount of enjoyment you experienced. A rating of 0 would mean that you had no sense of mastery or pleasure. A rating of 10 would mean that you experienced maximum mastery or pleasure.

| | Sunday | Monday | Tuesday | Wednesday | Thursday | Friday | Saturday |
|---|---|---|---|---|---|---|---|
| 8:00 A.M. | | | | | | | |
| 9:00 A.M. | | | | | | | |
| 10:00 A.M. | | | | | | | |
| 11:00 A.M. | | | | | | | |
| 12:00 P.M. | | | | | | | |
| 1:00 P.M. | | | | | | | |
| 2:00 P.M. | | | | | | | |
| 3:00 P.M. | | | | | | | |
| 4:00 P.M. | | | | | | | |
| 5:00 P.M. | | | | | | | |
| 6:00 P.M. | | | | | | | |
| 7:00 P.M. | | | | | | | |
| 8:00 P.M. | | | | | | | |
| 9:00 P.M. | | | | | | | |

**Figure 6–2.** Weekly activity schedule form.

*Note.* This form is also available in a larger format at https://www.appi.org/wright.

ing breakfast can be a big feat and therefore might receive a rating of 8 or 9. Juliana's activity monitoring example is presented in Figure 6–3. For her, returning phone calls was an important accomplishment, since she had managed to avoid them for several months. Therefore, when she was able to make some calls, she gave herself a mastery rating of 8 on a 0–10 scale. In the past, Juliana would have rated returning phone calls only 4 for mastery because it took so little effort.

When symptoms of depression are moderate to severe, low ratings of pleasure should be expected for two reasons: 1) there is usually little involvement in activities that most people would consider highly pleasurable, and 2) the capacity for experiencing joy or pleasure is usually blunted. If an event that would normally make the patient laugh or smile elicits no more than an intellectual understanding that the stimulus was amusing, this event is likely to be given a low rating for pleasure. When this phenomenon occurs, it may be beneficial to develop more realistic expectations for feeling pleasure until the depression has improved. As an alternative to feeling disappointed with events and rating them 0, encourage the patient to at least give a low rating of 1–3 if any pleasant or positive feelings were experienced.

> In completing the activity schedule, Juliana gave having dinner with her parents a rating of only 1 for pleasure. When questioned about what elements of dinner she had enjoyed, she listed the comfort of being with her mother, the mashed potatoes with butter, and the banana pudding—a childhood favorite—she had had for dessert. When queried about why three different enjoyable things resulted in a rating of only 1 for pleasure, she reconsidered the rating and raised it to a 4. It was hard for her not to be conscious of her brother's absence during family meals, and thinking about his loss usually lowered her mood. But when she gave more consideration to the positive parts of the meal, it seemed more enjoyable overall. With this in mind, Juliana re-rated some of the other activities on her schedule and raised their pleasure ratings accordingly.

The questions in Table 6–2 are designed to help patients evaluate and change their activity levels to increase pleasurable or rewarding activities and improve mood. When reviewing the activity schedule form with patients, it is important to take a collaborative approach and use the questions in Table 6–2 to assist patients in reaching their own conclusions about the role of pleasurable and rewarding activities and to encourage them to make suggestions for changing their behavior.

> When reviewing the activity monitoring form she completed, Juliana discovered that there was a pattern of greatest pleasure when she was involved in activities outside the house or when she made an attempt to

**Weekly Activity Schedule**

**Instructions:** Write down your activities for each hour and then rate them on a scale of 0–10 for mastery **(m)**, or degree of accomplishment, and for pleasure **(p)**, or amount of enjoyment you experienced. A rating of 0 would mean that you had no sense of mastery or pleasure. A rating of 10 would mean that you experienced maximum mastery or pleasure.

| | Sunday | Monday | Tuesday | Wednesday | Thursday | Friday | Saturday |
|---|---|---|---|---|---|---|---|
| 8:00 A.M. | Wake up m-2 Get dressed p-0 | | | | Wake up m-3 Get dressed p-1 | | |
| 9:00 A.M. | Church with parents m-3 p-4 | | | | Walk the dog m-5 p-7 | | |
| 10:00 A.M. | | Wake up m-3 Get dressed p-1 | Wake up m-3 Get dressed p-1 | Wake up m-3 Get dressed p-1 | Therapy m-7 p-6 | | Wake up m-2 Get dressed p-1 |
| 11:00 A.M. | | Walk the dog m-4 Breakfast p-6 | Walk the dog m-4 p-5 | Walk the dog m-4 p-5 | | Wake up m-3 Get dressed p-1 | Walk the dog m-4 Breakfast p-5 |
| 12:00 P.M. | Lunch with parents m-4 p-2 | | | | | Walk the dog m-5 p-6 | Clean my room m-6 p-3 |
| 1:00 P.M. | | | Lunch m-2 p-2 | Lunch m-2 p-2 | | | Hand wash laundry m-7 p-4 |
| 2:00 P.M. | Read newspaper m-4 p-2 | Bring in the mail m-3 p-1 | Bring in the mail m-3 p-1 | Bring in the mail m-3 p-1 | Bring in the mail m-4 p-2 | Bring in the mail m-4 p-3 | |

**Figure 6–3.** Juliana's activity schedule.

| | Sunday | Monday | Tuesday | Wednesday | Thursday | Friday | Saturday |
|---|---|---|---|---|---|---|---|
| 3:00 P.M. | Read magazine m-4 p-4 | | | | | | |
| 4:00 P.M. | | Watch Oprah m-1 p-3 | Watch Oprah m-1 p-3 | Watch Oprah m-1 p-3 | Watch Oprah m-1 p-3 | Buy food for dinner m-6 p-2 | |
| 5:00 P.M. | | | | | | Walk the dog m-5 p-7 | Walk the dog m-5 p-7 |
| 6:00 P.M. | Walk the dog m-4 p-5 | Dinner with parents m-2 p-4 | Dinner with parents m-3 p-4 | Dinner with parents m-3 p-4 | Dinner with parents m-3 p-4 | Dinner alone m-5 p-3 | Cook/eat dinner alone m-5 p-4 |
| 7:00 P.M. | Dinner with parents m-2 p-4 | Walk the dog m-4 p-6 | Walk the dog m-4 p-6 | Walk the dog m-4 p-5 | Walk the dog m-5 p-7 | | |
| 8:00 P.M. | TV w/Mom m-2 p-4 | Make phone calls m-8 p-5 | | TV w/Mom m-2 p-5 | | TV alone m-2 p-2 | TV alone m-2 p-3 |
| 9:00 P.M. | | | | | | | |

**Figure 6–3.** Juliana's activity schedule. *(continued)*

**Table 6–2.** Activity monitoring

| |
|---|
| Are there distinct periods of time when the patient experiences pleasure or a sense of accomplishment? |
| What kinds of activities seem to give the patient pleasure or a sense of accomplishment? |
| Are these pleasurable or rewarding activities associated with changes in mood? |
| Can these pleasurable or rewarding activities be repeated or scheduled on other days? |
| Are there certain times of day or specific activities that appear to be low on mastery or pleasure? |
| Are these times of the day associated with low mood? |
| What can be done to improve activity patterns during those times of day? |
| Do the ratings tend to be higher for activities that involve other people? If so, can social contact be increased? |
| What kinds of activities did the patient do previously that provided pleasure or a sense of mastery that have been stopped or reduced? Are there opportunities for rekindling interest in these activities? |
| Are there any types of activities (e.g., exercise, music, spiritual involvement, art, crafts, reading, volunteer work, cooking) that the patient is ignoring but may interest her? Is she open to considering adding new or different activities to her weekly schedule? |

connect with friends (such as making phone calls). She gave one of her highest ratings for pleasure when walking her dog. In contrast, she noted that the lowest pleasure ratings were given when she was home alone with nothing to do. Because her involvement in productive activities had fallen to such a low level, she observed that her ratings of mastery were usually minimal. When reviewing the mastery ratings, Juliana complained that her life had no meaning. She had limited household responsibilities, was no longer in school, did not have a job, had lost touch with many of her friends, and had no clear prospects for becoming more involved in life. Thus she needed to find activities or commitments that would give her a sense of purpose and fulfillment.

In Video 13, Meredith and Dr. Wichmann reviewed an activity monitoring task during their third session. Meredith had completed her planned trip to the grocery (see Video 12) and recorded this activity and ratings on the activity schedule. When reviewing the form during the session, Meredith observed that she had felt a sense of mastery and pleasure from this activity and she was surprised by how good the activity made her feel. Although she found it somewhat challenging to go to the grocery store, her mood clearly improved after doing so. Meredith and Dr. Wichmann also reviewed other patterns of engaging in pleasurable activities and how they influenced her mood ratings. Finally, Dr. Wichmann asked Meredith if she had thought about engaging in any new activities.

> **Video 13.** Activity Scheduling: Dr. Wichmann and Meredith (9:32)

## Increasing Mastery and Pleasure

If you and the patient have determined that there are deficits in experiences of mastery or pleasure in the course of day-to-day life, you can help make improvements by assisting the patient to schedule activities between sessions that will make him feel good about himself. Begin by asking the patient to generate a list of pleasurable activities, based on his previous experiences. The patient may also want to include activities from the monitoring exercise that had the highest ratings of pleasure. Then you may brainstorm with the patient to list some new activities that may be worth trying (see the questions in Table 6–2).

Some patients may have difficulty identifying pleasurable activities even after reviewing the activity schedule or when asked about their prior experiences. For these patients, it may be helpful to review a list of potentially pleasurable activities using a questionnaire, such as the Pleasant Events Schedule (MacPhillamy and Lewinsohn 1982; available at: www.healthnetsolutions.com/dsp/PleasantEventsSchedule.pdf). Once the patient has identified some of these activities, then the patient and therapist collaboratively determine which of these activities to add to the daily routine.

Next, use the activity monitoring exercise to help the patient determine the types of activities that seem to produce feelings of mastery. For example, Juliana's activity schedule (see Figure 6–3) shows higher mastery scores when she was responsible for making her own dinner and when she did her own chores. Using guided discovery, you can assist the patient in recognizing that continuing current activities that are high on mastery, or modifying current activities, may increase their value to the patient and improve mood. If the patient has completed a goal list, efforts toward reaching any of the stated goals can be added to the activity schedule.

After completing the schedule, elicit the patient's expectations for success in changing his level of activity and the likelihood of engaging in the activity. Ask about any barriers or obstacles that may affect the patient's ability to follow the activity schedule as planned. Then work with the patient to devise a strategy for overcoming these obstacles. Armed with this information, assign the new schedule for the following week and ask the patient to rate each event for mastery and pleasure. Review the plan at the next session and modify it as needed. Usually activity scheduling is used in the early parts of therapy and can be discontinued when the patient is able to initiate pleasurable and achievement-oriented activities spontaneously. However, we sometimes use activity scheduling later in therapy when there are persistent problems with anhedonia, organizing effective behavioral plans, or procrastination.

## Working With Difficulties in Activity Scheduling

### Case Example

Charles is a 75-year-old man who lost his wife to cancer when he was 63. Life was great before his wife died. They traveled a lot together, took cruises, and went to movies and the theater. Charles had a good deal of grief after his wife died, but he rallied and threw himself into his work as a sales manager for an auto dealer. He still misses his wife greatly, but he was able to move on after her death without falling into a deep depression.

He has a history of one previous depression in his 40s when he lost his job as a manager in the auto industry. At that time, he went to a primary care doctor and was prescribed an antidepressant that was effective for relieving his depression. Then he found a job as a car salesman. He continued to sell cars but reduced his work hours until age 73, when he retired fully because he was having trouble being on his feet at the dealership. Arthritis in his knees and feet were giving him much pain after an hour or two of work.

After retiring, Charles began to slide into depression. Most of his friends were coworkers at the dealership. He kept in contact with them for a few months, but then felt that he was just an "old guy" and was getting in their way. So he stopped visiting the dealership or going out with them after they finished work as he had done in the past. His energy slipped, and he pulled back from a host of previously satisfying activities, including woodworking and watching movies. About once a month, he used to drive 4 hours to his son's house for a long weekend, but he stopped doing that. Other behavior changes included not eating regularly or well and not preparing food (he used to bake and cook for family and friends). Charles also has backed away from socializing with others. He thinks it is too much trouble to go, so he has refused invitations.

Charles had been asked to do a homework assignment by his therapist, Dr. Chapman. The assignment was to monitor and record his activities for 1 day using an activity schedule. They had also talked about some positive activities such as going out to dinner with a friend or doing some woodworking. In Video 14, Dr. Chapman reviews the activity schedule that Charles had recorded for 1 day. Although there were pleasure ratings for the activities, there were no mastery ratings. When Charles was asked

| | Pros/Benefits | Costs/Cons |
|---|---|---|
| **Change** | 1. Companionship with friends<br>2. Get shop in order<br>3. Get house cleaned | 1. My friend could be busy or not be responsive to my call.<br>2. I'll get more tired from effort of cleaning and sorting through my messes. |
| **Stay the same** | 1. Requires less effort<br>2. I don't have to see people and explain why I've been staying away from them. | 1. I'll remain depressed and lonely.<br>2. I won't get anything accomplished.<br>3. People will give up on me if I continue to ignore them. |

**Figure 6–4.** Charles's decisional balance worksheet.

about the difficulty in completing the mastery ratings, Charles indicated that he didn't "see the point" of rating activities such as eating a meal, which involved little sense of mastery.

Overall, Charles seemed to be stuck in his low activity pattern and unimpressed with the value of activity scheduling in making any differences. Thus, Dr. Chapman introduced a decisional balance worksheet (Figure 6–4) that included the costs and benefits of engaging in additional activities as well as not engaging in any new activities (or not changing behavior). Using guided discovery, he assisted Charles in completing this worksheet.

After completing the exercise, Dr. Chapman asked Charles for his conclusions about the benefits and the cons of making changes in his behavior. Charles saw the benefits of changing his behavior and decided that he would contact a friend next week. He also agreed to complete the activity schedule, including mastery and pleasure ratings, for 1 day as a homework assignment. Watching the next video will help you troubleshoot problems in using activity schedules.

**Video 14.** Difficulty Completing an Activity Schedule: Dr. Chapman and Charles (8:03)

Troubleshooting Guide 3 includes some guidelines and suggestions for responding to homework noncompletion. When addressing problems with completing homework, it is important that the therapist be nonjudgmental and not blame or label the patient for being "noncompliant." It is more helpful for the therapist to be supportive, understanding, and empathic when discussing homework assignments, as well as to take a collaborative, problem-solving approach by following some or all of the guidelines described in Troubleshooting Guide 3.

## Troubleshooting Guide 3
### Difficulties Completing Homework Assignments

1. **Patient doesn't understand the rationale for homework.** Take time to explain the value of homework again. Clarify misunderstandings. Give examples of how others have used homework to their benefit.

2. **Patient doesn't think that homework is helpful.** Check out the patient's reactions to your assignments. Are they seen as meaningful, yet doable? If you aren't suggesting assignments that are viewed as helpful, step back and rethink your treatment plan. Also, be sure to check homework from previous sessions at each subsequent session. If you don't do so, patients will conclude that you do not think that homework is very important.

3. **The homework assignment didn't seem feasible to the patient.** Be careful in assigning too much reading, an entire week of an activity schedule, or a effortful task to a patient with deep depression and limited energy. Recalibrate homework assignments so they are realistic and consistent with the patient's abilities, motivation, and situational factors.

4. **Patient didn't fully understand the assignment, forgot parts of it, or had difficulty concentrating on the activity.** Was the assignment specific and clearly stated? Is the patient keeping a notebook or other record of assignments? Because patients with depression may have problems with concentration and comprehension, ask for feedback about their understanding. Ask for the main take-home points at the end of sessions. And ask patients to repeat the steps they have planned to do for homework. Use memory aids such as sticky notes, prompts from mobile devices, or daily schedules to assist patients with remembering and completing homework.

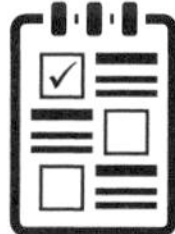

## Troubleshooting Guide 3 *(continued)*
### Difficulties Completing Homework Assignments

5. **Likelihood of completing the homework was not assessed.** If you suggest a homework exercise that the patient is unlikely to do, the chances of success have been compromised from the start. When assigning or reassigning homework, assess the likelihood that the patient will actually complete the assignment: 80%? 10%? If the patient indicates that she is unlikely to complete the assignment, troubleshoot reasons for the low estimate and/or generate alternative homework.

6. **Patient has negative thoughts about homework in general or the specific assignment.** Most adult patients will not have negative reactions to use of the word *homework*. They will understand that you are suggesting practical exercises that can help them cope better with their problems. However, alternative terms for homework may be useful when treating patients who are of school age or who have a negative view of their school experiences. You can call the assignment an action plan or a self-help exercise. Also, be sure to emphasize collaboration in generating assignments so patients don't think that they are being told to do things. When patients contribute to the design of homework assignments, they may be more likely to complete them. Specific homework tasks should be suggested by the patient as often as possible.

   Examples of maladaptive thoughts about homework include "I was never any good in school....I can't do this"; "I have to do the homework perfectly or not at all"; "I can't do anything right....why should I try?" When you identify these types of reactions to homework assignments, you can work to modify the cognitions with thought records, examining the evidence, or other CBT methods.

   Another useful strategy is to normalize homework noncompletion. Discuss how commonly people have such problems, and explain that you aren't expecting perfection in doing assignments. State that if difficulties are encountered, you will understand and will help the patient use the experience as a learning opportunity.

## Troubleshooting Guide 3 *(continued)*
### Difficulties Completing Homework Assignments

7. **Obstacles such as busy schedules, lack of family support, or situational stressors repeatedly derail patient from doing homework exercises.** You may need to spend more time troubleshooting ways to overcome obstacles. Could you sharpen the focus on goals that are more realistic or achievable? Could you look for activities that are less likely to be affected by these obstacles? Could the patient enlist support of friends or others to follow through with exercises? If these actions don't offer much help, remember that you can do homework in sessions. You can use cognitive-behavioral rehearsal to spot obstacles that could be overcome and build skills for completing the exercises.

8. **Patient has a long-standing pattern of procrastination and difficulty completing tasks.** If procrastination is a chronic problem, you can apply core CBT methods to help the patient become more active and productive. For example, elicit and attempt to modify cognitions associated with procrastinating behavior (e.g., "I'll mess it up anyway, so why try.... It will be too hard.... I've tried before and not succeeded.... Everyone else has their act together"). Assess basic behaviors such as organization of daily activities and scheduling. Then assist the patient with organizing realistic plans to complete homework exercises. Use homework exercises as opportunities to alter procrastination habits. For example, coach the patient on the step-by-step methods for graded task assignments discussed in the next section of this chapter.

**Learning Exercise 6–1.** Activity Scheduling

1. Complete at least 1 day of an activity schedule for your own life. Review the ratings of mastery and pleasure.
2. Practice introducing an activity schedule in a role-play exercise with a colleague.
3. Use activity scheduling in your clinical practice.

## Graded Task Assignments

*Graded task assignment* (GTA) is a method for making overwhelming, unmanageable, or complex tasks more feasible by breaking them down into smaller and more easily accomplished tasks. GTA can be used in conjunction with activity scheduling to increase mastery experiences and is particularly helpful when patients have fallen behind on chores (e.g., household maintenance or yard work), when they have put off difficult tasks that have looming deadlines (e.g., paying bills or filing taxes), or when goals they wish to accomplish are complicated and require lengthy efforts (e.g., getting in shape, earning a General Educational Development [GED] certificate or college degree, filing for divorce). If the perceived magnitude or complexity of the tasks has kept patients from taking action, GTA may be the answer.

Begin GTA by eliciting patients' perceptions of the tasks that require attention. Listen for negative automatic thoughts and evaluate their validity before beginning GTA. Catastrophic thoughts and black-and-white thinking can interfere with initiative. Ask patients to write down their modified thoughts and to review this cognitive analysis before initiating behavioral exercises. Suggest that they hold on to this written record as a handy reminder in case negative thoughts return. An example from the treatment of Robert illustrates the value of eliciting automatic thoughts about taking behavioral actions.

### Case Example

*Therapist:* When you think about filing your taxes, what goes through your mind?

*Robert:* I go blank. I don't know where to start.

*Therapist:* Take a moment and imagine yourself at home and seeing a commercial for a tax service on television. What would you be thinking?

*Robert:* I feel this tightness in my throat. I want to change the channel.

*Therapist:* Change the channel because you imagine what?

*Robert:* I know I have to file my taxes. I didn't turn them in last year, and I know the IRS [Internal Revenue Service] is going to go after me if I turn in this year's report. I don't know how to get started. I don't have the forms. I can't ask anyone else to help because I would have to tell them that I never filed taxes last year. That would be too embarrassing. It's all too much for me right now.

*Therapist:* So when you are reminded that you have to file your taxes, you get pretty upset.

*Robert:* You got that right.

*Therapist:* And when you get upset, what happens to your motivation to begin working on the taxes?

*Robert:* I don't want to deal with it. I put it off for another day.

*Therapist:* If you thought you had the ability to handle the stress of doing the taxes, would you want to start tackling the problem?

*Robert:* I have to do something about it.

*Therapist:* What would happen if we could find a way to make it easier for you?

*Robert:* If it were easier, I think I might be able to handle it. But it's not easy.

*Therapist:* I think I know a way to help.

Robert was overwhelmed by the thought of filing taxes, partly because he was uncertain where to begin. He had also made a number of assumptions about the reactions others would have if he asked for help. The therapist started working with Robert by modifying the belief that he couldn't ask for help. When this was accomplished, they were able to break the task down into smaller parts and make a schedule for their completion.

The behavioral component of GTA involves listing the specific components of a larger task and then placing them in a logical order. Because there are usually many ways to tackle an uncompleted task, it often helps to discuss several possible approaches before creating a specific action plan.

Robert thought it might be best to begin by finding someone to help him with his taxes. His sister, Celeste, thought it would be better for Robert to organize his materials and collect the proper tax forms before asking someone for help. His mother, Brenda, suggested he start by calling the IRS to find out if it would be better to turn in last year's tax return first or work on the one for this year. After discussing these options with his therapist, Robert decided to follow his first inclination and ask for assistance. He was so overwhelmed with the task, he did not think he could initiate things on his own. So he decided to ask Celeste for help as his first step.

The remaining steps involved finding the materials he had at home, organizing them, downloading the appropriate form from the IRS Web site, scheduling time with Celeste to begin filling out the forms, completing the forms, and calling the IRS to discuss last year's taxes. Because he wasn't certain about the order of the steps and thought it was possible that there were other things he needed to do, Robert asked Celeste for advice about the order of the remaining tasks and for suggestions about any other steps that might be needed.

When patients report on their progress at subsequent therapy sessions, you should praise their efforts and inquire about how their actions made them feel about themselves. Reinforce the cognitive-behavioral model, explaining once again that positive changes in action will help improve mood, strengthen self-esteem, and create optimism about future efforts. Ask about their motivation to take on the next step, and elicit and modify negative thoughts if necessary. After the first few items from the GTA have been assigned, some patients may feel enough momentum building to follow through with the other tasks without assistance from the therapist. Others will require continued coaching from the therapist to maintain progress. As energy and motivation levels return to normal, GTA may no longer be needed to initiate activity.

There will be times when GTA is not successful. A common reason is that the steps are too complicated for the patient to accomplish or require more energy than the patient possesses. In these cases, such tasks may be broken down into smaller subtasks. You will need to match the complexity or scope of the subtask to the energy level and the time available to the patient. Another common reason that GTA fails is that the person is flooded with negative automatic thoughts that discourage or interfere with his taking action. When tasks are difficult, initial attempts to carry them out may be less than completely successful. The person who is prone to black-and-white thinking may not give herself credit for progress made toward a goal. Instead, partial success is viewed as failure. When designing a GTA intervention, caution should be taken to keep each step within the capacity of the patient. When in doubt, it is better to make a task too easy to accomplish than too difficult.

To learn more about how to implement GTAs, watch Video 15, an engaging scene from Dr. Chapman's treatment of Charles. Despite many attempts and good intentions, Charles has not been able to get back to work in his woodshop—a pursuit that previously gave him great satisfaction. He is overwhelmed by the condition of the shop and has been stalled in efforts to make objects such as toys for a grandchild, a previous homework assignment. In this video, you'll see how to effectively blend cognitive and behavioral methods to construct a GTA that works.

**Video 15.** Developing a Graded Task Assignment: Dr. Chapman and Charles (7:43)

## Behavioral Rehearsal

Any behavioral plan that you want the patient to complete outside therapy can be rehearsed or practiced first during a treatment session to 1) assess the patient's understanding of the rationale for the plan, 2) check on the patient's ability and motivation to carry out the activity, 3) practice behavioral skills, 4) provide feedback on the skills, 5) identify and address potential roadblocks, and 6) coach the patient on ways to ensure that the plan will have a positive outcome.

Behavioral rehearsal has many applications in CBT. For example, you might practice breathing training for reducing anxiety, exposure protocols for overcoming panic and avoidance, or strategies for stopping compulsive rituals (see Chapter 7, "Behavioral Methods II: Reducing Anxiety and Breaking Patterns of Avoidance"). Behaviors that may enhance adherence to medication regimens (e.g., using effective communication with the prescribing physician, organizing a complex medication regimen, implementing a reminder system) also could be rehearsed in a treatment session. Other opportunities for using behavioral rehearsal might include role-playing a plan worked out in a problem-solving exercise (see Learning Exercise 6–2 below) or practicing skills for managing social anxiety (e.g., how to make small talk).

**Learning Exercise 6–2.** Task Completion

1. In a role-playing exercise with a colleague, target a challenging or difficult task.
2. First practice using the GTA method to work out a plan to complete the task.
3. Then use behavioral rehearsal to build skills or spot potential problems in carrying out the plan.
4. Role-play another behavioral rehearsal exercise.

## Problem Solving

When people have difficulties solving their problems, it may be partly due to either a *performance* deficit or a *skill* deficit. Those with performance deficits possess adequate problem-solving skills but—due to depression, anxiety, extreme stress, or feelings of helplessness—have difficulty accessing and utilizing those skills. In contrast, people with skill deficits may be unable to analyze the nature of a problem and cannot seem to come up with reasonable ideas to solve it. Individuals with skill deficits often have had trouble solving problems in many different areas of their lives or have repeatedly chosen solutions that have failed or made matters worse. People with performance deficits can be helped by identifying and modifying, whenever possible, the factors that keep them from using their existing skills. However, patients with skill deficits may require basic training in problem-resolution methods.

**Table 6–3.** Obstacles to effective problem solving

| | |
|---|---|
| **Cognitive impairment** | Poor concentration, slowed thinking, impaired decision making |
| **Emotional overload** | Feeling overwhelmed, dysphoric, anxious |
| **Cognitive distortions** | Negative automatic thoughts, cognitive errors (e.g., catastrophizing, all-or-nothing thinking, magnification), hopelessness, self-criticism |
| **Avoidance** | Procrastination, forgetfulness |
| **Social factors** | Contradictory advice from others, criticism, lack of support |
| **Practical problems** | Insufficient time, limited resources, problem being beyond control |
| **Strategy factors** | Trying to find the perfect solution, looking for one overall solution that will solve several related problems |

## Working With Problem-Solving Performance Deficits

Some of the more common factors that interfere with effective problem solving are listed in Table 6–3. This list includes obstacles that may be associated with the symptoms of a mental or physical illness. For example, depression often impairs concentration and interferes with the cognitive functioning needed to solve problems. Other roadblocks occur when patients do not have the resources to properly address their problems (e.g., financial, intellectual, or physical limitations) or when they search for ideal or perfect solutions when such standards are not attainable.

### *Cognitive Impairment*

When reduced attention span and impaired concentration keep a person from being able to focus on a problem, stimulus control measures may be needed. Stimulus control procedures involve arranging the physical environment so that stimuli that might interfere with accomplishing a goal are limited or avoided, while environmental factors that can facilitate goal attainment are identified and promoted. If concentration is a problem, environmental noise and confusion can distract the person from a task, whereas peace and quiet can facilitate completion of the task.

#### Case Example

Jonathan was so concerned that he would not be able to pay all his bills that he was losing sleep, was distracted at work by worries about his finances, and was experiencing frequent headaches. He needed to solve the problem by figuring out what bills needed to be paid, which ones could be delayed, when they were due, and the total amount that he owed. He had been working on his bills while sitting at the kitchen table after dinner, but he had not been able to concentrate well enough to get the job done. When his therapist asked what was happening around him while he tried to pay bills, Jonathan described a noisy dining room table with the dinner dishes being cleared by his wife. The television was on, and his children were watching a comedy and laughing hysterically. Although he wished they would be quiet, he knew they were just kids, and the sound of their laughter did him some good. The therapist concluded that Jonathan's environment was not conducive to concentration and problem solving.

Jonathan needed a place to work that was free of extraneous visual and auditory stimuli. He needed a physical space with enough room to sort through his bills; the tools to accomplish the task; and enough time and energy to complete the task. These conditions were hard to come by during the workweek because his house was small, there were no quiet places to work on the bills, and he was always tired at the end of the day. After the therapist explained the principles of stimulus control, Jonathan concluded that he needed to set aside time early on Saturday morning to pay his bills. He chose a time before the children would be awake and before his wife would start to make breakfast.

### *Emotional Overload*

Efforts to diminish the intensity of emotion can also facilitate problem solving. Cognitive restructuring methods described in the next section, "Cognitive Distortions," are among the primary problem-solving techniques used to reduce distracting or painful emotions. A variety of other ideas can be tried, such as relaxation exercises, prayer, meditation, listening to music, physical exercise, massage, yoga, or self-care behaviors that induce a temporary feeling of well-being. These might include going for a walk, taking a warm bath, eating a favorite food, or sitting in a garden. The goal is to reduce tension—not to encourage avoidance of the task. When the person feels calmer, he can begin to tackle the problem. If he becomes overwhelmed again, a brief break should be taken to reduce tension.

### *Cognitive Distortions*

The key to using cognitive restructuring methods (see Chapter 5, "Working With Automatic Thoughts") for problem solving is teaching patients how to carry the lessons of therapy into real-life situations. After learning in treatment sessions how to recognize negative automatic thoughts and how to correct cognitive distortions, patients can start to apply this knowledge toward conceptualizing and coping with their environmental problems. A good illustration of the usefulness of cognitive restructuring is the application of methods for spotting and correcting cognitive errors. Patients with depression may magnify the seriousness of their problems, minimize their resources or strengths for coping with the difficulty, take excessive blame for the situation (i.e., personalization), and give global meaning to a problem when it can have circumscribed significance. If the person can recognize and revise these cognitive errors, he will be able to develop a clearer picture of the challenges he faces and the opportunities he has to solve the problem.

### Avoidance

Techniques described elsewhere in this chapter (see "Activity Scheduling" and "Graded Task Assignments" above) can be used effectively to help people overcome avoidance. In Chapter 7, "Behavioral Methods II: Reducing Anxiety and Breaking Patterns of Avoidance," we discuss other behavioral methods that can help patients cope with avoidance problems associated with anxiety disorders. All of these behavioral methods involve organizing a plan that is systematic, that overcomes helplessness or paralyzing fear, and that utilizes gradual or stepwise methods of taking action.

### Social Factors

When people seek out advice from significant others, they may receive a variety of suggestions that have the potential of being helpful. However, advice also can be conflicting, ineffective, or harmful. To help the patient sort out the advice received, you can recommend that he analyze the pros and cons of each suggestion made by others, as well as any ideas that he has come up with himself. Craft a solution that offers the most advantages and the fewest disadvantages. The potential for disappointing others by not taking their advice can create a new problem for the indecisive patient with low self-esteem. Therefore, you may need to coach the patient in skills for communicating effectively with these people.

Some of the most difficult barriers to problem solving are 1) lack of social support; 2) criticism and disparagement from family members, friends, or others; and 3) active efforts of other people to block problem resolution. Examples of the latter would be a spouse in a divorce case who refuses mediation and appears determined to cause the most distress possible to the patient; a child who continues to use illicit drugs despite intense efforts by the patient to help him get treatment; and a boss who is extremely critical and is unwilling to give the patient any constructive ideas for meeting his expectations. Some of these types of problems cannot be solved easily, if at all. Therefore, the strategy should include a realistic assessment of the chances of any change occurring, the resources the patient may have to respond to the challenge, and alternative ideas that may not have been tried previously. Advice from an expert may be needed. The patient also may benefit from reading books, viewing videos, attending support groups, consulting a counselor in an employee assistance program, or using other methods to get ideas on how to manage the situation.

### *Practical Problems*

When functioning has declined during a lengthy episode of depression, it is not unusual to find that the patient has developed significant practical problems, especially when symptoms have been severe enough to interfere with her ability to sustain employment. Financial difficulties can quickly mount. Medical problems can be neglected due to lack of health insurance. Housing may be in jeopardy because of an inability to continue making rent or mortgage payments. The desperation communicated by patients in these situations can be disheartening for therapists. If your cognitions begin to echo the patient's hopelessness, you can lose your ability to be objective and creative with problem solving. Therefore, when faced with a patient with limited resources to solve his problems, it is important to process your own negative automatic thoughts about the bleakness of the situation.

If you can retain a reasonable degree of optimism that solutions can be found, you will be more likely to help the patient persevere. Help her brainstorm ideas for facing the problem. If ideas do not come easily, ask the patient what she would have done about this same problem at a time in her life when she was not depressed. Or ask her what a thoughtful and supportive advisor might recommend. Don't allow the patient to discount solutions as quickly as they are generated. Keep a running list of ideas, and wait until the brainstorming has been completed to evaluate their potential.

When people are depressed, they often feel alone in their misery. They forget that there are people in their world who could provide assistance if they knew there was a need. Most patients would agree to help others in similar situations. If solutions considered by the patient do not include asking for help from family, friends, faith communities, or social service agencies, encourage her to think about these possibilities. Embarrassment or pride can keep people from asking for help. But when times are desperate, the patient may need to temporarily forgo a self-reliant style of problem solving.

### *Strategy Factors*

When depressed or anxious, some people discard obvious solutions because they seem too simple. Or they look for solutions that are perfectly thought out or are guaranteed to succeed. Sometimes they look for the magic solution that will resolve several issues simultaneously.

### Case Example

Olivia lost her job and had been looking for a replacement. She had two children in elementary school. The three of them lived with her elderly grandmother, who had recently developed some health problems. Olivia needed to make enough money to support her children, but she also needed a job that was close to their school so that she could get to them in the event of an emergency. She needed a compassionate boss who would allow her extra time at lunch to look in on her grandmother. Olivia did not want to hire a home health aide to assist her grandmother, and she preferred to put her children in an after-school program rather than in private day care. A job near the school would make it possible for her to meet her children at the time the program closed. The children's father finished work earlier in the day, but Olivia did not trust him to pick them up on time. Olivia had marketable skills and could find a job in the larger city a little farther from her home. She could ask her sister to help with the grandmother rather than take on the full responsibility for her care, but she felt obligated to do it herself because her grandmother had been so helpful to her in times of need. Thinking about how to make all the pieces come together exhausted Olivia. As a result, she gave up reading the want ads and immersed herself in doing household chores.

The answer to a dilemma like Olivia's is to help her change problem-solving strategies. Instead of trying to find one large solution, work with her to sort out the problems and find a solution that covers as many areas as possible. Draw out her underlying problem-solving skills, identify key resources and supports, and coach her on ways of simplifying the plan or taking it one step at a time.

## Working With Deficits in Problem-Solving Skills

Problem-solving skills are usually learned during childhood and refined during early adulthood when an individual is grappling with life transitions and psychosocial stressors. If good role models were available, the person probably learned by watching these people systematically work through problems and generate solutions. If the patient had early life experiences in which she was able to solve problems effectively, she may have developed the self-confidence and competence needed to take on future difficulties. Unfortunately, patients may not have acquired effective problem-solving skills—perhaps because they had ineffective role models, they were protected by parents who solved problems for them, or they were too depressed when they were growing up to fully develop these skills. When the patient has had limited experience in effectively conceptualizing and managing problems, CBT can be used to teach basic skills for problem resolution.

One useful way of helping patients gain these skills is to model problem-solving strategies in treatment sessions. For example, the steps listed in Table 6–4 might be used to assist patients with organizing a plan to tackle one of the difficulties on their problem list. The suggested structure helps patients organize their thoughts, approach the problem in an objective fashion, and see the process through to completion.

1. **Slow down and sort it out.** When patients describe their psychosocial difficulties in treatment sessions, they may jump from topic to topic. As they describe one problem, another comes to mind. Without realizing it, they present a disjointed list of issues, all of which may seem equally pressing and stressful. They may see links between the problems and layers of complexity that combine the facts of the situation, the people involved, the deeper meanings behind them, and implications for the future. When problems are reported in this fashion, the notion of resolving these difficulties can seem distant or hopeless.

   The first order of business is to slow down the process by defining the number and magnitude of problems and the urgency of resolving them. You can ask the patient to keep a written list of problems in his treatment notebook. After the patient is finished recording the problems, ask him to summarize by reading back the list. Empathize with him about how distressing it must be to face so many challenges at one time. Then go on with the next steps in the problem-solving process.
2. **Pick a target.** Teach the patient how to organize the list by prioritizing problems. For example, ask him to cross off the list any problem that has already been resolved or is currently dormant. Next ask the patient to eliminate items over which he has no control or problems that belong to others and cannot be resolved by him. Help the patient to separate the remaining items into difficulties that must be addressed in the near future and ones whose resolution could be delayed for some time. Then ask the patient to consider the most pressing problems and place them in order of priority based on importance or urgency. The final part of this step is to select one item from the top two or three as the beginning target for therapy.
3. **Clearly define the problem.** If problems can be stated in clear terms, patients may be more likely to generate specific solutions. You can assist patients with defining problems accurately by teaching them the principles of goal setting and agenda setting described in Chapter 4, "Structuring and Educating." It also may be helpful to ask questions

**Table 6–4.** Problem-solving steps

1. Slow down and sort it out.
2. Pick a target.
3. Clearly define the problem.
4. Generate or brainstorm potential solutions.
5. Select the most reasonable solution.
6. Implement the plan.
7. Evaluate the outcome and repeat the steps if needed.

that help patients sharpen their definitions. Examples of these types of questions would be "How could you define this problem so that you would know if you were making progress to cope with it?" "How could you state this problem in just a few words so that other people would know exactly what you are facing?" and "There seem to be lots of different issues involved in this problem. How could you define the problem so that you can zero in on the central issue?"

4. **Generate potential solutions.** There are usually many different ways to solve any given problem. People sometimes lock onto the first solution that comes to mind and become convinced that it is the only way to cope. However, their selected solution may not be practical, effective, or possible to implement. Finding it difficult to change direction, they may flounder or completely give up on attempting to resolve the problem. Try to help the patient learn to be creative in looking for solutions. For example, use the brainstorming technique or ask Socratic questions that stimulate creativity. Patients might consider ideas such as a) utilizing the assistance of others; b) doing research by reading, checking the Internet, or searching for community resources; c) delaying implementation of the plan; and d) considering not solving the problem at all but learning to live with it. Adding your own suggestions to the list also may help, but only after the patient has come up with a number of possibilities.
5. **Select the most reasonable solution.** Help the patient eliminate from the list any solutions that the patient concludes are unrealistic, are not likely to be useful, cannot be easily implemented, or could cause more problems than they solve. Ask the patient to pick the solution that she thinks is most likely to succeed and that she is willing to implement. Sometimes patients will make a choice that in your best judgment will fail. Instead of discouraging the patient by telling her your opinion, help her choose one or two other possibilities and then evaluate

the advantages and disadvantages of each. As the solutions are compared, the most appropriate choice usually becomes evident. Retain the original list of options in case they are needed at a later date.

6. **Implement the plan.** Once a solution has been selected, increase the chances of success by having the patient select a day and time to try out her plan. Role-play or rehearsal methods can be used to coach patients on problem-solving skills. Troubleshoot by inquiring about circumstances that could interfere with success, and develop a plan for coping if these problems should occur.
7. **Evaluate the outcome and repeat the steps if needed.** Despite great planning, solutions will sometimes fail. There may be unforeseen circumstances or elements of the problem that were not fully considered. When there are difficulties in carrying out a plan, help patients evaluate their automatic thoughts about their efforts to solve the problem, and assist them with correcting any distortions. In addition, review the manner in which the solution was implemented, to determine whether further skills training may be required. Revise the plan if necessary, and try again.

Occasionally, some therapists may assist patients by using problem-solving themselves during the session. Although doing so often results in an effective or reasonable solution to the patient's problem, it is ineffective for teaching or coaching patients to learn and use problem-solving skills on their own. Therapists should help patients to learn and apply effective problem-solving skills so that they can apply these skills in the future and not just for resolving the current problem.

## Summary

When patients have problems with low mood or lack of interest associated with reduced activity levels, low energy, and poor task completion, behavioral methods can help restore healthy functioning. The easiest technique to implement is a behavioral action plan—a simple exercise in which the therapist and patient choose one or two concrete actions that appear to be immediately doable and are likely to improve mood or self-esteem. Activity scheduling, a more systematic method of recording and shaping behavior, is often quite useful when patients are experiencing moderate to severe reductions in energy and interest. Another behavioral technique, GTA, can help patients organize a step-by-step plan to manage difficult or challenging tasks or to reverse patterns of procrastination and avoidance.

Behavioral rehearsal is commonly used in CBT to help patients develop action plans, build skills, and spot potential roadblocks in advance. This technique involves practicing behavioral methods in treatment sessions and then carrying out the plan for homework. Problem solving is another key behavioral method for helping patients cope with their stressors. Although some patients have good basic problem-solving skills and only need help in overcoming obstacles to using these strengths, others may need to be educated on the principles of effective problem solving. The behavioral methods described in this chapter can have a positive impact on a patient's activity level, mood, effectiveness in managing challenges, and hope for the future.

## References

Beck AT, Rush AJ, Shaw BF, et al: Cognitive Therapy of Depression. New York, Guilford, 1979

Beck AT, Greenberg RL, Beck J: Coping With Depression. Bala Cynwyd, PA, Beck Institute for Cognitive Therapy and Research, 1995

MacPhillamy DJ, Lewinsohn PM: The Pleasant Events Schedule: studies on reliability, validity, and scale intercorrelations. J Consult Clin Psychol 50:363–380, 1982

Wright JH, Thase ME, Beck AT, et al (eds): Cognitive Therapy With Inpatients: Developing a Cognitive Milieu. New York, Guilford, 1993

Wright JH, Thase ME, Beck AT: Cognitive-behavior therapy, in The American Psychiatric Publishing Textbook of Psychiatry, 6th Edition. Edited by Hales RE, Yudofsky SC, Roberts L. Washington, DC, American Psychiatric Publishing, 2014, pp 1119–1160

# Behavioral Methods II 7

## Reducing Anxiety and Breaking Patterns of Avoidance

The cognitive and behavioral features of anxiety disorders—unrealistic fears of objects or situations, overestimates of risk or danger, underestimates of ability to manage or cope with feared stimuli, and repeated patterns of avoidance—are outlined in Chapter 1, "Basic Principles of Cognitive-Behavior Therapy." We turn now to explaining the theoretical background for using behavioral techniques in anxiety disorders and to discussing specific methods for overcoming problems such as phobia, panic, and obsessive-compulsive disorder (OCD). The focus is on general principles and techniques that can be used for anxiety disorders, posttraumatic stress syndrome (PTSD), and OCD.

## Behavioral Analysis of Anxiety Disorders and Related Conditions

The behavioral methods typically used in cognitive-behavior therapy (CBT) for anxiety disorders, PTSD, and OCD were originally derived from the learning theory model that shaped the early development of behavior therapy (see Chapter 1, "Basic Principles of Cognitive-Behavior Therapy"). As behavior therapy and cognitive therapy matured, these two approaches were merged into the comprehensive cognitive-behavioral approach that we describe in this book. To explain the rationale for behavioral methods for anxiety disorder and related conditions, we briefly detail the concepts that underlie contemporary use of these interventions. Readers who would like to delve more deeply into the theoretical and empirical basis for CBT of anxiety disorders can consult the excellent book *Cognitive Therapy of Anxiety Disorders: Science and Practice,* by Clark and Beck (2010).

Patients with anxiety disorders usually report intense subjective experiences of fear accompanied by physical symptoms of arousal when exposed to a threatening stimulus. For example, if a person who has a phobia for heights is facing the prospect of climbing a tall ladder, he may have anxiety-provoking automatic thoughts (e.g., "I'll pass out....I'll fall....I can't stand it....I have to get down right away") and intense emotions and physiological activation (e.g., anxiety, sweating, fast heartbeat, quickened breathing, clamminess).

The emotional and physiological responses to feared stimuli are usually so aversive that the sufferer will do whatever is necessary to avoid experiencing these situations again. For example, persons with simple phobias will avoid heights, closed spaces, elevators, or other triggers for their anxiety; those with social phobia will stay away from events or places where they may feel exposed to social pressures; and people who have panic disorder with agoraphobia will take great care not to experience the situations that trigger their fear. Patients with PTSD will try to insulate themselves from the conditions that remind them of traumatic experiences (e.g., they will stop driving, will not return to work, or will avoid dating or having close interpersonal relationships).

Because avoidance is rewarded with emotional relief, the avoidant behavior is more likely to occur again when the person is faced with the same or similar circumstances. To illustrate, a socially phobic person decides not to go to a party and then feels immediate relief from anxiety. His avoidance is reinforced, so the next time an invitation is received for a social event, he is likely to continue the pattern of avoidance as a way of controlling the anxiety associated with anticipated social scrutiny. Each time he avoids social situations, his phobic behavior and his dysfunctional cognitions about social performance are further reinforced, and his symptoms become more deeply entrenched.

Videos 1 and 2, which you viewed earlier in the book (see Chapter 2, "The Therapeutic Relationship: Collaborative Empiricism in Action"), show therapeutic engagement and cognitive restructuring interventions used in the treatment of Kate, a woman with panic symptoms, agoraphobia, and a fear of driving. Additional videos from the treatment of Kate are featured later in this chapter. Kate had intense anxiety and panic associated with driving across bridges. Because her therapist recognized that avoidance was perpetuating her fear, he encouraged her to use behavioral methods to expose herself to the feared situation.

Another example of the reinforcing power of avoidance is observed in OCD. When obsessional thoughts occur in persons with OCD, compulsive rituals are often used to stop the thoughts. When the obsession is counteracted (and thus avoided) with the compulsive behavior, anxiety is reduced. Therefore, the compulsive act is reinforced as a coping strategy because it dampens or turns off the aversive obsessional thought. Because of the reinforcement, the next time the obsession occurs, the compulsive ritual is likely to be repeated.

In summary, the key features of the contributions of the CBT model for anxiety disorders are as follows: 1) unrealistic fears of objects or situations; 2) a pattern of avoidance of the feared stimulus reinforces the patient's belief that she cannot face the object or cope with the situation; and 3) the pattern of avoidance must be broken for the patient to overcome the anxiety.

Studies of cognitive processes in anxiety disorders (see Chapter 1, "Basic Principles of Cognitive-Behavior Therapy") and the development of cognitive methods for anxiety have enriched the behavioral model in several important ways. First, a number of investigations have shown that the automatic thoughts of persons with anxiety are characterized by illogical reasoning (e.g., magnification of the risk in situations, minimization of estimates of the person's ability to cope, catastrophic predictions of deleterious effects of being in the situation). Second, a developmental perspective suggests that fearful cognitions may be shaped by many life experiences, including teachings of parents and other significant people, which influence core beliefs about risk, danger, and the person's ability to manage these exigencies. Finally, many anxiety disorders (especially generalized anxiety disorder and panic disorder) and related conditions cannot be traced back to a single fearful stimulus that set off a pattern of conditioned stimuli and avoidance. Therefore, a more complex formulation—which may include the effects of learning experiences during growth and development, the impact of automatic thoughts and core beliefs, and other potential influences (e.g., the entire gamut of biopsychosocial factors as discussed in Chapter 3, "Assessment and Formulation")—is recommended for treating anxiety disorders and OCD with CBT. We focus here on describing the behavioral elements of the overall CBT model. Cognitive interventions for anxiety are detailed further in Chapter 1, "Basic Principles of Cognitive-Behavior Therapy"; Chapter 5, "Working With Automatic Thoughts"; and Chapter 8, "Modifying Schemas."

## Overview of Behavioral Treatment Methods

The two most commonly used behavioral procedures are *reciprocal inhibition* and *exposure*. Reciprocal inhibition is defined as a process of reducing emotional arousal by helping the patient experience a positive or healthy emotion that counteracts a dysphoric response. A common method of implementing reciprocal inhibition is to induce deep relaxation of voluntary musculature, thereby producing a state of calm largely incompatible with intense anxiety or arousal. When this method is practiced regularly, the power of the stimulus to evoke fear and avoidance can fade or be eliminated.

Exposure works in a different way. As a coping strategy, exposure has effects that are the opposite those of avoidance. If a person intentionally exposes himself to a stressful stimulus, he is likely to experience fear. However, fear is generally time limited because physiological arousal cannot be maintained at a heightened state indefinitely. Fatigue occurs, and in the absence of new sources of arousal, the person will begin to adapt to the situation. For example, if a person who is afraid of heights is taken to the top floor of a tall building and asked to look out the window, he will be frightened, even panicked. But eventually the fear response will be depleted and a normal homeostatic state will return. With repeated exposures, the physiological response to the feared situation should decrease as the person concludes that the stimulus can be faced and managed.

Cognitive restructuring techniques can aid the process of uncoupling a fearful response from a stressful stimulus by facilitating the relaxation response and by promoting involvement in exposure-based interventions. Methods that reduce or turn off negative thoughts can lower tension levels, thereby helping the person enjoy the physical and emotional sensations of relaxation.

An example of a cognitive restructuring method that can help in the unpairing of anxiety responses from their stimuli is decatastrophizing. Decatastrophizing helps the patient to 1) systematically evaluate the likelihood of an imagined catastrophic outcome occurring on exposure to the stimulus, 2) develop a plan to reduce the probability that such an outcome will occur, and 3) create a strategy to cope with the catastrophe should it occur. Procedures for decatastrophizing are described more fully later in this chapter (in the section "Step 3: Basic Skills Training").

## Sequencing Behavioral Interventions for Anxiety Symptoms

The sequence of behavioral interventions is similar in the treatment of different types of anxiety disorders, PTSD, or OCD. First the therapist assesses symptoms, anxiety triggers, and existing coping strategies. Then specific targets of intervention are defined to guide the course of therapy. Next the patient is taught basic skills for coping with the thoughts, feelings, and behaviors that characterize the anxiety disorder. Finally, these skills are used to assist patients in systematically exposing themselves to anxiety-provoking situations.

### Step 1: Assessment of Symptoms, Triggers, and Coping Strategies

In assessing anxiety disorders, it is important to clearly delineate 1) the events (or memories of events or streams of cognitions) that serve as triggers for the anxiety response; 2) the automatic thoughts, cognitive errors, and underlying schemas involved in the overreaction to the feared stimulus; 3) the emotional and physiological responses; and 4) habitual behaviors such as panic or avoidance symptoms. Thus all elements of the basic cognitive-behavioral model are evaluated and considered in developing the formulation and treatment plan. General assessment methods used in CBT are discussed in Chapter 3, "Assessment and Formulation." The major form of assessment is a careful interview targeted at uncovering the key symptoms, triggers for anxiety, and salient cognitions and behaviors (see Video 1).

Specialized diagnostic and rating measures also may be useful in the assessment phase of working with patients with anxiety disorders, PTSD, and OCD. Self-report measures (e.g., Generalized Anxiety Disorder 7-Item Scale [GAD-7; Spitzer et al. 2006]; Beck Anxiety Inventory [BAI; Beck et al. 1988]; Penn State Worry Questionnaire [PSWQ; Meyer et al. 1990]) and clinical rating scales (e.g., the Yale-Brown Obsessive Compulsive Scale [Y-BOCS; Goodman et al. 1989]) can be used to measure the severity of anxiety or OCD symptoms. Sources for these scales are shown in Table 7–1.

The thought change record described in Chapter 5, "Working With Automatic Thoughts," can be a helpful tool for assessing anxiety-provoking situations because it provides a structure for documenting triggering events as well as automatic thoughts associated with those events. Identification of places, situations, and people that elicit anxiety will aid in

**Table 7–1.** Measures for anxiety disorders and related conditions

| Rating scale | Application | Source | Reference |
|---|---|---|---|
| Generalized Anxiety Disorder 7-Item Scale | Anxiety | www.phqscreeners.com | Spitzer et al. 2006 |
| Beck Anxiety Inventory | Anxiety | www.pearsonclinical.com | Beck et al. 1988 |
| Penn State Worry Questionnaire | Anxiety | http://at-ease.dva.gov.au/professionals/files/2012/11/PSWQ.pdf | Meyer et al. 1990 |
| Yale-Brown Obsessive Compulsive Scale | Obsessive-compulsive disorder | https://psychology-tools.com/yale-brown-obsessive-compulsive-scale | Goodman et al. 1989 |

preparation for exposure interventions. Spotting cognitive errors can give the therapist leads for possible cognitive restructuring interventions. Another useful strategy is to ask patients to make notes of things they encounter that cause anxiety and to rate the intensity of the reaction on a scale of 0–100, with 100 indicating the most extreme emotion. These types of ratings can be used for baseline assessments and for measuring progress in achieving treatment goals.

Assessment of the behavioral component of the anxiety response should go beyond identifying avoidance reactions to include a more detailed analysis of actions the patient takes to cope with the anxiety. For example, there may be healthy coping strategies that are being used (e.g., problem solving, employing a sense of humor, meditation) that could be strengthened or given more emphasis. However, patients with anxiety disorders frequently engage in *safety behaviors*—actions that may fall short of outright avoidance but still perpetuate the anxiety reaction. To illustrate, a person with social phobia may be able to force himself to go to occasional parties, but he copes with anxiety by going immediately to the buffet and gulping down more food than he would ordinarily eat, staying by his partner's side so that she can do all the talking, and going to the bathroom much more frequently than needed to get away from the crowd. Although he is attending the party, he is engaging in safety behaviors that are part of his pattern of avoidance. To be successful in overcoming problems such as the social anxiety experienced by this patient, the therapist will need to obtain a full picture of coping strategies, both maladaptive and adaptive, and design interventions that will help the patient identify all of the avoidant behaviors and expose himself to the full experience of facing and managing the feared situation.

One especially important type of safety behavior occurs when a patient has involved family members, friends, or others in helping her cope. Sometimes support from others can be quite useful in overcoming anxiety, but there is a risk that the attempts of others to help can inadvertently reward or reinforce avoidant behavior and thus perpetuate the patient's anxiety symptoms. For example, if Kate had her family or coworkers drive her to work consistently, she would not be directly addressing her avoidance and would be less likely to overcome her problem with driving across bridges. Also, there could be positive reinforcement for continuing the assistance because she would be spending additional time with family or coworkers.

When you plan interventions for anxiety symptoms, you will need to take environmental contingencies into consideration. If the full range of reinforcers of anxiety are not considered, your efforts at helping the patient achieve more independence from fear could easily be thwarted by subtle safety behaviors that escape your notice or by a well-intentioned family member or friend who facilitates avoidance as a coping strategy.

## Step 2: Identifying Targets for Intervention

It is not unusual for an individual to have multiple manifestations of anxiety. What often works best is to start by targeting a symptom or goal that is most easily accomplished, so that the patient can build confidence by having early success. Also, lessons learned from experiences in managing one feared situation can often be generalized to provide effective coping strategies for other anxieties.

Sometimes patients choose to start by tackling their most challenging problem because it is vitally important to them or because environmental pressures are forcing them to make progress quickly (e.g., anxiety about a job interview when the patient is unemployed and running out of money). If in your judgment the patient will need some further experience before being able to effectively address the situation, you can break the overall problem into pieces. In a manner similar to the graded task assignment approach described in Chapter 6, "Behavioral Methods I: Improving Mood, Increasing Energy, Completing Tasks, and Solving Problems," target a circumscribed part of the problem for immediate attention. Whether you begin by attacking the most difficult situation or you ease the patient into exposure therapy in a step-by-step fashion, the basic skills training described below can give patients tools to overcome their anxiety.

## Step 3: Basic Skills Training

Several core CBT skills can help patients successfully engage in exposure-based interventions for anxiety disorders. We detail five of these methods below: relaxation training, thought stopping, distraction, decatastrophizing, and breathing training.

### *Relaxation Training*

The goal of relaxation training is to help patients learn to achieve a relaxation response—a state of mental and physical calmness. Muscle relaxation is one of the principal mechanisms for achieving the relaxation response. Patients are taught to systematically release tension in muscle groups throughout the body. As muscular tension is decreased, the subjective feeling of anxiety is usually reduced. A common method for teaching patients deep muscle relaxation is to follow the steps outlined in Table 7–2. Resources such as recordings and apps are available online for promoting deep muscle relaxation. Because these resources may vary widely in content and quality, we recommend that clinicians check out options themselves to choose a few that they think best fit the needs of their patients. A starting point for choosing resources might be to check out a review of best apps for anxiety (e.g., see www.healthline.com).

**Learning Exercise 7–1.** Relaxation Training

1. Try out the relaxation instructions in Table 7–1 on yourself. Work on achieving a state of deep muscle relaxation.

2. Then practice the induction procedure with one or more of your patients with anxiety symptoms.

### *Thought Stopping*

Thought stopping is different from most cognitive interventions in that it does not involve an analysis of negative thoughts. Its aim is to stop the process of negative thinking and replace it with more positive or adaptive thoughts. Thought stopping may be helpful for some patients with anxiety disorders such as phobias and panic disorder. However, some studies of patients with OCD have shown an intensification of obsessions when the patient makes a conscious effort to suppress them (Abramowitz et al. 2003; Purdon 2004; Rassin and Diepstraten 2003; Tolin et al. 2002). Therefore, if thought stopping is not useful in helping the patient reduce

**Table 7–2.** A method for relaxation training

1. **Explain the rationale for relaxation training.** Before beginning the relaxation induction, give the patient an overview of the reasons for using relaxation training. Also briefly explain the overall method.
2. **Teach patients to rate their level of muscle tension and anxiety.** Use a 0–100 scale, where a rating of 0 is equivalent to no tension or anxiety and 100 represents maximum tension or anxiety.
3. **Explore the range of muscle tension.** Because the focus of relaxation training is primarily on reducing muscular tension, it often helps to ask the patient to try to tighten one fist to the maximum level (100) and then let it completely relax to a rating of 0 or to the lowest level of tension he can achieve. Then the patient can be asked to try to tighten one hand to the maximum level while relaxing the other hand as much as possible. This exercise usually shows the patient that he can gain voluntary control over his state of muscle tension.
4. **Teach the patient methods for reducing muscle tension.** Starting with the hands, try to help the patient reach a state of full relaxation (rated as a 0 or close to 0). The primary methods used in cognitive-behavior therapy are a) exerting conscious control over muscle groups by monitoring tension and telling oneself to relax the muscles, b) stretching the targeted muscle groups through their full range of motion, c) gentle self-massage to soothe and relax tight muscles, and d) use of calming mental images.
5. **Help the patient systematically relax each of the major muscle groups of the body.** After the patient has achieved a state of deep relaxation of the hands, ask him to allow the relaxation to spread through the entire body, one muscle group at a time. A commonly used sequence is hands, forearms, upper arms, shoulders, neck, head, eyes, face, chest, back, abdomen, hips, upper legs, lower legs, feet, and toes. However, any sequence can be chosen that you and the patient believe will work best for him. During this phase of the induction, all of the methods from step 4 that have proved helpful can be repeated. We often find that stretching allows the patient to find especially tense muscle groups that may require extra attention.
6. **Suggest mental images that may assist in relaxation.** Mental images that you suggest (or that are evoked by the patient) can divert attention from worrisome thoughts and help him to concentrate on achieving the relaxation response. For example, you might say, "Picture your tensions melting away and dripping onto the floor like ice melting slowly." Use a calm, soothing, and genuine vocal tone as you suggest these images.
7. **Ask the patient to practice the relaxation induction method regularly.** Usually it takes a considerable amount of practice before patients can master the deep relaxation technique. Therefore, it is often useful to suggest that patients perform relaxation exercises for homework assignments. When relaxation is part of the treatment plan for anxiety disorders, it is also important to check on the patient's progress in using this technique in subsequent sessions.

worrisome thoughts, try another technique. A typical procedure for thought stopping is as follows:

1. **Recognize** that a dysfunctional thought process (e.g., excessive worrying, exaggerated fears, rumination) is active.
2. **Give self-instructions to interrupt the thought process.** Patients who find this method useful are able to make a conscious decision to shift their thinking away from the anxiety-ridden thought content. Some may find it helpful to tell themselves, "Stop!" or "Don't go there!"
3. **Consider imagining a pleasant or relaxing scene.** Examples are a vacation, sports, or music memory; the face of a pleasant person; or a photograph or painting the person has seen. The positive image can be amplified by deep muscle relaxation and by embellishing the image with details such as the time of day, weather conditions, and sounds associated with the image.

Each step can be rehearsed in session by asking the patient to first generate the upsetting thought(s) and then implement the thought-stopping strategies. Ask the patient for feedback on his experience, and then make any needed adjustments to the procedures. For example, if the positive image was difficult to create or sustain, choose another scene or modify the image to make it more vivid.

### *Distraction*

The imagery technique described in the above section, "Thought Stopping," is a commonly used CBT distraction method. Imagery also can be used to augment other behavioral interventions, including breathing training (see Video 16 in the section "Breathing Training" later in this chapter). When using imagery, try to help the patient generate several positive, calming scenes that she can use to relax and, at least temporarily, defuse the intensity of anxiety-ridden thoughts. Myriad other possibilities exist for helping patients use distraction to lessen the impact of intrusive or worrisome thoughts. Commonly used distractions are reading, going to a movie, working on a hobby or craft project, socializing with friends, and spending time on the Internet. When distraction is employed, the therapist needs to be careful to monitor the activities so that they are not being used as safety behaviors to avoid feared situations or to escape from the exposure-based methods described later in this chapter. Effective use of distraction should facilitate participation in exposure and other behavioral interventions by reducing the frequency or intensity of automatic thoughts and lowering physical tension and emotional distress. Some studies have suggested that distraction may be more useful than thought stopping for reducing obsessional thoughts in OCD (Abramowitz et al. 2003; Rassin and Diepstraten 2003).

## *Decatastrophizing*

The general principles for using decatastrophizing methods are explained in Chapter 5, "Working With Automatic Thoughts," and are depicted in part in Video 2. This vignette shows Dr. Wright working with Kate on her fear of passing out if she drives across a bridge. This sample of dialogue from the session gives an example of steps that can be taken to modify catastrophic predictions. With many patients, efforts to modify dysfunctional cognitions can unlock their potential for using behavioral methods to master anxiety.

*Kate:* Well, I don't want to drive if I'm afraid I'm gonna pass out.

*Dr. Wright:* Is that a recurrent thought that you have?

*Kate:* Pretty much.

*Dr. Wright:* Right.... Now let's take a look at that and check out to see whether it will continue or not—or how accurate it is. Let's see, you've driven lots of times in your life already, haven't you? Even though you've been anxious sometimes?

*Kate:* Yeah.

*Dr. Wright:* So, how old are you now? You're early 50s—52, I think it was. And you started driving at about what age?

*Kate:* Like 16, 17.

*Dr. Wright:* OK. And so you've been driving for...what, 36 years?

*Kate:* (*laughs*) Yeah.

*Dr. Wright:* And as you were having this thought....what do you think the likelihood was in your mind that you would actually pass out?

*Kate:* I would say...the likelihood?...I would say about 90%.

*Dr. Wright:* Oh, 90% sure that you were going to pass out?

*Kate:* Well, that I could, yeah.

*Dr. Wright:* Going back to the numbers of years you've been driving—36 years....Roughly, how many times have you driven daily over those years, just to give us an average?

*Kate:* Well, probably one or two every day.

*Dr. Wright:* So we add it all up, I wonder how many times that you have actually driven a car since you've been 16.

*Kate:* (*sighs*) Well, it's gotta be in the thousands.

*Dr. Wright:* Right, at least 10,000. If we did twice a day, it would be 20,000 or more. Have you ever passed out in those 20,000 or so times of driving?

*Kate:* No.

*Dr. Wright:* You've never passed out?

*Kate:* No...but I feel like I'm gonna.

*Dr. Wright:* You feel like it, but it hasn't happened. And so, we have this 90% estimate that it's going to happen, and yet we have the 0% actually happening. What do you think? Is there another estimate you could make that would be more on target?

*Kate:* Well…I mean, you're right (*nodding*). I've driven for a long time.… I've *often* felt like I was gonna pass out.

*Dr. Wright:* Yes.

*Kate:* But I haven't done it.

*Dr. Wright:* So what's the true risk for you?

*Kate:* So…let's say maybe like 5%.

*Dr. Wright:* 5%? Yeah…so, we went from 90% to 5% by thinking it through—which is great!

*Kate:* (*laughs*) It's sort of embarrassing.

*Dr. Wright:* But still, we're at 5%—and we have the actual experience of 0%.

*Kate:* Yeah.

*Dr. Wright:* I think what we're seeing here is something that happens with lots of people that have anxiety just like you. For one reason or another, whether it's the way their brains are wired or the experiences they've had in life, they get to the point where they overestimate the risk of something bad happening. So, when they think of driving or going up on an elevator, whatever it is that they are fearful of, they have an estimate that's way over what anyone who doesn't have that anxiety problem would give to the experience. But you're still giving it 5%. So we have a way to go.

*Kate (nodding):* Yeah.

*Dr. Wright:* The point here is not to say that there's no risk ever of things happening that are bad, but that if we can be realistic about it, it helps us manage the anxiety.

*Kate:* OK.

Here are some procedures that you can use to help patients reduce their catastrophic predictions:

1. **Estimate the likelihood** that the catastrophic event or outcome will occur, as shown in Video 2. Ask patients to rate their belief on a scale from 0% (completely unlikely) to 100% (absolute) certainty. Note the answer for future outcome assessments.
2. **Evaluate the evidence** for and against the likelihood that a catastrophic event will occur. Monitor patients' use of cognitive errors, and use Socratic questions to help patients discriminate between fears and facts.
3. **Review the evidence list** and ask patients to reestimate the likelihood of the catastrophe occurring. Usually there should be a lowering of the original value from step 1. If the probability estimate increases (the worry becomes more believable), inquire about the pieces of evidence from step 2 that made the feared outcome seem more likely. Apply cognitive restructuring methods from Chapter 5, "Working With Automatic Thoughts," if necessary.

4. **Create an action plan** by brainstorming strategies to reduce the likelihood that the catastrophe will occur. Have the patient write down the actions she could take to improve on or prevent the feared outcome. For example, Kate could work on an action plan to use if she were feeling light-headed or dizzy when driving. She could use the calming breathing exercises explained later in this chapter and/or pull over to the side of the road until she felt better.
5. **Develop a plan for coping** with the catastrophe if it should occur. In Kate's case, passing out while driving would be a true catastrophe. Fortunately, the chances are very tiny that this would happen without any warning that she could heed to make herself safe. For other patients who have fears of "catastrophes" that are more likely to occur (e.g., a patient with social phobia who clutches and doesn't know what to say at a party, a person who has a panic attack during an important business meeting and has to leave the room), it can be very useful to imagine the "worst-case scenario," and build a plan for successfully managing this feared event.
6. **Reassess** the perceived likelihood of the catastrophic outcome. Compare this assessment to the original ratings and discuss any differences.
7. **Debrief** by asking the patient what it was like to talk about his catastrophic thoughts in this way. Reinforce the value of decatastrophizing as part of the treatment plan.

## *Breathing Training*

Breathing training is often used in the treatment of panic disorder because irregular breathing and hyperventilation are frequent symptoms of panic attacks. Hyperventilation typically reduces $PCO_2$ (a measure of carbon dioxide in blood) by overbreathing (Meuret et al. 2008). Although there has been debate about the specificity of methods for regulating breathing and $PCO_2$ levels (one study found that either lowering or increasing $PCO_2$ was effective for panic disorder; Kim et al. 2012), research studies have documented the effectiveness of breathing training (Kim et al. 2012; Meuret et al. 2008, 2010) and this method remains a key feature of the CBT approach to panic disorder.

A frequently used strategy for breathing training for panic attacks begins with simulating the experience of hyperventilation and panic. The therapist may demonstrate overbreathing and then ask the patient to increase the respiration rate before reducing it. The patient may be instructed to breathe rapidly and deeply for a short time (maximum of a minute and a half) to replicate the respiration experience of a panic attack. The next step is to ask the patient to attempt to breathe slowly until he regains normal control over his respiration. Most patients with panic disorder report that this exercise closely approximates the feeling of a panic attack. Thus it is helpful to allay catastrophic fears about possible outcomes by explaining what is happening physiologically when a person hyperventilates.

Therapists can help patients learn to control their breathing by teaching methods for slowing respirations such as counting breaths, using the second hand of a watch to time breaths, and using positive imagery to calm anxious thoughts. However, caution needs to be taken not to encourage overly deep breathing. Such breathing patterns can worsen panic through continued hyperventilation. Video 16 shows Dr. Wright simulating the hyperventilation that often occurs in panic attacks and asking Kate to practice this method between sessions. Note how Dr. Wright works on normalizing breathing patterns and using positive imagery to enhance the effects of controlling the rate of respiration.

**Video 16.** Breathing Training for Panic Attacks: Dr. Wright and Kate (7:48)

Once mastered in session, breathing training exercises are recommended for use as homework. They should be rehearsed daily until confidence is gained in using the technique. Patients should also be asked to attempt to use this method in anxiety-provoking situations, with the caveat that their expectation for control of anxiety should be tempered until the skill has been fully developed.

**Learning Exercise 7–2.** Breathing Training

1. After viewing Video 16, practice breathing training by role-playing with a colleague.
2. Rehearse overbreathing and then slowing the breathing rate to about 15 breaths per minute.
3. Practice using imagery to reduce anxiety and facilitate breathing training.

## Step 4: Exposure

Exposure to anxiety-provoking stimuli is usually the most important step in using CBT for anxiety disorders, PTSD, and OCD. To counter the reinforcement cycle caused by avoidance, the patient is assisted in confronting stressful situations while using the cognitive restructuring and relaxation methods described above in "Step 3: Basic Skills Training." Although some anxiety symptoms such as simple phobias can be treated in a single session with *flooding* therapy (i.e., the patient is encouraged to directly face the feared stimulus while the therapist models coping with the situation), most exposure therapies use the *systematic desensitization* method. This procedure involves the development of a hierarchy of feared stimuli that is used to organize a graded exposure protocol for overcoming anxiety a step at a time. The remainder of this chapter is devoted to providing details on the specific methods of exposure therapy and related techniques.

## Developing a Hierarchy for Graded Exposure

The success of systematic desensitization, or graded exposure, often hinges on the quality of the hierarchy that is developed for this procedure. Some suggestions for developing effective hierarchies are noted in Table 7–3.

Video 17 shows Dr. Wright and Kate constructing a hierarchy to help her overcome avoidance of driving across bridges and other driving activities that trigger anxiety. He starts by explaining the rationale for the hierarchy and then generates several items that Kate rates fairly low on a 0–100 distress scale. After identifying some driving activities that would cause distress ratings of 90–100, they complete the hierarchy with a full range of possible targets for exposure therapy (see Figure 7–1). Note how they develop the hierarchy in a collaborative style.

Often there will be ratings of hierarchy items that can be explored with cognitive methods to enhance the patient's understanding of the CBT model for anxiety and promote participation in exposure therapy. In this video illustration, Dr. Wright draws Kate's attention to the relatively low rating of 20 given to her routine 3-mile drive to her current office. In contrast, she gave a higher distress rating to a shorter and less frequently taken drive. Using Socratic questioning, he helps Kate learn that repeated experience drops anxiety levels, while avoidance often increases anxiety. They use this insight to reinforce the value of exposure methods.

**Video 17.** Exposure Therapy for Anxiety: Dr. Wright and Kate (10:00)

When you view the video, you will see that Dr. Wright asked Kate if she could forecast an exposure activity that would be "over the top" for her—an activity that would cause so much anxiety that a rating of 100 on the current hierarchy would be too low to capture the intensity of the

**Table 7–3.** Tips for developing hierarchies for graded exposure

1. **Be specific.** Help the patient write out clear, definitive descriptions of the stimuli for each step in the hierarchy. Examples of overgeneralized or ill-defined steps are "Learn to drive again"; "Stop being afraid of going to parties"; and "Feel comfortable in crowds." Examples of specific, well-delineated steps are "Drive two blocks to the corner store at least three times a week"; "Spend 20 minutes at the neighborhood party before leaving"; and "Go to the mall for 10 minutes on a Sunday morning when there are very few people there." Specific steps will help both you and the patient make good decisions about the plan for progressing through the hierarchy.
2. **Rate the steps for degree of difficulty or amount of expected anxiety.** Use a scale of 0–100, with 100 representing the greatest difficulty or anxiety. These ratings will be used to select the steps for exposure at each session and to measure progress. The usual effect of progressing through a hierarchy is to have significant reductions in the ratings for degree of difficulty or anxiety as each step is mastered.
3. **Develop a hierarchy that has multiple steps of varying degrees of difficulty.** Coach the patient on listing a number of different steps (typically 8–12) that range in degree of difficulty from very low (ratings of 5–20) to very high (ratings of 80–100). Try to list steps throughout the entire range of difficulty. If the patient lists only steps with high ratings or can think of no midrange steps, you will need to assist him in developing a more gradual and comprehensive list.
4. **Choose steps collaboratively.** As with any other cognitive-behavior therapy assignment, work together with the patient as a team to select the order of steps for graded exposure therapy.

experience. After thinking for a moment, Kate replied that driving across the big bridge in her sister's convertible would be rated 140 on the distress scale. The strategy of asking patients to generate ideas for activities that would justify over-the-top anxiety ratings can have several benefits: 1) ratings for other items on the hierarchy may be revised downward and thus appear to be more manageable; 2) spotting activities that cause extreme fear may stimulate the patient to think of other, less anxiety-provoking items for the hierarchy; and 3) the over-the-top items can eventually be added to the list of exposure activities and help the patient to fully confront the feared stimuli.

Did you spot any of Kate's safety behaviors in Video 17? One obvious safety behavior is keeping her eyes closed as a passenger when her husband is driving on the expressway. Although Dr. Wright did not specifically address safety behaviors in this brief video segment, he planned to look for these behaviors and incorporate them into the exposure plan as they worked together to reach her goals.

| Activity | Distress rating (0–100) |
|---|---|
| Drive around block in my neighborhood | 10 |
| Drive 3 miles to my current office | 20 |
| A short drive from office to pick up lunch for coworkers | 35 |
| Ride with husband on expressway (with my eyes closed) | 35 |
| Drive over a short bridge over a little creek | 40 |
| Ride with husband on expressway (with my eyes open) | 50 |
| Drive over small bridge close to my house | 60 |
| Drive on expressway by myself on Sunday morning (when there isn't much traffic) | 70 |
| Drive on expressway by myself at a busy time | 85 |
| Drive over the big bridge to my new office (when it is sunny) | 90 |
| Drive over the big bridge to my new office (when it is raining) | 100 |

**Figure 7–1.** Kate's exposure hierarchy.

The exposure therapy with Kate went smoothly. However, hierarchical exposure doesn't always progress so well. Troubleshooting Guide 4 may give you some ideas for overcoming barriers to success with exposure-based treatment.

## Imaginal Exposure

There are two types of exposure, *imaginal exposure* and *in vivo exposure*. When imagery is used for graded exposure, the therapist asks the patient to try to immerse himself in the scene and to imagine how he might react. The imaginal exposure is typically started in sessions and continued by the patient for homework. Cues are given to help the patient experience the anxiety-related stimuli as vividly as possible. The imaginal exposure technique was used to help Raul, a man who developed PTSD after a work accident.

## Troubleshooting Guide 4
### Challenges in Exposure Therapy

1. **Missed/avoided appointments.** Are the patient's anxiety and avoidance interfering with regular attendance at therapy sessions? This problem can be seen in persons with agoraphobia and difficulty traveling out of a restricted "safety zone." For a patient with this roadblock to therapy, a temporary work-around can be to perform the session by telephone, e-mail, or telemedicine. Of course, CBT methods should be used to help the patient work toward attending sessions in person. Otherwise, the alternative method of attending could become part of a continued pattern of avoidance. Another step to take is to reassess the therapeutic relationship and your preparation of the patient. Have you paid enough attention to forging a collaborative relationship? Have you fully explained the rationale for exposure therapy?

   Some other options to consider are as follows: 1) elicit and modify dysfunctional cognitions about exposure therapy (e.g., "It will be too much for me....I won't be able to stand the anxiety...It's no use, I'll never change"); 2) employ motivational interviewing to build up the patient's commitment to therapy; 3) temporarily use a safety behavior, such as a family member or friend transporting the patient to appointments.

2. **Repeated noncompletion of exposure-based homework assignments.** When patients don't follow through with their exposure work between sessions, a good question to ask yourself is "Have I been pitching the assignments at the best level for this patient?" Perhaps you have been moving too fast or pushing too hard. Or you have been moving too slowly. You might need to recalibrate the hierarchy. Identify smaller steps, or be more creative in designing steps that are meaningful and doable.

   If patients aren't completing their assignments, discuss the issue with them. Ask about obstacles to participation in exposure. Then help them generate ideas for overcoming these obstacles. For example, a patient might report, "I'm too busy with work. And when I get home, I need to spend time with my family." A solution might be for the patient to develop a schedule with her partner's support for 20-minute blocks of time to do exposure activities between sessions.

## Troubleshooting Guide 4 *(continued)*
### Challenges in Exposure Therapy

The strategies outlined for missed or avoided appointments also can be applied to noncompletion of homework. To illustrate, a patient who has difficulty performing exposure activities at home might schedule a brief phone appointment with the therapist to promote participation in the assignment.

3. **Difficulty generating hierarchies.** If the patient can't detail a full series of steps for exposure therapy, there are several strategies you might try.

   You could suggest brainstorming, in which you free up the patient's imagination to write down any idea, even if it seems peripheral, undoable, or too easy. Sometimes such ideas can be springboards for productive entries in a hierarchy.

   Another strategy is for you to take the lead in making creative suggestions. When you make suggestions, try to phrase them as questions to stir the patient's interest and involvement in the process.

   A third tack is to use items the patient has already identified as a starting place for finding related activities for the hierarchy. For example, consider a man with agoraphobia who has identified shopping at a grocery store as an item for his hierarchy. The therapist might ask what the rating would be if the shopping was done at 7 A.M. on a Sunday morning when there are few other people in the store compared to a Saturday afternoon at 1 P.M. when crowds could be expected. Other layers for the hierarchy could be found by detailing conditions such as having a family member or friend along versus going alone, or shopping briefly for a small number of items versus spending 30 minutes or more to fill the shopping cart.

## Troubleshooting Guide 4 *(continued)*
**Challenges in Exposure Therapy**

4. **Difficulty arranging exposure experiences.** If patients have been struggling with common experiences in everyday life, such as crowded places, social occasions, or driving, exposure experiences can usually be arranged without great difficulty. When the trigger for anxiety is less common or more challenging to weave into a systematic hierarchy, therapists can turn to videos and computer tools to produce some of the stimuli. A person with a blood phobia could view videos on the Internet of increasingly vivid scenes depicting blood (e.g., blood cells under a microscope, a drop of blood from a minor cut, bleeding from a deeper cut, open heart surgery) as a preparation for in vivo exposure (explained and illustrated later in this chapter). A patient with fear of flying could watch videos with varying degrees of realism of the flying experience to ready him for taking actual flights.

   Virtual reality (VR)–facilitated exposure therapy can be an excellent way to provide engaging exposure experiences in therapist's offices or in the home setting. VR programs have been developed for fear of flying, height phobia, fear of public speaking, war-related PTSD, and other problems with anxiety-driven avoidance. Programs for VR are described in Chapter 4, "Structuring and Educating," and sources for computer tools for CBT are listed in Appendix 2.

5. **Skill deficits of patients.** Because of long-standing avoidance patterns, many patients may not have fully developed the skills they need to perform in feared situations. A person with public speaking anxiety probably has not had adequate learning experiences in how to deliver an effective presentation. A patient with social phobia likely has not mastered the skill of making small talk at parties or other social occasions. A person with height phobia may not know much about how to use ladders safely or how to hike on precipitous trails. When your patient has skill deficits, you can suggest readings (e.g., books on how to make small talk), classes (e.g. Toastmasters training or public speaking courses), or online resources (e.g., videos on how to start and carry out effective conversations with unfamiliar people, videos on ladder safety). You also can do role-playing in treatment sessions to build skills (e.g., participating in a job interview, speaking up at a work meeting, inviting someone to a social occasion).

**Troubleshooting Guide 4 *(continued)***
**Challenges in Exposure Therapy**

6. **Stalled progress.** When progress is slowed greatly or comes to a standstill, many of the methods detailed above may assist you and the patient with getting back on track. Two additional strategies could help you move beyond plateaus encountered in exposure therapy.

   First, we recommend you look more deeply for safety behaviors. Has the patient been employing safety behaviors that have reduced distress enough that motivation has ebbed? Have you failed to spot safety behaviors that need to be addressed in the exposure protocol? You can ask patients to demonstrate avoidance behaviors in session so you can see exactly how they manage feared situations. Perhaps you have missed important safety behaviors that could provide a key to future progress. You also could ask the patient to write out an imagined exposure activity in detail (as discussed in the next section, "Imaginal Exposure") to provide you with a more comprehensive and nuanced understanding of his behavior.

   Second, we suggest you evaluate the amount of pressure you are placing on the patient to complete the exposure assignments. If you expect too little and fall into an overly supportive style (e.g., commiserating excessively on the difficulties of doing assignments, having little optimism or energy for reviewing assignments and finding solutions to problems, habitually allowing sessions to drift away from the exposure work so the patient can ventilate about current stresses), you may be unwittingly contributing to the stalled progress. Patients with long-standing avoidance typically need solid doses of encouragement and a bit of a push from their therapists to make headway with exposure protocols. Otherwise, they may continue their avoidance patterns indefinitely.

   In Video 17, you saw Dr. Wright ask Kate to take on more of a challenge than she initially planned. Because they had a good therapeutic relationship and he leavened the intervention with kindness and humor, she readily accepted the suggestion. Pitching the expectations for exposure therapy at the most effective level is one of the core skills therapists need to learn in doing CBT for anxiety and OCD. Artful pitching of exposure therapy activities is demonstrated further in Videos 18 and 19, featured elements of the next part of this chapter.

## Case Example

Raul had fallen about 15 feet off a piece of equipment he was repairing when a coworker turned it on by mistake. Although his fractured ribs and leg had healed, he was unable to return to work because of fear of the work environment, flashbacks, and nightmares. He was promised a different job that did not involve any climbing or hazardous repair work. However, the idea of entering the workplace triggered severe anxiety.

Raul's therapist helped him develop a hierarchy for gradual exposure to the work situation. They began with imaginal exposure. Then with the assistance of Raul's supervisor, they organized an in vivo exposure plan in which he took a stepwise approach to getting back to work. A portion of the imaginal exposure component of treatment is illustrated below with dialogue from one of their sessions.

*Therapist:* Which of the early steps would you like to walk through here in the treatment session?

*Raul:* Let's try going through the door to the factory and signing in for work.

*Therapist:* OK. Try to picture yourself after you park your car. You're sitting in the parking lot. What do you see, how are you feeling, what are you thinking?

*Raul:* I'm gripping the wheel, hanging my head down, not looking at the factory. I'm thinking, I can't handle this.... Something else bad will happen.... I'll shake so hard, I'll look like a fool....

*Therapist:* What are you thinking of doing as you sit there in the car?

*Raul:* Turning around and going back home.

*Therapist:* What can you do to calm yourself and continue on your way into the factory?

*Raul:* Breathe easy, tell myself to stop the scary thoughts, remind myself that I only ever had one accident after working there for 15 years. The accident happened because I didn't use a safety harness and some guy didn't know I was working on the equipment. My new job is in quality control. I just need to sit in a lab and run tests. The chances of getting hurt there are very low.

*Therapist:* Now can you imagine yourself getting out of your car, going through the door, and signing in for work?

*Raul:* Yes, I want to do it.

The therapist went on to help Raul use imagery to walk around the factory to view and absorb the scenes he feared, to allow himself to experience them for longer periods of time, and to place himself in his new work environment—the quality control lab. Eventually Raul was able to use in vivo exposure to complete his recovery from PTSD triggered by his work accident.

Imaginal exposure can be particularly helpful in the treatment of PTSD, in which thoughts of the trauma and associated triggers are avoided and thereby retain their anxiety-provoking value. Imagery also can be beneficial in exposure therapy for OCD. Obsessional thoughts can be evoked in session and then quieted using cognitive methods, such as examining the evidence, and/or behavioral methods, such as relaxation or distraction. Exposure and response prevention protocols for compulsions can be worked through first with imagery to help the patient gain skills and confidence in being able to stop these behaviors.

Video 18 shows powerful methods of imaginal exposure for OCD. Dr. Elizabeth Hembree, an expert in treatment of OCD, is working with Mia, a woman with contamination fears and avoidance of objects she believes will make her ill. Video 18 opens with a review of Mia's homework. She has listened to a recording of an imaginal exposure from a previous session and has done some in vivo exercises, such as touching doorknobs without washing. For this session, Mia has prepared a script of an imaginal exposure to a dog leash, an object that she considers severely contaminated with dog hair, saliva, and feces.

Note how the imaginal exposure evokes very strong emotions and physiological responses. After Mia goes through the intense experience of living out the script in imagination, Dr. Hembree repeats the content. Then Mia immerses herself in the images once again. They repeat the procedure multiple times, with the goals of habituation to the stimuli and prevention of her usual avoidance behaviors, such as wearing gloves or washing her hands.

**Video 18.** Imaginal Exposure for OCD: Dr. Hembree and Mia (9:39)

For many patients with OCD, prolonged exposure, either in imagination or in vivo, may be required to change entrenched avoidance or compulsive behaviors. Psychologists or other nonphysician therapists may use sessions longer than 50 minutes to provide effective exposure therapy. However, psychiatrists rarely extend sessions to 90 minutes or longer. The psychiatrists who are authors of this book (J.H.W. and M.E.T.) often blend briefer exposure sessions with pharmacotherapy for OCD (see our book *High-Yield Cognitive-Behavior Therapy for Brief Sessions: An Illustrated Guide* [Wright et al. 2010] for details on using sessions of less than the traditional "50-minute hour"). In some cases, we have observed good results with shorter sessions of 20–25 minutes in persons who follow through with homework. But we also are prepared to schedule longer appointments or refer to other therapists if needed.

Because exposure therapy may be most effective if the patient can confront feared stimuli in real-life situations, it is advisable to engage the patient in subsequent in vivo exposure whenever possible. The case illustration of treating Raul's anxiety involved use of imagery as a method of preparing him for exposure to his real-life work setting. Other examples of using imagery to help patients make the transition to in vivo exposure include treatment of fear of flying (e.g., conducting imagery exercises in the office, followed by taking actual plane trips) and agoraphobia (e.g., practicing steps for going to a mall with imagery and then implementing the hierarchy in vivo).

## In Vivo Exposure

In vivo exposure involves direct confrontation with the stimulus that arouses fear in the patient. Depending on the resources of your clinical environment, it may be possible to conduct in vivo exposure during therapy sessions. Fear of heights, elevators, and some social situations can be re-created, and the therapist can accompany the patient as she engages in the exposure experiences. As demonstrated in the treatment of Mia, OCD with contamination fears is an important indication for in vivo exposure during treatment sessions. There are advantages and disadvantages to the therapist being present during in vivo exposure. The positive features of this approach include the opportunity for the therapist to 1) model effective anxiety management techniques, 2) encourage patients to confront their fears, 3) provide timely psychoeducation, 4) modify catastrophic cognitions, and 5) give constructive feedback. However, accompaniment by the therapist can make a threatening situation seem safer, just as having a friend or family member along can reduce levels of anxiety. Therefore, caution should be exercised so that the therapist's actions do not facilitate the pattern of avoidance. To complete the exposure process, more work will usually need to be done outside of sessions when the patient is unaccompanied.

Video 19 shows Dr. Hembree helping Mia perform in vivo exposure. This dramatic video demonstrates how therapists can prod patients to participate in exposure activities that they would ordinarily avoid, while retaining a solid and productive therapeutic relationship. Listen for Dr. Hembree's sincere words of encouragement such as "Wow, you're brave. Good for you!" Also, watch for Dr. Hembree's effective modeling of exposure to the "contaminated" dog leash when she shows Mia how to get "full body contact." Therapists who do in vivo exposure therapy need to be or become comfortable themselves with touching objects that are avoided by their patients.

▶ **Video 19.** In Vivo Exposure Therapy for OCD: Dr. Hembree and Mia (8:37)

After in vivo exposure in a therapy session, the patient should continue the exposure as homework assignments. Dr. Hembree asked Mia to spend an hour every day touching the dog leash, tying it around her waist, and using it to "contaminate" other things around her house. When you use homework for ongoing in vivo exposure, you should debrief the patient at the next session. Ask her to compare her predictions to the actual outcome. If the situation was less threatening and was handled better than anticipated, ask what she thinks this means for future efforts at coping with her anxiety. If the patient found that the situation was more difficult than anticipated or that she handled it more poorly than planned, make the next step easier to accomplish or review the methods used to control fear. If there were difficulties in applying coping strategies, practice them in session. If unanticipated obstacles made the situation more complex, try to help the patient find a way to surmount these problems.

## Response Prevention

*Response prevention* is a general term for methods used to help patients stop behaviors that are perpetuating their disorder. In CBT for anxiety disorders, PTSD, and OCD, exposure and response prevention are typically used together. For example, Mia repeatedly touched "contaminated" objects without washing her hands. Response prevention is an essential part of CBT for OCD rituals such as counting or engaging in repetitive behaviors (e.g., turning a light switch on and off 16 times before leaving a room, showering for 20 minutes in a ritual-bound order). Patients are encouraged to develop plans for gradual reduction in their rituals in which they will experience some anxiety for not completing their full rituals. Response prevention interventions in the treatment of OCD can be as simple as leaving the room where a compulsive ritual takes place (e.g., walking away from the sink after washing the hands once) or agreeing to participate in an alternative behavior. For checking behaviors around the house, the person can agree to leave his home after the first round of checks and not return home for a specified period despite feeling the urge to do so. Response prevention methods usually work best if they are determined collaboratively, instead of being a prescription from the therapist. The patient and therapist decide together on specific goals for response prevention, and then the patient logs his efforts to follow the plan.

## Rewards

Positive reinforcement may increase the odds that the rewarded behavior will occur again. Thus, in constructing exposure protocols, it may be helpful to consider the role of positive reinforcement in encouraging adaptive behaviors such as approaching feared situations. Family members and friends can praise the patient and provide rewards or incentives for accomplishing exposure goals. For example, they might go out to dinner with the patient to celebrate achieving an important milestone in the exposure process. Patients can also reward themselves for their accomplishments in combating fears. Rewards can be anything patients find pleasant or positive. The size of the reward should match the perceived size of the accomplishment. Smaller rewards such as food (e.g., eating a favorite ice cream) might be used for taking beginning or intermediate steps to face fears. Larger rewards (e.g., buying something special, taking a trip) could be planned for overcoming bigger hurdles.

**Learning Exercise 7–3.** Exposure Therapy

1. Ask a colleague to role-play a patient with an anxiety disorder, and/or do this exercise yourself for an object or situation that triggers your own anxiety.

2. Using the tips in Table 7–3, write out a hierarchy for exposure to a specific feared situation.

3. Identify at least eight separate steps, ranging from low to high degrees of difficulty.

4. Choose a beginning target for exposure therapy.

5. Use imaginal exposure to help prepare for in vivo exposure.

6. Try to spot potential problems in carrying out the plans for exposure, and coach the person (or yourself) in methods of overcoming these difficulties.

7. Keep practicing exposure therapy methods until you master this key behavioral technique.

## Summary

Cognitive-behavioral methods for anxiety disorders, PTSD, and OCD are based on the concept that persons with these conditions develop unrealistic fears of objects or situations, respond to feared stimuli with excessive anxiety or physiological activation, and then avoid triggering stimuli to escape from the unpleasant emotional reaction. Each time patients avoid an anxiety-provoking situation, they collect further evidence that they can't cope or manage. But if the pattern of avoidance can be interrupted, they can learn that the situation can be tolerated or mastered.

The behavioral interventions described in this chapter are directed primarily at stopping avoidance. Patients are taught how to reduce emotional arousal, how to moderate dysfunctional cognitions that amplify anxiety, and how to systematically expose themselves to feared situations.

A four-step process is used as a general template for behavioral interventions for anxiety disorders and related conditions: 1) assessment of symptoms, triggers for anxiety, and coping methods; 2) identification and prioritization of targets for therapy; 3) coaching in basic skills for managing anxiety; and 4) exposure to stressful stimuli until the fear response is significantly reduced or eliminated. These methods are first practiced in therapy sessions and then are applied in homework assignments to extend treatment gains into the patient's daily life.

## References

Abramowitz JS, Whiteside S, Kalsy SA, Tolin DF: Thought control strategies in obsessive-compulsive disorder: a replication and extension. Behav Res Ther 41(5):529–540, 2003 12711262

Beck AT, Epstein N, Brown G, Steer RA: An inventory for measuring clinical anxiety: psychometric properties. J Consult Clin Psychol 56(6):893–897, 1988 3204199

Clark DA, Beck AT: Cognitive Therapy of Anxiety Disorders: Science and Practice. New York, Guilford, 2010

Goodman WK, Price LH, Rasmussen SA, et al: The Yale-Brown Obsessive Compulsive Scale, I: development, use, and reliability. Arch Gen Psychiatry 46(11):1006–1011, 1989 2684084

Kim S, Wollburg E, Roth WT: Opposing breathing therapies for panic disorder: a randomized controlled trial of lowering vs raising end-tidal P(CO2). J Clin Psychiatry 73(7):931–939, 2012 22901344

Meuret AE, Wilhelm FH, Ritz T, Roth WT: Feedback of end-tidal pCO2 as a therapeutic approach for panic disorders. J Psychiatr Res 42(7):560–568, 2008 17681544

Meuret AE, Rosenfield D, Seidel A, et al: Respiratory and cognitive mediators of treatment change in panic disorder: evidence for intervention specificity. J Cons Clin Psychol 78(5):691–704, 2010 20873904

Meyer TJ, Miller ML, Metzger RL, Borkovec TD: Development and validation of the Penn State Worry Questionnaire. Behav Res Ther 28(6):487–495, 1990 2076086

Purdon C: Empirical investigations of thought suppression in OCD. J Behav Ther Exp Psychiatry 35(2):121–136, 2004 15210374

Rassin E, Diepstraten P: How to suppress obsessive thoughts. Behav Res Ther 41(1):97–103, 2003 12488122

Spitzer RL, Kroenke K, Williams JB, Löwe B: A brief measure for assessing generalized anxiety disorder: the GAD-7. Arch Intern Med 166(10):1092–1097, 2006 16717171

Tolin DF, Abramowitz JS, Przeworski A, Foa EB: Thought suppression in obsessive-compulsive disorder. Behav Res Ther 40(11):1255–1274, 2002 12384322

Wright JH, Sudak D, Turkington D, Thase ME: High-Yield Cognitive-Behavior Therapy for Brief Sessions: An Illustrated Guide. Arlington, VA, American Psychiatric Publishing, 2010

# Modifying Schemas 8

When you help people change schemas, you will be working at the bedrock of their self-concept and way of living in the world. Schemas are the core beliefs that contain fundamental rules for information processing. They provide templates for 1) screening and filtering information from the environment, 2) making decisions, and 3) driving characteristic patterns of behavior. The development of schemas is shaped by interactions with parents, teachers, peers, and other significant people in the person's life, in addition to life events, traumas, successes, and other formative influences. Genetics also plays a role in the production of schemas, by contributing to temperament, intellect, special skills or lack of skills (e.g., athletic prowess, body shape, attractiveness, musical talent, problem-solving ability), and biological vulnerability to both mental and physical illnesses.

There are several reasons why it is important to understand your patient's underlying schemas. First, a basic theory of cognitive-behavior therapy (CBT)—the stress-diathesis hypothesis—specifies that maladaptive core beliefs, which may lie under the surface and have relatively few

---

Items mentioned in this chapter that are available in Appendix 1, "Worksheets and Checklists," are also available as a free download in larger format on the American Psychiatric Association Publishing Web site: https://www.appi.org/wright.

negative effects during periods of normality, can be primed by stressful events to become potent controllers of thinking and behavior during illness episodes (Clark et al. 1999). Thus, efforts to revise dysfunctional schemas may have positive benefits in two principal domains: 1) relief of current symptoms and 2) improved resistance to stressors in the future. CBT has been shown to have strong effects in reducing the risk for relapse (Evans et al. 1992; Jarrett et al. 2001). Although the exact mechanisms for this feature of CBT are not known, it is presumed that schema modification may be involved.

Another reason for focusing treatment interventions on core beliefs is that patients typically have a mix of different types of schemas. Even patients with the most severe symptoms or profound despair have adaptive schemas that can help them cope. Although maladaptive schemas may seem to be in full charge during an illness episode, efforts to uncover and strengthen positively oriented beliefs can be quite productive. Therefore, it is important to explore and burnish the adaptive parts of patients' basic cognitive structures.

The cognitive-behavioral theory of personality, as articulated by Beck and Freeman (1990), specifies that self-concept, character types, and habitual behavioral patterns can be best understood by examining core beliefs. For example, a person with obsessive-compulsive personality traits might have deeply held schemas such as "I must be in control" and "If you want something done right, do it yourself." It is likely that this person would have a behavioral repertoire (e.g., rigidity, tendency to be controlling toward others, difficulty delegating authority) consistent with these beliefs. A person who has a cluster of dependency-related schemas (e.g., "I need others to survive"; "I'm weak....I can't make it on my own") might cling to others and lack assertiveness in interpersonal relationships. In contrast, a more adaptive group of schemas—such as "I can figure things out"; "I can handle stress"; and "I like challenges"—would be associated with effective behaviors for problem solving.

CBT for depression and anxiety is typically geared toward symptom relief instead of personality change. Nevertheless, an analysis of the core beliefs and compensatory behavioral strategies that contribute to the patient's personality makeup can help you build an in-depth formulation and help you design treatment interventions that take full account of the patient's vulnerabilities and strengths. In addition, some patients with depression and anxiety may have treatment goals that include elements of personal growth. They may want to become more flexible, break patterns of excessive dependency, or overcome long-standing problems with self-esteem. In such cases, the treatment process can be enriched by articulating and revising schemas that may block the way to achieving these goals.

**Table 8–1.** Methods for identifying schemas

| |
|---|
| Using various questioning techniques |
| Performing psychoeducation |
| Spotting patterns of automatic thoughts |
| Conducting a life history review |
| Using schema inventories |
| Keeping a personal schema list |

In Chapter 10, "Treating Chronic, Severe, or Complex Disorders," we briefly outline some recommended modifications of CBT for treatment of personality disturbances. If you are interested in learning more about CBT for personality disorders, we recommend the excellent books by Beck et al. (2014) and Young et al. (2003). Schema-focused CBT methods also are described in a self-help format in *Reinventing Your Life* (Young and Klosko 1994). Our primary emphasis here is on helping you learn how to identify schemas in patients with depression and anxiety and how to use CBT to modify these core beliefs (Table 8–1).

## Identifying Schemas

### Using Questioning Techniques

Guided discovery, imagery, role-play, and other questioning techniques used for automatic thoughts also are used to uncover schemas. However, it may be more challenging to implement successful questioning strategies when working on the schema level of cognitive processing. Because schemas may not be readily apparent to the patient or may not be revealed by standard questioning, a hypothesis should be developed about what core beliefs might be present. Then the therapist can frame questions that point in the direction of the presumed schemas. This type of guided discovery is shown in Video 20.

We will rejoin Dr. Sudak's therapy with Brian (shown earlier in Chapter 5, "Working With Automatic Thoughts") for an example of formulation-driven questioning. In this session, Brian reports an unsettling event at work. Renee, a coworker, stops by his desk to ask him if he would like to have lunch with her. Instead of greeting this invitation with pleasure, he is reminded of his "ex" and has the automatic thought "I just can't do it." Using a series of Socratic questions, Dr. Sudak helps Brian understand that his early experiences with a father who was usually "gone like the wind," in addition to a traumatic breakup with his girlfriend who cheated on him, led him to conclude that "people can't be counted upon." His current behavioral pattern in relationships is consistent with this belief. He builds walls around him like he is in "Fort Knox." As you will see in later videos of Brian's therapy in this chapter, finding the core belief "people can't be counted upon" opened possibilities for fundamental changes in his schemas about others and his ability to build meaningful relationships. As you watch the video, note how Dr. Sudak's formulation (see Chapter 3, "Assessment and Formulation") guides them to a damaging core belief.

▶ **Video 20.** Uncovering a Maladaptive Schema: Dr. Sudak and Brian (12:22)

Mood shifts can be good clues that a consequential schema is at work. These sudden displays of intense feelings can serve as excellent entry points for a series of questions directed at uncovering a core belief. In Video 20, you saw some intense displays of depressed mood that led to empathic and productive questioning from Dr. Sudak. Dialogue from the treatment of Allison, a young woman who was hospitalized because of a severe eating disorder, provides another example of leveraging mood shifts to uncover maladaptive schemas.

*Therapist:* How are you adjusting to being in the hospital?

*Allison:* Everybody has been nice. I like most of the nurses. (*Appears calm and mildly happy.*) But I can't stand it when they bring out the dinner cart. Why do they have all of that food? (*Mood becomes much more anxious.*)

*Therapist:* I noticed that you got pretty nervous when you talked about the food cart. What upsets you about the way they serve meals here?

*Allison:* Everybody eats so much food, and the server just piles it on. I can't stop myself if I get in that food line.

*Therapist:* Can you imagine yourself lined up to get served at the food cart? Try to picture yourself standing in line. What thoughts are going through your mind?

*Allison:* I'll eat everything on the cart; I'll totally lose control.

*Therapist:* How much control do you think you have over your behavior?

*Allison:* I have no control.

Another useful CBT method for uncovering schemas, the *downward arrow technique,* involves a series of questions that reveal increasingly deeper levels of thinking. The first questions are typically directed at automatic thoughts. However, the therapist infers that an underlying schema is present and constructs a chain of linked questions that build on a supposition (to be tested and modified later) that the patient's cognitions are providing an accurate representation of her true self. Most of the questions follow this general format: "If this thought that you have about yourself is true, what does it mean about you?"

Because the downward arrow technique requires the patient to assume (for the purposes of the intervention) that negative or hurtful cognitions are actually true, this method should not be attempted before a good therapeutic relationship has been established and there have been previous therapy successes in modifying maladaptive cognitions. The patient should be fully aware that the purpose of the questioning is to bring out core beliefs that will probably need to be changed, and that the therapist is not trying to convince her of the validity of troubling schemas. A kind and empathic tone of questioning, and sometimes a light touch of hyperbole or judicious humor, can help make the downward arrow technique work to best effect.

### Case Example

Maria is a 45-year-old woman who recently discovered her husband was having an affair. She had experienced two short-lived depressions earlier in her life after losses (breakup with a boyfriend before marriage, being fired from a job). This time, the depression was worse, and it showed no signs of subsiding. Although she did not have suicidal thoughts, her Patient Health Questionnaire–9 (PHQ-9) score was 20 (severe depression). Her self-esteem had been rocked by the infidelity and her husband's subsequent filing for divorce.

Maria's therapist had noticed patterns of recurrent automatic thoughts that she thought were linked to underlying schemas about acceptance and lovability and decided to use the downward arrow technique to draw these out. Employing a highly collaborative questioning style, she helped Maria find a core belief that had been activated by the relationship fracture. Several of the key questions and Maria's responses are diagrammed in Figure 8–1.

It may take a fair amount of practice before you become proficient at using the downward arrow technique. Building your knowledge of commonly held schemas can help you formulate directions for questioning. Gaining experience in knowing when to exert pressure to go further and when to back off will help you to be more effective in using inference chaining methods. It is important to keep the emotional tone at a plane that is conducive to learning and that is experienced as helpful by the patient. Yet the process of uncovering maladaptive schemas often generates painful affects.

Experienced cognitive-behavior therapists who use the downward arrow technique try to pitch the questions at just the right level to assist

*Maria:* The only two men I ever loved left me...broke my heart. There must be something wrong with me.

*Therapist:* When you say there's something wrong with you, I wonder if you have a basic belief about yourself that's making it hard to pull out of depression. If we could find the core belief, we would know what we need to change. So let's assume that your automatic thought is true. What could be wrong about you?

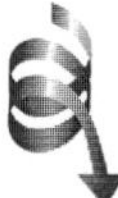

*Maria:* I'm no good at relationships.

*Therapist:* And what if that were true?

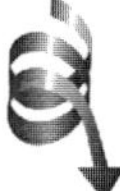

*Maria:* I'm bound to be unhappy. I'll never find a man who will stay with me.

*Therapist:* And what if that were true?

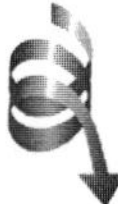

*Maria:* I'm unlovable.

**Figure 8–1.** The downward arrow technique.

the patient in revealing an important core belief—and to make the questioning process a highly therapeutic experience. We recommend that you practice the learning exercises for uncovering schemas and that you review the list of tips for using the downward arrow technique that are presented in Table 8–2.

**Learning Exercise 8–1.** Questioning Methods for Core Beliefs

1. Practice guided discovery for uncovering schemas by asking yourself a series of questions that start with one of your own situation-specific automatic thoughts and then reveal deeper levels of cognition. Try out the downward arrow technique on yourself. Use this method to get in touch with one or more of your personal schemas. If

**Table 8–2.** How to use the downward arrow technique

1. Start the questioning by targeting an automatic thought or a stream of cognitions that is causing distress. Choose an automatic thought that is likely to be driven by a significant underlying schema.
2. Generate a hypothesis about a possible schema or set of schemas that may underlie this automatic thought.
3. Explain the downward arrow technique so that the patient understands your intent in asking these difficult questions.
4. Be sure that you and the patient are fully collaborating in using this technique. Emphasize the collaborative empirical nature of cognitive-behavior therapy (CBT).
5. Anticipate timing and pacing concerns in advance. Ask yourself questions such as "Is this a good time to attempt to uncover this schema?" "Is the patient ready to come to grips with this core belief?" "How fast and how intensively should I ask questions that will lead the patient's thinking to this schema?" and "What signs would tell me to go slower or to end this line of questioning?"
6. Think ahead to what you will do after the schema is identified. What positive benefits will there be to revealing this schema? What will be the next steps after the core belief comes out? How will you help the patient make good use of knowing about this schema?
7. Use if-then questions that progressively reveal deeper levels of cognitive processing. For example, "I've heard you mention several times that you have trouble making friends. If it's true that you have trouble making friends, what does this tell us about the way that others may see you? How about the way you view yourself?"
8. Be supportive and empathic as core beliefs are uncovered. Convey an attitude that knowing about schemas will help the patient build self-esteem and learn to better cope with problems. Even if a negatively toned core belief is partially accurate, CBT can be directed at acquiring skills for tempering the maladaptive schema and its behavioral consequences.

possible, try to uncover a schema that has some maladaptive effects, in addition to a schema that is largely positive or adaptive. Write down the questions and your answers in your notebook.

2. Next, enlist a classmate or helper to role-play guided discovery and the downward arrow technique for identifying core beliefs, or practice these methods with patients you have in treatment.

3. Make a list of the strengths and weaknesses that you have in asking questions to uncover core beliefs. What are you doing well? What do you need to practice more

intensively? Are you able to develop an accurate formulation in a timely manner? Can you phrase questions in a way that instills hope while still getting to painful and troubling core beliefs? Are you paying enough attention to recognizing adaptive schemas? Identify any problems you are having in implementing questioning strategies for schemas, and discuss possible solutions with classmates, colleagues, or supervisors.

## Educating Patients About Schemas

Psychoeducation about schemas is typically implemented concurrently with the questioning methods described above in "Using Questioning Techniques." In addition to brief explanations in therapy sessions, we often recommend readings or other educational experiences to help patients learn about and identify their schemas. *Mind Over Mood* (Greenberger and Padesky 2015) contains exercises directed at teaching patients how to recognize their assumptions and core beliefs. *Breaking Free From Depression: Pathways to Wellness* (Wright and McCray 2011) includes examples of both adaptive and maladaptive schemas; such examples can help patients recognize their own basic rules of information processing.

The computer program *Good Days Ahead* (Wright et al. 2016) has a number of interactive scenarios designed to promote the discovery and modification of schemas. Computer-assisted CBT can be especially helpful in teaching patients about core beliefs because it uses stimulating multimedia learning experiences that can point the way to cognitions that may not be apparent on the surface. Also, computer-assisted CBT employs learning enhancement techniques that promote rehearsal and recall.

## Spotting Patterns of Automatic Thoughts

If recurrent themes can be recognized in automatic thoughts, this often indicates that a core belief is behind these clusters of more superficial, situation-specific cognitions. There are several good methods for finding schemas in patterns of automatic thoughts.

1. **Recognize a theme during a therapy session.** When using guided discovery or other questioning methods, listen for themes that play over and over. Exploring such themes can frequently lead to key schemas.

For example, this pattern of automatic thoughts—"Jim doesn't respect me....My children never listen to me....It doesn't matter what I do at work, they'll always treat me like I hardly exist"—might be stimulated by core beliefs such as "I'm a nothing" or "I don't deserve respect."

2. **Review thought records in a therapy session.** Thought records can be treasure troves for material that will help you find schemas. Compare several thought records that have been completed on different days to see if there are any recurrent patterns of automatic thoughts. Ask the patient to see if she can recognize consistent themes. Then use guided discovery or the downward arrow technique to uncover related core beliefs.
3. **Assign review of thought records for a homework assignment.** After examining a thought record in a treatment session and explaining the process of spotting schemas, ask the patient to look over additional thought records between sessions and to record any core beliefs that she can recognize. Such homework assignments can have many benefits, including a) identification of schemas that might not be apparent during a therapy session, b) increased awareness of the powerful effects of core beliefs, and c) acquisition of self-help skills for uncovering schemas.
4. **Review a written list (or a computer-generated inventory) of automatic thoughts.** If the patient has completed an automatic thoughts questionnaire or has recorded a comprehensive list of her common automatic thoughts, it may be useful to check over this inventory to see if any clusters of thoughts may be linked to core beliefs. Consider using this alternative procedure if you are having trouble identifying schemas through guided discovery and other questioning methods. Viewing a large number of automatic thoughts may help you and the patient spot beliefs that otherwise would have gone unrecognized.

We present a learning exercise here that you can use to practice finding underlying schemas in patterns of automatic thoughts. You also can use this exercise to help your patients gain skills in recognizing their core beliefs.

**Learning Exercise 8–2.** Finding Schemas in Patterns of Automatic Thoughts

Instructions: Match one number to each of the letters in the exercise.

| Automatic Thoughts | Maladaptive Schemas |
|---|---|
| 1. "Abby [daughter] will have a wreck if she doesn't watch out.... She has no idea how quickly she could get into trouble.... I wish she never had to learn to drive." | ____ A. I'm a loser. |
| 2. "I messed up again.... This job is too much for me.... I can't fool them any longer." | ____ B. I need to be perfect to be accepted. |
| 3. "Don't talk with me about trying to meet somebody.... It wouldn't work out.... I'm better off being alone." | ____ C. I must be on guard all the time or something terrible will happen. |
| 4. "I can't make mistakes on the test.... It will be worth it to study all weekend.... Jim will be proud of me." | ____ D. I will always be rejected. Without a man, I'm nothing. |

*Answers:* A: 2; B: 4; C: 1; D: 3.

## Conducting a Life History Review

Because schemas are shaped by life experiences, one valuable method of uncovering these basic rules is to ask the patient to go back in time to remember formative influences that may have promoted the development of either maladaptive or adaptive beliefs. This type of retrospective review can be accomplished through guided discovery, role-play, and homework assignments. As with other methods of identifying schemas, an in-depth formulation can help point you in directions that will yield results. Instead of doing a global review of developmental history, try to focus on interpersonal relationships, events, or circumstances that have previously been shown to be hot topics. For example, if your patient has already told you that he never felt comfortable around his peers and shied away from social experiences, you might focus your inquiries on especially memorable social interchanges from childhood or adolescence. Your goal with this line of questioning would be to elicit schemas about personal competence and acceptance by others.

Traumatic events, troubled relationships, or perceived physical or personality defects can be obvious targets for historical reviews of schema formation. However, it is important not to forget positive influences that may have promoted the development of adaptive beliefs. The following types of questions can be used to assist patients in getting in touch with life experiences that have played a role in schema development.

1. **Ask about influential people:** "Which people have made the biggest difference in your life?" "What have you learned from them about yourself?" "How have teachers, coaches, friends, classmates, or spiritual leaders influenced the way you think?" "How about people who have given you trouble or have put you down?" "How about people who have boosted your confidence or given you encouragement?"
2. **Ask about core beliefs that may have been shaped by these experiences:** "What negative messages did you get about yourself from all of the arguments with your family?" "How did your parents' divorce affect your self-esteem?" "What affirmative beliefs came out of your successes in school?" "What did you learn about yourself by going through the divorce and getting away from the abusive relationship?"
3. **Ask about interests, jobs, spiritual practices, sports, and other activities that are important to the patient:** "In what way have your interests and abilities in music changed how you see yourself?" "What core beliefs do you have about your work skills?" "How has your view of yourself been influenced by your spiritual beliefs?" "How about involvement in artistic pursuits, travel, or hobbies—could these activities have affected your self-concept?"
4. **Ask about cultural and social influences:** "What impact has your cultural background had on the way you see the world?" "How has growing up as a minority affected your self-concept?" "What beliefs might have been influenced by living in a small town your entire life and being so close to family and friends?"
5. **Ask about education, readings, and self-study:** "How did your time in school influence your basic beliefs?" "Which books have you read that you think might have changed the way you think about yourself?" "What ideas did you develop from reading that book?" "Can you remember any other learning opportunities that have made a difference in your attitudes about life?"
6. **Ask about the possibility of transforming experiences:** "Have you had any life-shaping experiences that you haven't told me about?" "Could there have been an event that opened your eyes to a whole new way of seeing the world?" "What attitudes or beliefs came out of that experience?"

## Using Schema Inventories

Inventories of commonly held core beliefs are another useful technique for helping patients identify their schemas. These instruments include the Dysfunctional Attitude Scale (Beck et al. 1991), a lengthy questionnaire primarily used in research; and another highly detailed scale, the Young Schema Questionnaire (Young and Brown 2001; Young et al. 2003). A briefer inventory of schemas was developed for the computer program *Good Days Ahead* (Wright et al. 2016). We provide this schema checklist in Learning Exercise 8–3 and in Appendix 1, "Worksheets and Checklists," so that you will have this tool available for clinical practice.

Schema inventories can be useful when patients are having difficulty recognizing their core beliefs. Seeing a variety of possible schemas can stimulate their thinking and can help them recognize beliefs that may be causing trouble or could be reinforced to build self-esteem. Taking a schema inventory is especially useful in generating a list of adaptive beliefs. In supervising trainees, we often find that insufficient attention is paid to identifying positive rules of thinking. Administering a schema inventory guarantees that you will spend some time scanning the patient's belief system for points of strength and for opportunities for growth.

Even when patients seem to readily identify their underlying core beliefs through guided discovery and other questioning techniques, administering a schema inventory can add depth to your formulation. We typically find that patients endorse both negative and positive schemas that we did not identify previously. In addition, discussion of reactions to completing a schema inventory can lead to discovery of other valuable information about core beliefs. Sometimes an underlying schema is not listed in the inventory, but the beliefs that are included trigger a series of thoughts that reveal one of the patient's most important underlying assumptions.

For the next learning exercise, we would like you to take this schema inventory adapted from some of our earlier work. Because the list was designed to be used for people with significant depression or anxiety, many of the dysfunctional schemas are expressed in absolute terms. However, our clinical experience and research with the inventory indicate that patients frequently endorse the maladaptive schemas on this list. We recommend that you start to administer a schema inventory to the patients you are treating with CBT and that you discuss the responses in your therapy sessions.

**Learning Exercise 8–3.** Taking an Inventory of Your Schemas

Instructions: Use this checklist to search for possible underlying rules of thinking. Place a check mark beside each schema that you think you may have. (This Schema Inventory is available online and can be printed for clinical use; click on the Appendix link at www.appi.org/wright.)

| **Healthy Schemas** | **Maladaptive Schemas** |
|---|---|
| ___ No matter what happens, I can manage somehow. | ___ I must be perfect to be accepted. |
| ___ If I work hard at something, I can master it. | ___ If I choose to do something, I must succeed. |
| ___ I'm a survivor. | ___ I'm stupid. |
| ___ Others trust me. | ___ Without a woman (man), I'm nothing. |
| ___ I'm a solid person. | ___ I'm a fake. |
| ___ People respect me. | ___ Never show weakness. |
| ___ They can knock me down, but they can't knock me out. | ___ I'm unlovable. |
| ___ I care about other people. | ___ If I make one mistake, I'll lose everything. |
| ___ If I prepare in advance, I usually do better. | ___ I'll never be comfortable around others. |
| ___ I deserve to be respected. | ___ I can never finish anything. |
| ___ I like to be challenged. | ___ No matter what I do, I won't succeed. |
| ___ There's not much that can scare me. | ___ The world is too frightening for me. |
| ___ I'm intelligent. | ___ Others can't be trusted. |
| ___ I can figure things out. | ___ I must always be in control. |
| ___ I'm friendly. | ___ I'm unattractive. |
| ___ I can handle stress. | ___ Never show your emotions. |
| ___ The tougher the problem, the tougher I become. | ___ Other people will take advantage of me. |
| ___ I can learn from my mistakes and be a better person. | ___ I'm lazy. |
| ___ I'm a good spouse (and/or parent, child, friend, lover). | ___ If people really knew me, they wouldn't like me. |
| ___ Everything will work out all right. | ___ To be accepted, I must always please others. |



## Keeping a Personal Schema List

We've made the point many times in this book that writing down material learned in therapy sessions and in homework assignments can be a critical step in being able to recall and effectively use CBT concepts. When you are working with core beliefs, it is especially important to emphasize the value of keeping a written record, either with pen and paper or electronically, and regularly reviewing these notes. Because schemas are often latent or below the surface of everyday thinking, awareness of core attitudes may erode quickly if not reinforced. In our clinical practices we have seen many situations where we have worked hard to identify a key schema in a therapy session, yet with the pressure of current environmental events and the passage of time, patients seem to "forget" about this core belief unless we draw their attention to it.

A customized schema list can be an excellent method of recording, storing, and reinforcing the knowledge that you and the patient have gained about core adaptive and maladaptive beliefs. In the opening phase of work on schemas, there may be only a few entries on this list. But as therapy proceeds, more schemas will be added, and maladaptive core beliefs will be changed with techniques described in the next section, "Modifying Schemas." Thus the personal schema list is a fluid entity that should show steady evidence of improvement throughout the course of CBT.

**Learning Exercise 8–4.** Developing a Personal Schema List

1. Use the methods described in this chapter to develop your own personal schema list. Try to write down as many adaptive and maladaptive schemas as possible.

2. Practice developing personal schema lists with one or more of your patients. Review the lists regularly in therapy sessions. Edit and modify the lists as progress is made to change schemas.

## Modifying Schemas

After you have helped your patient identify underlying schemas, you can begin to work on changing dysfunctional basic rules of thinking and behaving. When you are doing this, it is wise to remember that schemas often are deeply embedded and have been practiced and reinforced for many years. Therefore, it is unlikely that patients will change them dramatically by gaining insight alone. To modify these key operational principles, patients typically need to go through a concentrated process of examining the beliefs, generating plausible alternatives, and rehearsing the revised schema in real-life situations (Table 8–3).

### Socratic Questioning

Good Socratic questions often can help patients see inconsistencies in their core beliefs, appreciate the impact of schemas on emotions and behavior, and begin the process of change. One of the principal goals of Socratic questioning is to stimulate a sense of inquiry, thus moving the

**Table 8–3.** Methods for changing schemas

| |
|---|
| Socratic questioning |
| Examining the evidence |
| Listing advantages and disadvantages |
| Using the cognitive continuum |
| Generating alternatives |
| Cognitive and behavioral rehearsal |

patient away from a fixed, maladaptive view of self and the world to a more inquisitive, flexible, and growth-promoting cognitive style. Here are some suggestions for asking Socratic questions that may help patients be more open to revising their core beliefs.

1. **Develop a formulation to direct your line of questioning.** Have a good idea where you are heading. Chess masters plan many moves ahead and have a variety of strategies in mind to react to the possible actions of the other player. Act like a great chess player in planning ahead. Of course, your Socratic questions will be collaborative instead of competitive.
2. **Use questions to help patients see contradictions in their thinking.** Patients typically have a variety of core beliefs, some of which give them competing messages. In a classic videotape, Aaron T. Beck (1977) asked a patient who was facing a divorce to explain the contradiction between her belief that she could not live without her husband and another belief that she had been happier and healthier before she got married. These types of questions can lead to rapid breakthroughs in understanding and a willingness to engage in subsequent action plans to change.
3. **Ask questions that encourage the patient to recognize adaptive beliefs.** In general, it is more likely that adaptive beliefs will be fully endorsed, remembered, and acted on if the patient does a good deal of the work in uncovering positively toned schemas. Instead of telling patients that they have healthy attitudes or strengths to be used in fighting their problems, try to ask Socratic questions that get them highly involved in articulating adaptive core beliefs.
4. **Avoid asking leading questions.** Even if you have a good plan for what you would like the patient to see or do, don't ask questions in a manner that conveys that you already know the answers. Maintain the collaborative and empirical style of CBT. Remain open to following the train of the patient's thinking.

5. **Remember that questions that activate significant emotion may enhance learning.** If you can ask Socratic questions that either stimulate emotional arousal or sharply reduce emotional pain, the learning experience may be more meaningful and memorable for the patient.
6. **Ask questions that serve as a springboard for implementing other methods of changing schemas.** Good Socratic questions often prepare the way for other more specific methods of modifying core beliefs. Think of Socratic questions as keys that can unlock doors to learning. After you ask an effective Socratic question, be prepared to implement other methods such as examining the evidence, generating alternative beliefs, or using the cognitive continuum, all described in the next sections.

## Examining the Evidence

In Chapter 5, "Working With Automatic Thoughts," we explain how to examine the evidence for automatic thoughts. The procedures for examining the evidence for schemas are very similar. However, because maladaptive core beliefs are so long-standing and have often been reinforced by actual negative outcomes, criticism, dysfunctional relationships, or traumas, the patient may be able to generate considerable evidence that the belief is true. A man who believes that he is a loser may have had many instances of negative outcomes such as job losses, marital breakups, or financial problems. A woman who tells you that she is unlovable may recount a number of rejections in romantic relationships. Therefore, when examining the evidence for schemas, you may need to acknowledge that problems have existed and be empathic with the patient's life travails.

An exercise in examining the evidence is shown in Figure 8–2 from the therapy of Maria, the woman who has the schema "I'm unlovable" (see "Using Questioning Techniques" earlier in this chapter). The first step in this intervention is to help Maria recognize evidence for and against the belief. Then the therapist prompts her to spot cognitive errors in the evidence for the maladaptive schema. Finally, the therapist asks Socratic questions to assist Maria in modifying the belief. When you implement the method of examining the evidence with your patients, keep in mind the suggestions listed in Table 8–4.

The treatment of Allison, the 19-year-old woman with bulimia and depression described earlier in "Using Questioning Techniques," illustrates how an intervention to examine the evidence led to a productive homework assignment with specific behavioral goals. At this point in the treatment process, Allison's depression had improved and she was no lon-

Schema I want to change: I'm unlovable.

| Evidence for this schema: | | Evidence against this schema: | |
|---|---|---|---|
| 1. | My husband had an affair and left me. | 1. | Two men left me, but I think they both loved me for a while. There were at least 10 good years with my husband. |
| 2. | The only other man I loved also left me. I'm bound to get the same hurt if I try again. | 2. | I've blamed myself completely. Maybe it was partially their fault. |
| 3. | I always felt that I wasn't good enough. | 3. | My husband still says he cares about me and feels guilty for what happened. |
| 4. | I haven't dated many men. | 4. | Lots of other people love me (daughter, parents, sisters). My grandparents were very loving toward me. |
| | | 5. | Maybe there is another man who would be a better match and would stick by me. I'm basing my conclusions on just two chances at finding love. |

Cognitive errors: Ignoring the evidence, overgeneralizing, personalizing, all-or-nothing thinking.

Modified schema: I've been rejected twice but that doesn't mean I'm unlovable. I have strengths and deserve to be loved. I have a lot to offer in a relationship.

**Figure 8–2.** Examining the evidence for schemas: Maria's example.

ger suicidal. She had been discharged from the hospital and was continuing with outpatient CBT. Her therapist helped her develop a worksheet for the schema "I must be perfect to be accepted" (Figure 8–3). Note that Allison generated a fair amount of evidence against the statement and also added several observations about her cognitive errors. However, it appeared that she still needed more work on developing an alternative core belief. The blank worksheet for examining the evidence for schemas is available in Appendix 1, "Worksheets and Checklists," so that you can make copies to use with your patients.

## Listing Advantages and Disadvantages

Some maladaptive schemas are maintained through the years because they have a payoff. Even though the schema may be loaded with negative effects, it may also have benefits that induce the person to keep thinking and acting in the same dysfunctional way. Allison's schema, "I must be perfect to be accepted," is a good example of this type of core belief. Her drive for perfectionism had made her miserable, but she had also had

**Table 8–4.** How to examine the evidence for schemas

1. Briefly explain the procedure before beginning to examine the evidence.
2. Use an empirical approach. Engage the patient in a process of taking an honest look at the validity of the schema.
3. Write out the evidence on a worksheet. The first time through this procedure, it may work best for you to write down the evidence. Shift responsibility for writing to the patient whenever possible.
4. Worksheets can be initiated in therapy sessions and then completed for homework assignments, thus getting the patient fully involved in the process of generating and recording evidence.
5. Often evidence for schemas is absolutistic and is supported by cognitive errors and other dysfunctional information processing. Help the patient spot these errors in reasoning.
6. Where there is evidence that patients have had recurring problems with relationships, acceptance, competence, social skills, or other key functions, use this information to design intervention strategies. For example, a person with negative core beliefs about social competence may be helped by behavioral methods that break patterns of avoidance and teach skills needed to be facile in social settings.
7. Be creative in generating evidence against maladaptive core beliefs. Ask Socratic questions that stimulate different ways of viewing the situation. Because patients can have a fixed, negative view of themselves, your energy and imagination may be needed to help them find reasons to change.
8. Collect as much evidence as possible against dysfunctional schemas. This information will help patients refute core beliefs and will also provide important openings for other cognitive-behavior therapy interventions.
9. Use the method of examining the evidence as a platform for helping the patient make specific modifications in core beliefs. After examining the evidence with the patient, ask him to think about possible changes that will lead to healthier rules of thinking. Write these ideas down on the worksheet for examining the evidence, and follow up with other interventions described in this chapter.
10. Develop a homework assignment to build on the success of the exercise for examining the evidence. Possibilities might include adding more evidence to the worksheet, spotting cognitive errors, thinking of alternative schemas, or suggesting a behavioral assignment to practice acting in a new way that is consistent with the modified belief.

Schema I want to change: I must be perfect to be accepted.

Evidence for this schema:

1. My parents always pressured me to be the best at everything I do.
2. Men want thin women who look perfect.
3. When I got top grades in school, I won a scholarship. Everybody said I was a great student.
4. You need to excel to be popular. Who wants to be friends with somebody who is just average?

Evidence against this schema:

1. Even though my parents have high standards, I think they would accept me if I'm less than perfect. They aren't perfect themselves. I still love them, despite all of their flaws.
2. I have some friends who are overweight who have excellent relationships with their boyfriends.
3. Some of the happiest people I know aren't obsessed with perfection.
4. Other people who aren't perfect seem to be accepted for who they are. Maybe some people would be more comfortable having a relationship with a person who isn't perfect.

Cognitive errors: All-or-nothing thinking, magnifying, ignoring the evidence.

1. My parents have actually shown lots of caring and acceptance when I mess up or don't reach my goals. I know they would like me to be less obsessed about my weight.
2. There is a lot more to me than my weight or how flat my stomach is. I need to accept my other strengths.
3. I might make more friends if I didn't try so hard to be perfect. Setting such high standards may turn people off.

Now that I've examined the evidence, my degree of belief in the schema is: 30%.

Ideas I have for modifications to this schema:

1. I can strive for excellence but still accept myself when I don't reach perfection.
2. I will be happier and feel more accepted if I'm more realistic about reaching my goals.

Actions I will take now to change my schema and act in a healthier way:

1. I will write out a list of ways in which I am imperfect but am still a good person who deserves to be accepted.
2. I will purposely try to de-emphasize perfectionism in how I exercise by a) giving myself a day off at least twice a week and b) not counting or recording each repetition of work at the gym.
3. I will reduce perfectionism in my study habits by a) no longer logging the minutes I spend on each assignment, b) taking breaks from studying at least three times a week to do fun things (such as going to a movie or just goofing off with some friends), and c) changing my focus in study from always thinking about getting a perfect grade to enjoying the learning experience.

**Figure 8–3.** Worksheet for examining the evidence for schemas: Allison's example.

some major successes that were derived in part from her perfectionistic behavior. These double-sided schemas are very common, even in persons without any psychiatric symptoms. Perhaps you have some beliefs that have both advantages and disadvantages. Can you spot any of these schemas on your personal list?

**Learning Exercise 8–5.** Finding Schemas With Advantages and Disadvantages

1. Review your personal list of schemas from Learning Exercise 8–4.

2. Identify a schema that may have served you well but that also may have a downside. Perhaps a schema has influenced you to work hard but has also caused tension or has taken a toll on your social life. No one has a complete set of fully adaptive schemas, so try to find one that has had both positive and negative effects.

3. List the advantages and disadvantages for this core belief.

Clinical application of the technique of listing advantages and disadvantages involves many of the same kinds of steps used for examining the evidence. First, you should briefly explain the procedure so the patient will know where you are heading. Then ask a series of questions geared toward developing a written record of advantages and disadvantages. Next, use this analysis to consider modifications that will make the schema more adaptive and less of a burden. Finally, design and implement a homework assignment to practice new behaviors.

Comparing advantages and disadvantages of a schema has several potential benefits. The full spectrum of effects of the schema can be seen, and exploring these different effects may stimulate creative ideas for change. Of course, listing the deleterious effects of the schema can highlight the downside of continuing to hold the belief. But it is just as important to know about the advantages of the schema. Patients are unlikely to give up maladaptive schemas and associated behaviors that give them substantial positive reinforcement unless these advantages are also provided by the modified belief.

When we try to generate alternative schemas, we often suggest that patients think of changes that will eliminate or greatly reduce the negative effects of the previous schema while holding on to at least some of the benefits. Allison's schema about perfectionism was a logical target for this type of intervention. Listing advantages and disadvantages led to several good ideas for revisions in her core belief (Figure 8–4).

Schema I want to change: I must be perfect to be accepted.

| Advantages of this schema: | Disadvantages of this schema: |
|---|---|
| 1. I have always been at the top of my class in school. | 1. Perfectionism exhausts me. |
| 2. I've stayed thin. | 2. I have an eating disorder. |
| 3. I worked very hard to learn to play the violin and was named to the state orchestra. | 3. The only way I can feel happy is if everything is going just right. |
| 4. Many of my classmates looked up to me. | 4. Trying to be perfect distances me from others. They probably don't like me so much because it seems like I am trying to be better than them. |
| 5. I got a scholarship to go to college. | 5. I'm never really satisfied with myself. I think that I'm never good enough. |
| 6. I've never gotten into trouble, other than having psychiatric treatment. | 6. I can't relax and have fun. I get depressed a lot. I'm always tense and usually unhappy. |

Ideas I have for modifications to this schema:

1. I can choose my targets for trying to do my best. For example, I can continue to study hard and have goals for a successful career. But I can back off in other areas of my life.
2. I can develop interests and hobbies where I don't have to be the best and can still enjoy doing things.
3. I can relax around friends and family and hope that they will accept me without my having to accomplish so much or be a perfect person.
4. I am more likely to be accepted by others if I try to be successful but don't go overboard in a relentless pursuit of perfection.

**Figure 8–4.** Worksheet for listing advantages and disadvantages: Allison's example.

## Using the Cognitive Continuum

When schemas are expressed in absolute terms, patients may see themselves in an extremely negative light (e.g., "I'm a loser"; "I'm unlovable"; "I'm stupid"). If these types of schemas are present, the cognitive continuum technique can be used to help patients place their beliefs in a broader context and moderate their thinking.

In Video 21, Dr. Sudak uses the cognitive continuum to good effect in helping Brian change his schema "People can't be counted upon." After developing the continuum shown in Figure 8–5, Brian is able to revise the belief to "There are people you can count on.... There are people who aren't as reliable." When you view the video, note how Dr. Sudak designs a behavioral assignment that has excellent potential for solidifying the more adaptive schema while reducing Brian's loneliness and social isolation.

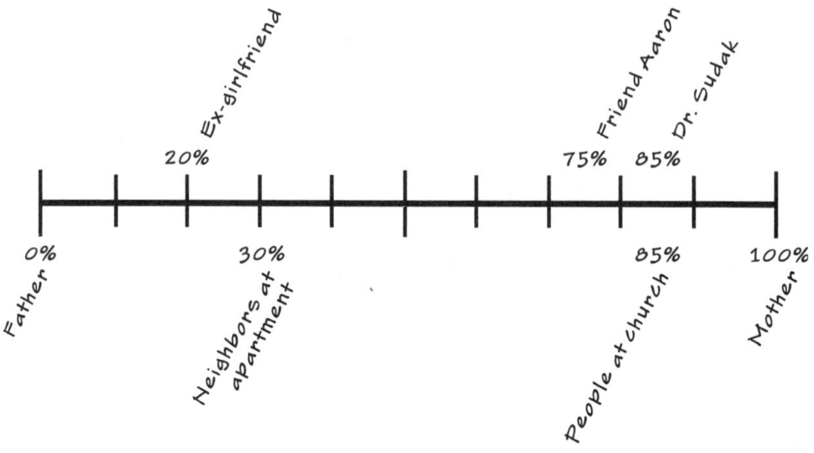


**Figure 8–5.** The cognitive continuum: Brian's example of how much he can count on people.

**Video 21.** Changing a Maladaptive Schema: Dr. Sudak and Brian (12:26)

## Generating Alternatives

Methods for changing core beliefs (e.g., Socratic questioning, examining the evidence, and listing advantages and disadvantages) described in this chapter often stimulate patients to consider alternative schemas. These key interventions can be very productive tools to help patients consider possible modifications in their basic rules of thinking. You also can adapt the techniques for finding rational alternatives to automatic thoughts (see Chapter 5, "Working With Automatic Thoughts") in your work with core beliefs. For example, you can encourage your patients to open their minds to a wide variety of possibilities by thinking like scientists or detectives—or to imagine that they are coaches who are building their strengths by helping spot positive but rational alternatives. The brainstorming method detailed in Chapter 5 can be particularly useful in generating alternatives to deeply held schemas. When we use this technique for revising core beliefs, we ask patients to try to step away from their old way of thinking and to consider a full range of potential changes.

Another way to help patients generate alternatives is to put a spotlight on the language of schemas. Consider, for example, the wording of these core beliefs: "I'm worthless"; "I'm no good at sports"; and "I will always be rejected." Pointing out the absolute terms in schemas and asking patients to consider using words that are less extreme is one way of generating healthier beliefs (e.g., "I've experienced rejections, but some family members and friends have stuck by me"). You can also help patients target if-then statements for change (e.g., "If people really knew me, they would know that I'm a fraud"; "If I don't meet all of his demands, he will leave me"; "If you get close to someone, they will always hurt you"). Educating people on the restricting nature of rigid if-then beliefs can prompt them to develop more flexible basic rules (e.g., "Getting close to someone has risks, but it doesn't always mean that I will get hurt"). Another technique that you might consider is to ask the patient to examine the wording of a core belief that may be offering some advantages but is having overall deleterious effects. Perhaps just changing one or two words will help the person to fine-tune the schema to a point where it is more adaptive or less damaging (e.g., revising "I must be in control" to "I like to be in control").

Some patients can productively use study, self-reflection, cultural activities, classes, and other growth-oriented experiences to explore possible changes in core beliefs. Readings might include inspirational, philosophical, or historical books that challenge the status quo of their thinking. Spiritual activities, theatrical or musical performances, the visual arts, stimulating public lectures, or adventures in the outdoors can provide opportunities for seeing the self and the world in different ways. These types of experiences may be especially useful for persons who are searching for a deeper sense of meaning or purpose in life. A few of the books that our patients have found most helpful include *Man's Search for Meaning* (Frankl 1992), *Full Catastrophe Living* (Kabat-Zinn 1990), *The Art of Serenity* (Karasu 2003), *The Mindful Way Through Depression* (Williams et al. 2007), and *Flourish* (Seligman 2012).

## Cognitive and Behavioral Rehearsal

The three most important words in predicting success in changing schemas are *practice, practice,* and *practice.* Because insight alone is rarely enough to reverse entrenched core beliefs, you will need to devise strategies to help your patients try out revised schemas in real-world situations, learn from their achievements and roadblocks, and build skills for acting differently. Typically, rehearsal of possible modifications of schemas begins in therapy sessions and then extends via homework assignments into daily life. We discuss basic methods for cognitive and behavioral rehearsal in Chapter 5, "Working With Automatic Thoughts," and Chapter 6, "Behavioral Methods I: Improving Mood, Increasing Energy, Completing

Tasks, and Solving Problems." To refresh your memory of how to perform rehearsal methods and to illustrate the use of this technique for schema change, we draw an example from Dr. Sudak's treatment of Brian.

Previous video illustrations in this chapter have shown Dr. Sudak helping Brian develop alternatives to his core belief "People can't be counted upon." In the next vignette, she works with Brian to put a healthier schema into action. By this point in therapy, Brian has made substantial gains and is ready to risk asking Renee, a coworker, for a date. However, he fears that something could go wrong. Renee could say no or tell him she is busy with something else. After Brian tells Dr. Sudak the worst outcome would be for Renee to accept and then cancel the date, they practice coping with this possibility.

**Video 22.** Putting a Revised Schema Into Action: Dr. Sudak and Brian (10:48)

Many effective strategies are available for practicing revised schemas. As shown in Video 22, Dr. Sudak used a role-play exercise to help Brian build skills in implementing a modified belief. Other commonly used methods include imagery, brainstorming, and making coping cards. Table 8–5 displays suggestions for rehearsing modified schemas and behavioral plans for implementing these beliefs.

## Growth-Oriented CBT

Although the goals of schema change are most commonly focused on symptom relief and relapse prevention, therapy can also be taken to another plane: working on personal meaning and growth. Even when patients are primarily concerned with relief of symptoms, it may be useful to look for core beliefs that may expand their potential for personal growth or may help them develop a full sense of purpose in life. Here are some examples of questions you might ask to find out if your patients have goals that may lead therapy in a growth-oriented direction: "When you get over the depression, will you still have some things you would like to work on in therapy?" "Do you have any additional goals for how your life might change after you retire (or your children leave home, or you get over the divorce, etc.)?" "You mentioned that you want to stop being a workaholic.... What goals would you have for your life if you weren't working most of the time?"

Allison, the young woman with depression and bulimia, was so fixated on her pursuit of perfection and her struggle to maintain control that she was missing out on many of the potentially meaningful things in her

**Table 8–5.** Tips for practicing new schemas

1. Develop a plan for trying out a new or revised schema. This plan should identify the modified core belief in addition to specific behaviors that will be undertaken to put the revised schema into action.
2. Use imagery and/or role-play to rehearse the plan in a therapy session. Identify automatic thoughts, other schemas, or dysfunctional behavioral patterns that may interfere with the plan for change.
3. Develop coping strategies for overcoming obstacles.
4. Develop a homework assignment to practice the new core belief and the adaptive behaviors in a specific real-life situation.
5. Coach the patient on ways to make the homework a productive experience.
6. Record the plan on a coping card.
7. Review the outcome of the homework in the next session, and make adjustments in the plan as necessary.
8. Keep the "practice, practice, practice" strategy in mind as you continue to help the patient modify schemas. Choose multiple targets for applying the principles for changing schemas.

world. However, when her symptoms began to subside, she was able to gain a richer perspective of the path ahead. Adaptive beliefs that had been obscured by her dysfunctional schemas could now be nurtured and strengthened (e.g., "I am a good friend"; "I would like to make a difference—to do something in my life that helps others"; "I love to be in nature, to appreciate the things around me").

The process of building growth-oriented schemas sometimes involves exploration of new terrain. Perhaps the patient has always thought that something was missing in his life, or that his life has not been centered on purposeful or meaningful things. Or perhaps a major loss has shaken his core values and constructs. In these types of situations, CBT can be directed toward helping the person grapple with existential questions and attempt to find ways to move beyond a loss, unlock potential, or commit to fresh ideas. In our book written for the general public, *Breaking Free From Depression: Pathways to Wellness* (Wright and McCray 2011), we suggest several practical ways of searching for meaning. These ideas, largely drawn from the work of Viktor Frankl (1992), can be assigned as self-help exercises for persons interested in building their sense of purpose or deepening their commitment to core values.

Some authors of articles and books on growth-oriented CBT have used the term *constructivism* or *constructivist cognitive therapy* to describe an approach in which the therapist helps the patient develop adaptive schemas that *construct* a new personal existence (Guidano and Liotti 1985; Mahoney 1995; Neimeyer 1993). The ultimate expression of constructivist cognitive therapy would be a treatment process in which a person is transformed to a higher level of personal authenticity and well-being. In our experience with CBT, such major transformations are uncommon. However, when persons continue in therapy beyond the symptom relief stage and work on reaching growth-oriented goals, the result can be very gratifying for both patient and therapist.

A full description of CBT methods for growth-oriented and constructivist cognitive therapy is beyond the scope of this basic text. However, we recommend that you consider dimensions of personal growth and meaning in developing formulations for treatment and that you devote at least a portion of the therapy effort to helping patients find adaptive core beliefs that can provide guidance for their future. In Chapter 10, "Treating Chronic, Severe, or Complex Disorders," we briefly describe approaches that can promote personal growth, such as well-being therapy and mindfulness-based cognitive therapy.

**Learning Exercise 8–6.** Modifying Schemas

1. Use a role-play exercise with a helper to examine the evidence for a schema and weigh its advantages and disadvantages.

2. Next use the techniques for generating alternatives described in this chapter.

3. Work out a plan for putting a modified schema into action. Include details on how the person will both think and act differently.

4. Then implement these methods for changing schemas in your work with patients.

5. Elicit at least one adaptive, growth-oriented schema from a patient, and develop a plan for putting this belief into action.

## Summary

Changing core beliefs can be a challenging task. However, therapeutic work on modifying schemas can lead to important gains in self-esteem and behavioral effectiveness. Because schemas are deeply embedded basic rules of thinking, the therapist may need to show ingenuity and persistence in bringing them to the surface. Some of the commonly used methods for uncovering core beliefs are Socratic questioning, spotting schemas in patterns of automatic thoughts, and the downward arrow technique. Keeping a written list of schemas can help the therapist and patient remain focused on the change process.

To loosen the grip of maladaptive schemas, CBT methods encourage patients to step back from their core beliefs and check them for accuracy. Techniques such as examining the evidence and listing advantages and disadvantages can promote a broader perspective and stimulate the development of new schemas. When potential revisions in core beliefs are generated in therapy sessions or in homework assignments, a specific plan should be designed for trying out the schema in real-life situations. Repeated practice is usually required to cement modified schemas and to replace older, maladaptive rules of thinking. For some patients, a growth-oriented phase of CBT can help them work on adaptive core beliefs that add depth to their self-concept and enhance their sense of well-being.

## References

Beck AT: Demonstration of the Cognitive Therapy of Depression: Interview #1 (Patient With a Family Problem) (videotape). Bala Cynwyd, PA, Beck Institute for Cognitive Therapy and Research, 1977

Beck AT, Freeman A: Cognitive Therapy of Personality Disorders. New York, Guilford, 1990

Beck AT, Brown G, Steer RA, et al: Factor analysis of the Dysfunctional Attitude Scale in a clinical population. Psychol Assess 3:478–483, 1991

Beck AT, Davis DD, Freeman A (eds): Cognitive Therapy of Personality Disorders, 3rd Edition. New York, Guilford, 2014

Clark DA, Beck AT, Alford BA: Scientific Foundations of Cognitive Theory and Therapy of Depression. New York, Wiley, 1999

Evans MD, Hollon SD, DeRubeis RJ, et al: Differential relapse following cognitive therapy and pharmacotherapy for depression. Arch Gen Psychiatry 49(10):802–808, 1992 1417433

Frankl VE: Man's Search for Meaning: An Introduction to Logotherapy. Boston, MA, Beacon Press, 1992

Greenberger D, Padesky CA: Mind Over Mood: Change How You Feel by Changing the Way You Think, 2nd Edition. New York, Guilford, 2015

Guidano VF, Liotti G: A constructivist foundation for cognitive therapy, in Cognition and Psychotherapy. Edited by Mahoney MJ, Freeman A. New York, Plenum, 1985, pp 101–142

Jarrett RB, Kraft D, Doyle J, et al: Preventing recurrent depression using cognitive therapy with and without a continuation phase: a randomized clinical trial. Arch Gen Psychiatry 58(4):381–388, 2001 11296099

Kabat-Zinn J: Full Catastrophe Living: Using the Wisdom of Your Body and Mind to Face Stress, Pain, and Illness. New York, Hyperion, 1990

Karasu TB: The Art of Serenity: The Path to a Joyful Life in the Best and Worst of Times. New York, Simon & Schuster, 2003

Mahoney MJ (ed): Cognitive and Constructive Psychotherapies: Theory, Research, and Practice. New York, Springer, 1995

Neimeyer RA: Constructivism and the cognitive psychotherapies: some conceptual and strategic contrasts. J Cogn Psychother 7:159–171, 1993

Seligman MEP: Flourish: A Visionary New Understanding of Happiness and Well-Being. New York, Atria Books, 2012

Williams M, Teasdale J, Segal Z, Kabat-Zinn J: The Mindful Way Through Depression: Freeing Yourself From Chronic Unhappiness. New York, Guilford, 2007

Wright JH, McCray LW: Breaking Free From Depression: Pathways to Wellness. New York, Guilford, 2011

Wright JH, Wright AS, Beck AT: Good Days Ahead. Moraga, CA, Empower Interactive, 2016

Young JE, Brown G: Young Schema Questionnaire: Special Edition. New York, Schema Therapy Institute, 2001

Young JE, Klosko JS: Reinventing Your Life: The Breakthrough Program to End Negative Behavior and Feel Great Again. New York, Plume, 1994

Young JE, Klosko JS, Weishaar ME: Schema Therapy: A Practitioner's Guide. New York, Guilford, 2003

# 9 Cognitive-Behavior Therapy to Reduce Suicide Risk

If a patient has given up all hope and can see nothing in the future except pain and despair, suicide may seem like a reasonable choice. Because hopeless cognitions can have such intensely negative consequences, their validity should be challenged with all of the skill and creativity that the therapist can muster. If the therapist does not aim toward assisting the patient to modify these hopeless cognitions, a tacit validation of the beliefs may occur, and the therapy process may be undermined. When a patient believes that recovery is possible or likely, has genuine reasons to live, and can see possible solutions for problems, he may be able to tolerate extreme levels of depression without seriously considering self-harm (Wright et al. 2009).

Several evidence-based treatments to prevent suicidal behavior have been tested in randomized controlled trials. Cognitive therapy for suicide prevention (CT-SP; Brown et al. 2005), brief cognitive-behavioral therapy (Rudd et al. 2015; Slee et al. 2008), dialectical behavior therapy (Linehan et al. 2006), and several other approaches (Bateman and Fonagy 1999; Guthrie et al. 2001; Hatcher et al. 2011) have shown positive effects for preventing suicide attempts or self-directed violence in adults. For example, individuals who recently attempted suicide and were treated with CT-SP were 50% less likely to try to kill themselves again within 18 months than individuals who did not receive the therapy (Brown et al. 2005). A primary feature of this treatment is to apply cognitive and behavioral strategies that directly target the prevention of suicidal behavior, as well as reduce the severity of hopelessness and depression. The Substance Abuse and Mental Health Services Administration's National Registry of Evidence-Based Programs and Practices has identified CT-SP (Brown et al. 2005) as a promising evidence-based treatment for reducing suicide risk.

In this chapter, we describe some of the key cognitive and behavioral strategies to reduce suicide risk based on CT-SP treatment. These strategies focus on engaging hopeless patients in cognitive-behavior therapy (CBT), explaining CBT to patients, developing a commitment to treatment, screening for and assessing suicide risk, developing a safety plan, identifying reasons for living and instilling a sense of hope, and applying other cognitive and behavioral strategies to reduce risk and prevent relapse of suicidal crises.

## Engaging Hopeless Patients in CBT

Many patients who are at risk for suicide are hopeless about the likelihood that things will ever improve and are thinking about giving up altogether. Although CBT strategies can be used to help patients identify hopeless cognitions and develop more realistic alternative responses to these cognitions, patients at risk for suicide may feel hopeless about the possibility that any psychiatric treatment will be helpful to them. Some patients may report that "nothing has worked." They have tried a litany of medications and psychotherapies and none of these previous treatments have relieved symptoms or kept them well. One approach for addressing patients' hopelessness is for the therapist to do a careful review of the adequacy or quality of these treatments, including patients' adherence with treatment recommendations, and then to help patients reevaluate their conclusions about the effectiveness of these treatments. However, this approach may not be effective if used early in treatment before patients have developed an understanding of cognitive-behavioral methods or before an effective therapeutic alliance has been established.

Given these concerns, it is often helpful to carefully listen to patients' concerns and to empathize with their struggles and challenges in obtaining or receiving treatments that could provide relief. Recognizing and acknowledging patients' feeling of hopelessness is a first step in engaging patients in the treatment process. After listening closely to patients' descriptions of their previous experiences in treatment, the therapist may assess the degree to which negative treatment experiences from the past are contributing to a negative attitude toward the current treatment, including CBT. Giving patients the opportunity to describe the helpful and unhelpful aspects of prior treatments allows clinicians to tailor the CBT intervention by emphasizing specific aspects of the intervention that are likely to increase treatment effectiveness. Once patients feel understood by their therapist, the therapist may also point out that hopelessness is a way of thinking that is commonly experienced by individuals who are depressed and that the focus of CBT is to assist them in addressing their hopelessness.

Another component of CBT that usually reduces hopelessness early in treatment is the structure of treatment. Patients who are overwhelmed and may think there is no way out of their dilemma can respond positively to setting realistic goals, keeping on track toward solving problems, and having an experience of working with a therapist who helps guide them toward reaching their goals.

## Providing Information About CBT

Educating patients about the structure and process of CBT and the limits of privacy and confidentiality is especially important with suicidal patients. Providing information about these issues and then giving patients with suicidal risk the opportunity to ask questions is critical given their propensity to feel hopeless about treatment or to drop out of treatment altogether. When describing the details of the format and structure of CBT, the therapist may outline the structure of a typical session, including conducting a mood check, assessing clinical symptoms including suicidal ideation and behavior, providing a summary of the previous session, setting a prioritized agenda, providing a summary of the current session, collaborating on a self-help assignment, and obtaining feedback regarding the helpfulness of the session. Educating patients about how CBT is practiced helps them to understand that their problems, including their reasons for wanting to kill themselves, can be addressed in a thoughtful and systematic manner.

## Developing a Commitment to Treatment

A crucial task during the initial CBT sessions is to obtain an explicit commitment to treatment, including patients' agreement to consistently attend and participate in the sessions, to work toward achieving the treatment goals, to complete homework assignments, and to actively participate in other aspects of treatment in order to better manage their suicidal crises and hopelessness.

An important strategy for enhancing motivation for treatment is to be explicit that a primary goal of treatment is to prevent suicide. In this regard, the therapist may ask patients to refrain from acting on their suicidal urges and to fully engage in the treatment process for a given number of sessions. The aim of this approach is to have patients fully commit to treatment for a period of time while they are learning specific coping skills to reduce risk and refrain from attempting suicide. Patients are informed that after they complete the agreed-upon number of sessions, the therapist and patient will evaluate whether or not treatment was helpful and make plans for further treatment if needed. In our experience, using these methods to increase patients' motivation for engaging in CBT treatment decreases the likelihood that they will drop out of treatment.

## Screening for and Assessing Suicide Risk

Assessing risk for suicide is an essential step in developing effective action plans that are geared to the level of risk. Patients who are at low risk may be treated routinely in outpatient medical settings, while patients who have higher levels of risk may require more intensive therapy, additional mental health or substance abuse treatment, or other levels of care, such as inpatient treatment programs, in order to help them remain safe.

Because suicidal individuals constitute a high-risk population, clinicians should conduct a comprehensive suicide risk assessment at the beginning of treatment, as well as screen for suicide risk at each subsequent CBT session. A comprehensive suicide risk assessment includes direct questioning about patients' current mental status, the administration of self-report measures, review of medical records, clinical observation of patients' behavior, and contacting patients' family members or friends, if available. The risk assessment should include questions about the content, frequency, duration, and severity of current suicidal thoughts, as well as any past suicidal ideation and behavior (including suicide attempts). Plans for suicide, intent to make a suicide attempt, and access to potentially lethal means are particularly important components of suicide risk assessment.

Risk factors associated with the patient's clinical condition include hopelessness and despair, major depression or other mood disorder, substance abuse or dependence, personality disorder, agitation or severe anxiety, social isolation or loneliness, problem-solving deficits, dysfunctional attitudes (such as perfectionism or perceived burden on family or others), highly impulsive behavior, homicidal ideation, aggressive behavior toward others, and chronic physical pain or other acute medical problems. Environmental stresses that can increase risk for suicide include recent life events such as a breakup of a relationship or other interpersonal loss, conflict or violence, legal problems, financial difficulties, unemployment, pending incarceration, and homelessness. Examples of risk factors from the patient's past history are physical or sexual abuse and suicide in a family member or friend.

Another vitally important series of questions should be directed at protective factors that decrease the risk of suicide. Questions about reasons to live are especially useful in assessing risk. If the patient can't identify meaningful reasons to live, risk may be quite high. In contrast, the patient who articulates powerful reasons to live may have a lower risk of suicide. As we note later in the chapter, generating reasons to live is one of the key CBT methods for reducing suicide risk. Other protective factors include expressions of hopefulness, having a responsibility to family or others, a supportive social network or family, spiritual or religious beliefs against suicide, a fear of death or dying due to pain and suffering, believing that suicide is immoral, and engaging in work or school activities.

The routine use of self-report measures, such as the Patient Health Questionnaire–9 (PHQ-9; www.phqscreeners.com) or the Beck Depression Inventory–II (BDI-II; Beck et al. 1996), can provide a useful method for screening for suicide risk. These measures may be administered before each CBT session to screen for level of suicide risk, as well as to assess the severity of depression. Additional assessment of suicide risk may then be conducted for patients who endorse items on the PHQ-9 or BDI-II that indicate presence of suicidal ideation or hopelessness.

For patients who have made a suicide attempt or report acute suicidal ideation, the therapist may conduct a detailed narrative interview about the suicidal crisis. The narrative interview allows for patients to "tell their story" of a recent suicidal crisis that includes the sequence of events, thoughts, feelings, and behaviors that led up to the crisis point. The narrative interview helps foster the therapeutic relationship, in addition to providing information for the CBT formulation and treatment plan. To begin the narrative interview, the clinician may ask, "What happened that led up to the suicidal thinking or behavior? What started or triggered the crisis?" During the narrative interview, it is helpful to avoid asking a lot of detailed questions that may divert the patient from the main points of her story. Instead, the therapist can use brief summaries to communicate understanding and empathy during this process.

## Safety Planning

Once the narrative interview has been completed, the therapist may introduce safety planning as a method for helping patients recognize the warning signs or triggers that were identified during the narrative interview. Careful guided discovery of the information obtained during the narrative interview will usually indicate how suicidal ideation occurs and then diminishes over time. The safety plan intervention is based on the observation that suicide risk ebbs and flows and that helping the patient apply specific skills during periods of increased risk can prevent suicide. This strategy leads to a prioritized written list of warning signs and coping strategies and resources to use during or before a suicidal crisis (Stanley and Brown 2012). The intent of the intervention is to help patients refrain from acting on the urge to kill themselves and to allow time for suicidal thoughts to diminish and become more manageable.

Safety planning was initially developed and conducted in clinical trials of CBT, including CT-SP with adult suicide attempters (Brown et al. 2005) and CBT for suicide prevention with adolescent suicide attempters (Stanley et al. 2009). Since then, safety planning has been developed further as a stand-alone intervention that can be used with or without other treatments, including CBT. The safety plan intervention, as described here, is used widely in many health care systems, including the Department of Veterans Affairs (Knox et al. 2012). The Suicide Prevention Resource Center and the American Foundation for Suicide Prevention have recognized the safety plan intervention as a best practice.

The safety plan includes a series of specific steps that are collaboratively developed with the patient. Patients are informed that if the completion of any step is not helpful in reducing suicide risk, then they should proceed to the next step(s) until the risk for suicide is lower. A brief guide for helping patients develop a safety plan (Brown and Stanley 2016) is shown in Table 9–1, and a worksheet for safety planning is included in Appendix 1, "Worksheets and Checklists." In training others to use the safety plan intervention, we have noted that the successful implementation of safety planning requires more than simply filling out the safety plan worksheet. Additional safety planning training and other resources are available at: www.suicidesafetyplan.com.

### Case Example

David is a 20-year-old engineering student who is in his senior year of college. His depression and anxiety have been at a moderate level of severity. He had a prior episode of depression when he was 17 years old. While in high school, he lived with his father, mother, and a younger sister. His fa-

**Table 9–1.** Safety planning steps

**Step 1. Identify warning signs.** Inform the patient that the purpose of identifying warning signs is to help him recognize when a crisis may escalate so that he knows to refer to his plan and take action to reduce risk. If the warning signs are vague, explain that it is important to be specific so he is more likely to recognize the beginning of the crisis.

**Step 2. Develop coping strategies.** Explain how distraction from suicidal thoughts can help to lower risk. Ask "What can you do if you become suicidal again to help yourself *not* to act on your thoughts or urges?" Identify at least three specific strategies unless individuals decline. Determine if these strategies are safe, will not increase distress, and are feasible. Assess barriers to using these strategies, if any, and use a collaborative, problem-solving approach to address potential roadblocks or identify alternative coping strategies that are more feasible.

**Step 3. Identify social contacts and social settings.** Explain that if Step 2 does not lower risk, the patient should go to Step 3. Ask the patient to identify individuals who would help distract him from his problems and who could help him feel better. Also, identify social settings that may help distract him from his problems. Determine the likelihood that he would be able to talk with someone or go somewhere during a time of crisis. Assess the barriers to using these strategies and identify ways to resolve roadblocks or identify alternatives.

**Step 4. Contact family members or friends.** Explain that if Step 3 does not lower risk, the patient should go to Step 4. Ask patients to determine family members or friends who could be contacted for help during a crisis. Assess the likelihood that the patient will be able to reach out to each identified person. If doubt is expressed about contacting others, assess the barriers and address potential roadblocks or identify others to contact.

**Step 5. Contact professionals or agencies.** Explain that if Step 4 does not lower risk, the patient should go to Step 5. Identify any mental health professionals who can be contacted during a crisis. Explain how to contact the Suicide Prevention Lifeline (1-800-273-8255) or go to a hospital or urgent care setting during a crisis. Assess the likelihood the patient will contact each professional, agency, or crisis line; identify potential obstacles, and problem-solve.

**Step 6. Make the environment safe.** Explain that making the environment safer will help to lower the risk of acting on suicidal feelings. Ask patients whether they have access to a firearm. If individuals have identified other potentially lethal methods, then determine if they have access to them. For each lethal method, collaboratively develop a plan to make the environment safer so that they will be less likely to use this method. If doubt is expressed about limiting access to these methods, identify the pros and cons of having access to this method and whether there is an alternative way of limiting access so that the environment is safer. For firearms, consider asking a family member or friend who would be authorized to possess a firearm to remove it or consider locking up the firearm and ammunition separately.

**Table 9–1.** Safety planning steps *(continued)*

| |
|---|
| **Step 7. Identify and build up reasons to live.** Use the methods described in the section "Reasons for Living" later in this chapter. Spend enough time with the patient to recognize and amplify these especially valuable protective factors against suicide. |

ther is a civil engineer who spends many hours working. His mother is a schoolteacher. David noted that his father pushed him to excel in school, and when he didn't do well, he would be berated for not studying hard enough or taking his schoolwork seriously. His mother was supportive, but when David and his father argued, his mother was careful not to take sides. As a result, David responded poorly when he did not obtain the grades he desired. He studied for long hours and reported high anxiety and difficulty sleeping before taking his exams.

At one point when he was in high school, David obtained a poor grade on a math exam. He felt ashamed and predicted that his poor grade would keep him from getting into college. A sense of hopelessness gained force, and he subsequently took an overdose of acetaminophen. After telling his mother about the suicide attempt, he was taken to a hospital, where he was admitted. A brief hospital stay with prescription of escitalopram and supportive therapy was helpful in reducing symptoms of depression and thoughts of suicide.

Now in his last year of college, David is struggling again with depression and anxiety. He lives on campus and has a roommate who has become a good friend. And he has made other friends and developed interests in singing and volunteer work. However, he constantly worries about whether he will do well on exams. Recently, he obtained a low grade on one of his tests, and he began to feel hopeless and suicidal again. He did not have any intent to die or specific plans to kill himself. But recognizing that he was not doing well, he sought CBT to help with depression and anxiety and to reduce the chances of escalation of his suicidal thoughts.

In Video 23, David and Dr. Brown focus on David's recent feelings of anxiety and depression that were triggered by receiving a low grade. After addressing David's expectations for treatment, Dr. Brown conducted a comprehensive risk assessment followed by a narrative interview of the most recent setback in college and his recurrent thoughts of suicide. The video shows them developing a safety plan including identifying reasons to live. The following piece of dialogue from Video 23 gives an example of performing step 1 of safety planning (Table 9–1). Take time now to watch the entire video so you can see how to develop a full safety plan.

▶ **Video 23.** Safety Planning: Dr. Brown and David (8:37)

*Dr. Brown:* So thank you, David, for telling me your story. As you noticed, that crisis got more intense and then it came back down. One of the things that I'd like to do is identify some of the warning signs or triggers of that crisis. I want to record these on your safety plan so that you'll know when to use the safety plan. So what were some of the warning signs that you had?

*David:* Um...When I heard about the test score and not being able to make the grade, I just felt like a complete failure. It was so overwhelming because I put out my best and I didn't get the results I was looking for. So what good am I? My first thought was that my parents are so disappointed that I can't tell them. I was feeling overwhelmed and anxious about that—and just so ashamed that this was how things turned out.

*Dr. Brown:* That's a good summary. So let's write down, specifically, what they were. What should be first?

*David:* I guess when I start to feel overwhelmed or anxious.

*Dr. Brown:* So, "overwhelmed...anxious" (*writing*).

*David:* Or ashamed.

*Dr. Brown:* "Ashamed" (*writing*). What else?

*David:* Not being able to tell my parents. I'm usually very open and can talk to them about anything, but...when I need to shut down, and I feel like I can't share those things with them.

*Dr. Brown:* So "I can't tell my parents" (*writing*). And what else?

*David:* And just overall feeling like a failure.

*Dr. Brown:* "Feeling like a failure" (*writing*). So whenever you have any of these warning signs, you'll know to look at your safety plan. That's a cue to you to use it.

(*David nods.*)

*Dr. Brown:* So the first thing I want to talk about is when you go to that dark place, you're feeling overwhelmed, anxious, ashamed, having these other thoughts, and maybe feeling like giving up, that's when you use some strategies to help you get through the crisis or keep it from escalating. So what I'd like to do next is...see if we can brainstorm some strategies to take your mind off of your problems, kind of get away from that crisis for even a little while. What have you done in the past that's helped you deal with a crisis like this?

This sample of dialogue shows how both therapist and patient can work collaboratively on the safety plan and how it is important to use the patient's own words when completing it. Once the safety plan has been developed, review the steps of the plan with the individual and ask about the likelihood of using it. Also, determine where the safety plan will be kept so that the patient is likely to use it during a crisis. Finally, give the completed safety plan to the patient and retain a copy in the medical record. Explain how the safety plan can be reviewed later in treatment to determine how helpful it was for lowering risk, and how it can be revised, if needed, to be more useful.

## Reasons for Living

Earlier in this chapter, we emphasized the importance of asking for reasons for living as a way of assessing suicide risk. Questions about reasons for living also can be highly therapeutic because they can break through the negatively biased, hopeless thoughts of persons considering suicide and open their thinking to life-sustaining forces such as relationships with loved ones, spiritual or religious beliefs and values, unmet goals and aspirations, and enduring commitments.

As part of his work with inpatients who have just attempted suicide or who have very serious suicidal thoughts and plans, one of the authors (J.H.W.) typically begins to generate a list of reasons to live during the first session, asks the patient to post the list on the wall of his hospital room, enlists nurses and other staff to discuss these reasons with the patient, and adds depth to the list at subsequent visits. If the patient gives a reason such as "my grandchildren," the therapist might ask questions that build detail and strengthen the meaning of the reason. "What about your grandchildren makes you want to live…to overcome your suicidal thoughts? How do you see yourself with your grandchildren in the future? What would you be missing if you took your own life? What impact would your suicide have on them? Tell me about your grandchildren and why they are important to you."

A list of reasons to live is an important part of safety planning, as shown in Video 23. When Dr. Brown asks David about reasons to live, his first reply is "My family." Dr. Brown then asks "Anybody in particular?"—a prompt that yields results. David says: "My little sister…I'm like the world to her…She looks up to me.…I don't want to lose that." They go on to identify other reasons to live, including "my best friend"; "a lot of things I haven't gotten to do yet, like take a trip to China to see family"; and "joy in singing, I wouldn't want to give that up." The video segment ends after David talks about his joy in singing, but Dr. Brown went on to ask more questions to firm up David's resolve to live.

In cases where patients are unable to identify any reasons to live, or struggle to generate a substantive list, the therapist may need to suggest examples that may uncover reasons that have been obscured by depression or substance abuse. For example, inquiries could be made about activities that the patient used to enjoy. Another strategy is to ask about reasons they might have had to live before they became depressed or how they might see things differently if the depression or current life problems were resolved.

David's safety plan, including his reasons to live, is shown in Figure 9–1.

Step 1. Identify warning signs.

- Feeling overwhelmed and anxious
- Feeling ashamed
- Not being able to tell my parents
- Feeling like a failure

Step 2. Develop coping strategies.

- Singing by myself
- Cooking foods that remind me of home
- Pottery

Step 3. Identify social contacts and social settings.

- Spend time with roommate, Charlie

Step 4. Contact family members or friends.

- Call my best friend, Vanessa
- Visit with my sister or mother

Step 5. Contact professionals or agencies.

- Dr. Brown at office or answering service if office is closed*
- University of Pennsylvania Emergency Psychiatric Service*
- Suicide Prevention Lifeline 1-800-273-TALK (8255)

Step 6. Make the environment safe.

- I have no access to firearms.
- I'll give my medication to my roommate, who can dispense it daily.

Step 7. Identify and build up reasons to live.

- My family...my little sister
- My best friend
- Take a trip to China and other things I haven't done yet
- Joy in singing
- Volunteer work
- Having a family of my own

**Figure 9–1.** David's safety plan.

*Actual phone number of Dr. Brown and emergency psychiatric service would be entered here.

## Developing a Hope Kit

Patients also may be encouraged to develop a *hope kit,* a collection of items that reminds them of their reasons for living. To construct a hope kit, patients should review the reasons for living that were previously identified and then locate something as simple as a shoebox, envelope, or scrapbook where they can store mementos such as pictures, letters, postcards, prayers or poems, music, pieces of fabric, or other objects. Hope kits also can be built on computers, smartphones, and other devices. We have found that hope kits are quite enjoyable for patients and are one of the most useful strategies learned in CBT to address suicidal thoughts and behaviors. Moreover, during the course of constructing a hope kit, patients often find that they are able to identify reasons for living that they previously overlooked.

## Modifying Automatic Thoughts and Core Beliefs

Another fundamental part of CBT for suicide risk is to use the methods described in Chapter 5, "Working With Automatic Thoughts," and Chapter 8, "Modifying Schemas," to help patients develop skills to modify negative thoughts and schemas associated with suicide risk. We do not detail these methods here because they were fully explained earlier in the book. One example of a core CBT method that is particularly useful in suicide risk reduction is the use of coping cards. These cards contain adaptive coping statements that patients can review during a time of distress. We have found that coping cards are most likely to be located and used when they are developed during the session and then reinforced at subsequent sessions. An automatic thought that has occurred during a suicidal crisis may be written at the top of the card, and the alternative, more balanced response can be written on the remainder of the card. For example, a suicide-related thought might be "I can't take it anymore." The more balanced or adaptive statement could be "I know that I experience periods of time that are very difficult, but these feelings do not last for a long time, and I have been able to recover from them on my own.…I can call my friend Larry when I am feeling this way.…He helps me take my mind off my troubles when he comes over to visit."

## Behavioral Methods for Reducing Suicide Risk

The strategies described in Chapter 6, "Behavioral Methods I: Improving Mood, Increasing Energy, Completing Tasks, and Solving Problems," and Chapter 7, "Behavioral Methods II: Reducing Anxiety and Breaking Patterns of Avoidance," can provide additional resources for you to tap when working with patients at suicide risk. For example, you might initiate a behavioral action plan to help move a patient out of the depths of hopelessness. If she begins to take action that reduces distress, or shows a glimmer of pleasure and sense of accomplishment, her hope for future gains may improve. An anxiety-reducing method such as relaxation training could be used as a distraction from suicidal thoughts and as a way of easing painful emotions. A problem-solving initiative could help her find ways to cope with a stressor associated with suicidal thinking. Cognitive and behavioral methods you have learned from earlier work with this book and other training experiences can be put to excellent use in preventing relapse—the next section of this chapter.

# Consolidating Skills and Preventing Relapse

## Consolidating Key Skills

A few weeks before ending or tapering treatment, clinicians should ask patients to review and organize any notes that they have taken so they can easily refer to them in the future. If patients have not taken notes throughout the sessions, they might focus on making a therapy notebook or hope kit during the last few sessions. The clinician and patient can review and summarize the important points they have learned during therapy. Sometimes patients will resist writing or may not be able to write. In this case, the therapist can provide a written or audio-recorded summary of the skills they have learned.

## Guiding a Relapse Prevention Task

Following consolidation of specific skills, the therapist should introduce a *relapse prevention task* consisting of several guided imagery exercises in which patients imagine past suicidal crises, as well as crises that may occur in the future. The primary aim of this intervention is to have patients develop a detailed plan for how they could cope with potential triggers or crises. Thus, patients have an opportunity to practice their coping skills in a safe environment before applying them in a state of distress. The relapse prevention task also facilitates "overlearning" a specific skill so that patients remember to use it during a crisis. In addition, this task can help in assessment of treatment progress and provides valuable information on whether or not therapy can be reduced in frequency or stopped. If patients have difficulty successfully completing the relapse prevention task, then more work needs to be done in therapy, and the end of treatment is delayed until these skills can be applied during crisis periods.

### *Consent and Preparation*

Before conducting the relapse prevention task, the clinician should prepare patients to experience painful memories and aversive emotions. First, the clinician obtains verbal consent from patients to conduct the task. Patients are advised that this task has the potential to elicit unpleasant feelings, but the clinician will guide them through the activity and assist them in resolving such emotions by the end of the session. In addition, it is important to provide a sound rationale for this task in order to motivate patients to actively engage in this potentially aversive procedure. Patients are informed that by imagining the suicidal crisis and reliving the emotional turmoil they experienced, they will learn whether they can implement the coping strategies discussed in therapy. After a discussion of the risks and benefits of completing this task, some patients may prefer not to do it. In this case, the patients' preference is respected, but the clinician may review the coping skills that patients have learned and the manner in which they might apply these skills in the future.

## *Sequence of Guided Imagery*

With the patient's consent to proceed with the relapse prevention task, the clinician uses imagery methods (described in Chapter 5, "Working With Automatic Thoughts") to help the patient develop vivid images of the events leading up to the suicidal crisis. Patients are encouraged to close their eyes and describe the sequence of events out loud to the clinician and attempt to reexperience the emotions and thoughts that occurred at the time of the crisis. Then the clinician leads the patient through a similar task, but this time encourages the patient to describe the scenario using cognitive and behavioral skills to cope with the event and mitigate suicide risk. Next, patients are instructed to imagine in detail a future suicidal crisis and outline the manner in which they would apply the skills learned in treatment to cope with any suicidal thoughts that might be activated. After completing these guided imagery exercises, the clinician debriefs the patient, commending him for successfully engaging in such a difficult activity, and obtains feedback on whether that task was helpful for reducing future risk. If suicidal ideation emerged during the task, then the clinician assesses suicide risk near the end of the session and uses the strategies presented in this chapter to address it (for example, reviewing the safety plan). The clinician also may pose additional crisis scenarios to ensure that the patient has adequate flexibility in applying the skills learned in treatment to specific situations. We have found that new information about the suicidal crisis is often revealed during this task. Patients may feel more secure in revealing such information after a strong therapeutic alliance has been established.

**Learning Exercise 9–1.** Using CBT Methods to Reduce Suicide Risk

1. Enlist a colleague to role-play a patient with suicidal thoughts. Use the safety planning worksheet (see Appendix 1, "Worksheets and Checklists") to develop a safety plan. Be sure to add layers of depth to the reasons for living and take precautions to reduce access to means of committing suicide. Troubleshoot difficulties in developing an effective plan.

**Table 9–2.** Tips for working with suicidal patients

1. Therapists should be aware of their personal reactions when treating suicidal patients. Such reactions may include feeling overwhelmed, fearful, uncomfortable, or anxious about being responsible for someone's life; connecting with patients' profound psychological pain and suffering; or anticipating a legal liability regarding their welfare.
2. Therapists who experience such reactions in working with suicidal patients should identify their automatic thoughts and emotions and use cognitive-behavior therapy methods, such as examining the evidence, to think as rationally and effectively as possible about treating those at suicide risk. They should also employ positive coping behaviors such as those described in the section "Therapist Fatigue or Burnout" in Chapter 11, "Building Competence in Cognitive-Behavior Therapy."
3. Therapists should always maintain the belief that suicide is not an acceptable solution for life's problems. Being understanding and empathic is essential in treatment of suicidal patients. But therapists need to be careful not to fall into the trap of being swayed by the patient's hopelessness.
4. Therapists need to seek consultation with their supervisors or peers when they experience fearful, angry, or hopeless reactions when working with suicidal patients. Therapists who are feeling "stuck" when treating suicidal patients are likely to communicate their frustration or fear to patients. If therapists have no hope for helping their patients, how can they expect that patients will have hope about being helped?

2. Use CBT methods for suicide prevention with one or more patients with significant suicidal thoughts.

3. Perform a relapse prevention task with your patient. Consider future triggers for increased suicidal thinking and help the patient develop a coping plan for reducing risk of self-harm.

## Coping With the Rigors of Treating Suicidal Patients

One of the problems that can be encountered by clinicians who work with high-risk patients involves feeling overwhelmed or even hopeless about successfully treating the patient. This problem may arise when working with patients who have chronic or reoccurring episodes of suicidal thoughts or who make repeated suicide attempts or intentionally injure themselves. Table 9–2 provides some suggestions for coping with the difficulties of working with suicidal patients.

We encourage you to use a team approach, if possible, when providing CBT for suicidal patients. In this context, treatment teams typically consist of the therapist, supervisor, and case manager or other providers who are involved in the patients' mental health care. In our experience, therapists find case managers to be especially helpful because they assist the therapist in maintaining contact with patients by reminding them of their appointments, providing referrals for mental health and social services, and serving as a supportive contact person (Brown et al. 2005). If you are not working in a clinical environment that uses treatment teams, it can be helpful to communicate regularly with other providers or professionals, such as primary care doctors; pastors, rabbis, or imams; or other therapists who are providing a network of support and care for the patient.

## Summary

This chapter describes how CBT can be adapted for patients who are at risk for suicide. The innovative aspects of treatment with high-risk patients involve an understanding of the patient's motivations for suicide, screening and conducting a comprehensive suicide risk assessment, developing a collaborative safety plan, identifying reasons for living, constructing a hope kit, and consolidating CBT skills and practicing them to prevent future suicidal behavior. We recommend that clinicians adopt these strategies as core elements of their work with patients who are thinking of suicide.

## References

Bateman A, Fonagy P: Effectiveness of partial hospitalization in the treatment of borderline personality disorder: a randomized controlled trial. Am J Psychiatry 156(10):1563–1569, 1999 10518167

Beck AT, Steer RA, Brown GK: The Beck Depression Inventory, 2nd Edition. San Antonio, TX, Pearson, 1996

Brown GK, Stanley B: The Safety Plan Intervention (SPI) Checklist. University of Pennsylvania and Columbia University, 2016

Brown GK, Ten Have T, Henriques GR, et al: Cognitive therapy for the prevention of suicide attempts: a randomized controlled trial. JAMA 294(5):563–570, 2005 16077050

Guthrie E, Kapur N, Mackway-Jones K, et al: Randomised controlled trial of brief psychological intervention after deliberate self poisoning. BMJ 323(7305):135–138, 2001 11463679

Hatcher S, Sharon C, Parag V, Collins N: Problem-solving therapy for people who present to hospital with self-harm: Zelen randomised controlled trial. Br J Psychiatry 199(4):310–316, 2011 21816868

Knox KL, Stanley B, Currier GW, et al: An emergency department–based brief intervention for veterans at risk for suicide (SAFE VET). Am J Public Health 102 (suppl 1): S33–S37, 2012 22390597

Linehan MM, Comtois KA, Murray AM, et al: Two-year randomized controlled trial and follow-up of dialectical behavior therapy vs therapy by experts for suicidal behaviors and borderline personality disorder. Arch Gen Psychiatry 63(7):757–766, 2006 16818865

Rudd MD, Bryan CJ, Wertenberger EG, et al: Brief cognitive-behavioral therapy effects on post-treatment suicide attempts in a military sample: results of a randomized clinical trial with 2-year follow-up. Am J Psychiatry 172(5):441–449, 2015 25677353

Slee N, Garnefski N, van der Leeden R, et al: Cognitive-behavioural intervention for self-harm: randomised controlled trial. Br J Psychiatry 192(3):202–211, 2008 18310581

Stanley B, Brown GK: Safety Planning Intervention: a brief intervention to mitigate suicide risk. Cogn Behav Pract 19(2):256–264, 2012

Stanley B, Brown G, Brent DA, et al: Cognitive-behavioral therapy for suicide prevention (CBT-SP): treatment model, feasibility, and acceptability. J Am Acad Child Adolesc Psychiatry 48(10):1005–1013, 2009 19730273

Wright JH, Turkington D, Kingdon DG, Basco MR: Cognitive-Behavior Therapy for Severe Mental Illness: An Illustrated Guide. Washington, DC, American Psychiatric Publishing, 2009

# 10 Treating Chronic, Severe, or Complex Disorders

After completing your initial training in cognitive-behavior therapy (CBT)—which is usually best accomplished through supervised work with patients with major depressive disorder or one of the common anxiety disorders—it is time to gain experience working with patients with more complex problems. A number of research studies have documented the utility of CBT and related models of therapy for patients with severe or treatment-resistant disorders such as chronic depression, schizophrenia, bipolar disorder, and personality disorders.

For these populations of patients with conditions that are more difficult to treat, several common elements guide therapy. These include the following:

- The cognitive-behavioral model and all aspects of CBT are fully compatible with appropriate forms of pharmacotherapy.
- Regardless of the level of severity or impairment, the therapeutic relationship is characterized by the collaborative empirical stance.
- Homework assignments build directly on the material addressed within sessions.
- Therapeutic strategies target aspects of problematic cognitions, affects, or behaviors.

- When indicated, family members and significant others may be invited to join the therapy team to facilitate progress in therapy.
- Outcomes are assessed and methods of therapy are adjusted to maximize the chances for improvement.

In this chapter, we briefly review CBT and related models of therapy that have been adapted for use with patients who have severe, chronic, or treatment-resistant psychiatric conditions. The emphasis is on discussing empirical evidence for these approaches and providing general guidelines for working with patients with more complex or disabling illnesses. Books and treatment manuals for CBT of problems such as schizophrenia, bipolar disorder, and personality disorders are listed in Appendix 2, "Cognitive-Behavior Therapy Resources."

## Severe, Recurrent, Chronic, and Treatment-Resistant Depressive Disorders

Traditional models for the treatment of depressive disorders either implicitly or explicitly suggest that severe or chronic depression is largely biological in nature and therefore is more likely to require somatic forms of therapy (American Psychiatric Association 1993; Rush and Weissenburger 1994; Thase and Friedman 1999). Although the results of some early studies suggest that severely depressed outpatients may be less responsive to CBT than patients with milder depression (Elkin et al. 1989; Thase et al. 1991), severe depression is not a contraindication to CBT alone. In fact, results of several meta-analyses of individual patient data derived from comparative clinical trials suggested that more severely depressed patients are as likely to respond to CBT as to pharmacotherapy with antidepressants (DeRubeis et al. 1999; Weitz et al. 2015). In addition, a number of studies have demonstrated that the addition of standard CBT to pharmacotherapy resulted in significant improvement in the outcomes of patients with severe, recurrent, treatment-resistant, or chronic forms of major depressive disorder (Hollon et al. 2014; Rush et al. 2006; Thase et al. 1997, 2007; Watkins et al. 2011; Wiles et al. 2013; Wong 2008).

### Standard Cognitive-Behavior Therapy

Several modifications of standard CBT have been recommended for patients with markedly severe or chronic depressive disorders (Fava et al. 1994; Thase and Howland 1994; Wright et al. 2009). Standard CBT methods are fully described along with video examples in *Cognitive-Behav-*

**Table 10–1.** Potential targets for cognitive-behavior therapy of treatment-resistant depression

| |
|---|
| Hopelessness |
| Suicide risk reduction |
| Anhedonia |
| Low energy |
| Anxiety |
| Negative automatic thoughts |
| Maladaptive beliefs |
| Interpersonal problems |
| Nonadherence to pharmacotherapy |

*ior Therapy for Severe Mental Illness: An Illustrated Guide* (Wright et al. 2009). These modifications are designed to adapt commonly used methods for CBT, as originally conceptualized by A.T. Beck and colleagues (1979)) and described in this book, for treatment of chronic and severe depression. These adaptations center on several observations: 1) patients with more-difficult-to-treat depression can become discouraged, hopeless, or burned out with treatment; 2) chronic depression is associated with significant suicide risk; 3) persons with treatment-resistant depression are usually plagued by slowed thinking and activity, low energy, and anhedonia; 4) symptoms such as anxiety and insomnia may require special attention; and 5) chronic depression is frequently associated with major interpersonal and social problems such as marital conflict, job loss, or financial difficulties. Targets for CBT are summarized in Table 10–1.

Addressing hopelessness and demoralization with CBT techniques and the methods for suicide risk reduction detailed in Chapter 9, "Cognitive-Behavior Therapy to Reduce Suicide Risk," are key elements of the CBT approach to chronic depression. Also, treatment modifications can include an early emphasis on behavioral strategies such as scheduling of activities and pleasant events, especially when the patient is deeply depressed and is having difficulty with intense anhedonia and very low energy. Therapists can use cognitive restructuring to address maladaptive thought patterns, but they may need to work intensively to help the patient carry out these interventions in therapy sessions and then in homework assignments. Problem-solving methods can also be targeted toward social and interpersonal difficulties.

The timing and pacing of CBT sessions for severely depressed patients should fit their level of symptoms and capacity to participate in therapy. For some patients, twice-weekly sessions can be undertaken early in the treatment process. If concentration is a significant problem, frequent brief sessions of 20–25 minutes may be more helpful than conventional sessions of 45–50 minutes. Methods for shorter CBT sessions are described in *High-Yield Cognitive-Behavior Therapy for Brief Sessions: An Illustrated Guide* (Wright et al. 2010).

## Well-Being Therapy

Fava and colleagues (Fava 2016; Fava and Ruini 2003; Fava et al. 1997, 1998a, 1998b, 2002) have developed well-being therapy (WBT), a variant of CBT, as a method of treating chronic depression and reducing risk of relapse. They describe two primary conceptualizations of well-being: hedonic and eudaimonic (Fava 2016; Fava and Ruini 2003). From the *hedonic* perspective, well-being is associated with positive emotions such as happiness and pleasure, in addition to satisfaction with various domains of a person's life. The *eudaimonic* perspective is concerned with fulfillment of potential and achieving self-realization. In WBT, these perspectives are combined as therapists help patients take positive actions in six key domains: environmental mastery, personal growth, purpose in life, autonomy, self-acceptance, and interpersonal relationships.

The core methods of WBT are closely related to standard CBT. For example, behavioral methods such as activity scheduling, graded exposure, and problem solving are used to foster environmental mastery and personal growth. Examining the evidence or other cognitive techniques are used to generate more positive thoughts and emotions. However, WBT adds specific methods that are not typically used in standard CBT. For example, in the early phases of WBT, patients are asked to keep a well-being log. This method is similar to the thought change record used in standard CBT, but the focus is on identifying states of well-being, not on distressing thoughts and emotions. Patients are coached on trying to spot feelings of well-being and to link these experiences with events in their lives. After patients build skills in these basic logging functions of WBT, they move on to well-being diaries that identify the thoughts or behaviors that interrupt or derail the states of well-being. When they are able to recognize interfering thoughts (e.g., negative automatic thoughts, maladaptive core beliefs) or behaviors (e.g., excessive focus on control or work, procrastination), they are encouraged to become an "observer" who suggests ways to nurture and sustain the well-being experiences.

After patients learn how to identify and sustain states of well-being, the next phase of WBT is to work on the six domains of functioning (Fava 2016). Standard CBT methods are the basic platform for modifying cognitions or behaviors that are interfering with progress in any of the domains. However, the therapist may employ a variety of other methods, such as those described by Viktor Frankl (1959) for finding meaning and purpose or interpersonal therapy strategies for enhancing positive relationships with others. The major difference with standard CBT is the increased attention to promotion of personal growth, self-realization, and living a purposeful life.

## Cognitive Behavioral Analysis System of Psychotherapy

McCullough (1991, 2001) suggested a different set of modifications of CBT for work with patients with chronic depressive disorders. His approach, systematized as the cognitive behavioral analysis system of psychotherapy (CBASP; McCullough 2001), is based on observations that persons with chronic depression develop persistent difficulties with effectively defining and solving interpersonal problems. The CBASP method involves teaching patients how to effectively manage social situations, in addition to revising dysfunctional cognitions. However, less attention is paid to cognitive restructuring than in the standard CBT approach used in other studies of CBT for treatment-resistant depression (Thase et al. 2007; Watkins et al. 2011; Wiles et al. 2013; Wong 2008). One large study of chronic forms of depression found a robust additive effect for the combination of CBASP and pharmacotherapy (Keller et al. 2000), whereas a study using a more complex medication strategy failed to document added benefit (Kocsis et al. 2009). Readers interested in CBASP are referred to McCullough 2001 for a detailed explanation of how to implement this treatment method for chronic depression.

## Mindfulness-Based Cognitive Therapy

Another approach, mindfulness-based cognitive therapy (MBCT), was developed by John Teasdale, Zindel Segal, and J. Mark Williams (Segal et al. 2002; Williams et al. 2007) to complement conventional CBT strategies for relapse/recurrence prevention. Like more traditional approaches to relapse prevention, the MBCT model posits that people who are vulnerable to depression are prone to respond to relevant stressors or cues by automatic cognitive processes (e.g., automatic negative thoughts or activation of depressive core beliefs). In contrast to conventional CBT, a primary goal of MBCT is to teach individuals to observe and accept these negative cognitions without judging them or trying to correct them (Segal et al. 2002).

Building on the methods of mindfulness-based stress reduction popularized by Kabat-Zinn (1990), MBCT teaches individuals to use meditation and related strategies to heighten awareness of the thoughts and feelings that have habitually been associated with depressive states and to practice acceptance. Sometimes referred to as gaining meta-cognitive awareness, this decentering strategy helps the individual perceive and accept thoughts and feelings as both impermanent and objective occurrences in the mind, not factual statements about his or her true self. Beyond experiential evidence that this approach can reduce distress and decrease or prevent depressive symptoms, studies using neuroimaging of those who practice mindfulness meditation show improvements in mechanisms related to emotion regulation and attentional control (e.g., see Ives-Deliperi et al. 2013).

MBCT is typically conducted in groups that can range from a more traditional size (e.g., four to six participants) to an auditorium full of participants. The best-studied protocols for MBCT for depressive relapse prevention are typically 8 weeks long, with sessions ranging from 1 to 2 hours. Some programs begin therapy with an all-day introductory workshop. As in conventional CBT, there is great emphasis on the value of homework to practice skills in real-world situations. Evidence is emerging to suggest that the amount of time spent practicing MBCT strategies is a key moderator of therapeutic benefit.

With respect to efficacy for prevention of depressive relapses or recurrences, a meta-analysis was conducted on results of 9 controlled studies with a combined total of 1,258 patients (Kuyken et al. 2016). The authors found that MBCT significantly reduced the risk of depressive relapse as compared to those who did not receive MBCT. Nevertheless, results of a large study by Huijbers et al. (2016) indicate that MBCT does not fully normalize the risk of relapse/recurrence following discontinuation of antidepressants. Patients withdrawn from antidepressants showed more than a 25% greater risk of relapse/recurrence than did those who remained on medication.

## Bipolar Disorder

Converging lines of evidence have established that 1) only a minority of patients with bipolar disorder respond to standard pharmacotherapies with long periods of remission; 2) nonadherence with medication regimens is a major cause of relapse; 3) stress increases the likelihood of illness episodes, whereas social support has beneficial effects; and 4) most people with bipolar disorder must cope with high levels of stress because of marital or relationship difficulties, unemployment or underemployment, periods of outright disability, and other problems that impair quality of life. Thus there are multiple reasons to evaluate the potential benefits of CBT and other psychotherapies for people with bipolar disorder.

The overall results of research studies on the effectiveness of CBT for bipolar disorder have been positive. Although a large study (Scott et al. 2006) found that CBT was more helpful than treatment as usual only for those patients with fewer than 12 previous episodes, and another trial (Parikh et al. 2012) reported that CBT was no better than psychoeducation, most investigations have observed benefits in reducing patients' symptoms, shortening the time to recovery, and/or improving functioning (Gregory 2010; Isasi et al. 2010; Jones et al. 2015; Lam et al. 2003; Miklowitz et al. 2007a, 2007b; Szentagotai and David 2010). For example, the multicenter Systematic Treatment Enhancement Program for Bipolar Disorder (STEP-BD) study found that CBT improved total functioning, relationship functioning, and life satisfaction to a greater extent than pharmacotherapy alone (Miklowitz et al. 2007b); and Jones et al. (2015) reported enhanced recovery and increased time to relapse in patients with bipolar disorder.

Comprehensive methods of CBT for bipolar disorder have been developed by Basco and Rush (2007) and Newman et al. (2002). These methods are explained and shown in videos in *Cognitive-Behavior Therapy for Severe Mental Illness: An Illustrated Guide* (Wright et al. 2009). CBT of bipolar disorder begins with the assumption that pharmacotherapy with a mood stabilizer (and possibly an atypical antipsychotic medication) is a necessary precondition for effective therapy; psychotherapy thus is viewed as having a treatment-enhancing or adjunctive role. Although an attempt might be made to use CBT alone for bipolar depressed patients who refuse pharmacotherapy, we recommend concomitant use of lithium, divalproex, or another mood stabilizer or atypical antipsychotic medication with proven prophylactic effects against mania.

The goals of CBT for bipolar disorder are summarized in Table 10–2. Each goal is discussed further in the text below.

The first goal is to provide **psychoeducation** about bipolar disorder. The psychoeducational process includes teaching the patient about 1) the biology of bipolar disorder, 2) pharmacotherapy of this condition (if the clinician is a physician or nurse practitioner), 3) the effects of stress on symptom expression, 4) the impact of alterations in sleep and activity on well-being, and 5) the cognitive and behavioral elements of both depression and mania.

Involvement in **self-monitoring** is the second goal of CBT for bipolar disorder. Early in the course of therapy, patients are taught to monitor several manifestations of their illness (e.g., symptoms, activities, and moods). Self-monitoring has several purposes: 1) to help separate features of the illness from normal moods and behaviors, 2) to evaluate how the illness affects the patient's day-to-day life, 3) to develop an early

**Table 10–2.** Goals of cognitive-behavior therapy for bipolar disorder

1. Educate the patient and family about bipolar disorder.
2. Teach self-monitoring.
3. Routinize circadian rhythms.
4. Develop relapse prevention strategies.
5. Enhance adherence to pharmacotherapy regimens.
6. Relieve symptoms with cognitive and behavioral methods.
7. Develop a plan for long-term management of bipolar disorder.

warning system for signs of relapse, and 4) and to identify targets for psychotherapeutic intervention.

Because people with bipolar disorder are prone to living rather chaotic, disorganized lifestyles and having sleep difficulties, the third goal of CBT focuses on efforts to **promote regularity** in the daily schedule. Activity monitoring and scheduling can include goals of having consistent bedtime and wakening times 7 days a week, in addition to regular times for meals and other common activities.

**Developing relapse prevention strategies** is a critical fourth goal of CBT for bipolar disorder. One method used to promote relapse prevention is the production of a customized symptom summary worksheet that clearly delineates the changes that the patient and his family observe when he is beginning to exhibit early warning signs of mania or depression. This document is used as an early warning system to spot shifts in mood or behavior before a severe episode occurs. The therapist then helps the patient devise specific cognitive and behavioral strategies that are targeted toward limiting or reversing the progression of symptoms. For example, an inclination to think of schemes to rapidly make money might be countered with a list of advantages and disadvantages of pursuing these ideas and a behavioral plan to report these ideas to the therapist before taking any action.

A symptom summary worksheet for a man with hypomanic and manic symptoms is shown in Figure 10–1. This 33-year-old man with bipolar disorder was able to write down specific changes that typically occurred when he began to cycle into a manic episode. Detailed instructions on using this technique and other CBT methods for relapse prevention can be found in Basco and Rush (2007).

The fifth goal of CBT for bipolar disorder is one of the most important: **enhancing adherence to pharmacotherapy regimens**. From the CBT perspective, nonadherence is a common and understandable problem

| Mild symptoms | Moderate symptoms | Severe symptoms |
|---|---|---|
| I start thinking of ideas and schemes to make a lot of money, but I don't do anything about it. | I am actively searching for inventions or investments that will make a lot of money or make me famous. | I try to withdraw funds from my IRA, get loans, or find some other way to get money to invest in a big deal or to start a new business. |
| I may have trouble falling asleep because my mind is full of ideas, but I try to sleep 7 hours so I can be rested to go to work. | I delay going to bed for 1–2 hours past the normal time. I'm too occupied with other things to want to sleep. | I only sleep 2–4 hours a night. |
| I feel more lively than usual. I don't care as much about my everyday problems. I want to party. | I go out a lot at night and ignore the work reports and planning documents I should be doing at home. I don't drink to excess, but I do have three to four beers when I go out with friends. | I spend way too much money entertaining, going out to fancy restaurants, etc. I've taken off on a whim to fly to New York City for a weekend and have charged beyond my limit on credit cards. |
| My mind feels more creative than usual. Ideas come easily. | My mind is going too fast. I don't pay attention to other people. I make mistakes at work because I don't pay attention. | I'm really juiced up. I'm thinking of so many different things that I'm jumping all over the place. |
| I'm a little more irritable than normal. I don't have much tolerance for people who I think are lazy. I'm more critical of my girlfriend than usual. | I get into lots of arguments at work and with my girlfriend. | I'm insufferable. |
| People I know well (my girlfriend and my mother) tell me that I need to slow down. They can tell that I'm speaking more rapidly or that I seem charged up. | I'm definitely speaking more rapidly and loudly than normal. Others seem to be irritated with the way that I talk to them. | I'm talking a mile a minute. I'm often impolite. I interrupt others and can shout in conversations. |

**Figure 10–1.** A patient's symptom summary worksheet: an example of hypomanic and manic symptoms.

that frequently complicates treatment of chronic disorders. Treatment adherence can be enhanced by identifying obstacles to regular medication taking and then systematically addressing these roadblocks. Troubleshooting Guide 5 gives useful tips for promoting treatment adherence for all psychiatric disorders.

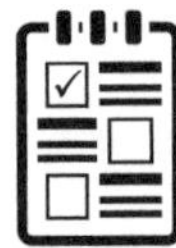

## Troubleshooting Guide 5
### Problems With Adherence to Pharmacotherapy

1. **Adherence not assessed regularly.** You might be surprised to learn how often people miss doses of medications. Studies have found that patients with either bipolar disorder or unipolar depression have nonadherence rates of about 50% (Akincigil et al. 2007; Keck et al. 1997). Thus, it is a good idea to inquire about adherence on a routine basis, even with patients you assume are taking medication as prescribed. Ask questions that invite the patient to talk about medication taking in a collaborative manner. For example, you could ask, "How is your medication taking going?… How about problems in taking the medication regularly?… What percent of the medication do you think you take each week?"

2. **Patient has negative thoughts about taking medication.** Encourage your patient to be open to the possibility that irregular medication taking might represent one of those chains of "thoughts/feelings/behaviors" that can be addressed in therapy. A homework assignment could be used to keep track of such thoughts and to examine them using standard CBT methods (e.g., checking for cognitive errors, using a thought change record). Some of the most common thoughts associated with adherence issues include "I feel fine, so I don't need to take this medication anymore.…I should be able to do this on my own.… I hate this medication because it causes [fill in the blank with the most disagreeable side effects]."

3. **Medication isn't helping.** One of the most frequently cited reasons for nonadherence is the patient's conclusion that the medication is not working or is unlikely to work. If the pharmacotherapy regimen isn't effective, the clinician (if a prescribing provider) needs to consider modifications of the treatment plan. However, patients may benefit from further education about giving certain medications time to work. They can be encouraged to discuss their concerns about effectiveness before stopping treatment on their own. And hopeless or excessively pessimistic views of the potential benefits of medication can be modified with CBT methods.

**Troubleshooting Guide 5 *(continued)***
**Problems With Adherence to Pharmacotherapy**

4. **Patient criticizes self because of nonadherence and may be ashamed to admit problems with taking medication.** It is usually helpful to normalize adherence difficulties. Discuss how common such problems are in taking medicine for a wide range of ailments. You might use appropriate personal revelation to show how you also have had times of less than perfect medication taking. Perhaps you could share a story about taking a short course of antibiotics and having some doses left over at the end of 7–10 days. It may be useful to think about adherence to taking medication along a continuum of success, not measured in shades of black or white.

5. **Patient has trouble with complicated medication regimen.** The greater the number of medications prescribed and the greater the frequency that medications are to be taken, the greater the likelihood of errors, mistakes, and omissions. In current practice, most patients with bipolar disorder are taking two, three, four, or even more psychotropic medications. Look together for ways to streamline the regimen. And if you are not the prescriber, determine if your patient might need help in negotiating changes.

6. **Forgetting.** When forgetting is an issue, work with your patient on solutions. For example, once-a-day medications can be taken together with a regular event such as brushing teeth (morning or bedtime) or breakfast. Daily or weekly pill containers can be used. And most people will have access to one or more forms of technology that can be harnessed to provide relatively unobtrusive prompts.

The sixth goal is **relief of symptoms through cognitive-behavioral interventions**. The methods used for addressing depressive symptoms are the same as in standard CBT. In treating hypomanic symptoms, the therapist may focus on using behavioral strategies to treat insomnia, overstimulation, hyperactivity, and pressured speech. For example, CBT methods for insomnia (e.g., reducing distractions in the sleeping environment, providing education on healthy sleep patterns, and using thought stopping or diversions to decrease the rate of intrusive or racing thoughts) have been shown to be effective in restoring normal sleep patterns (Siebern and Manber 2011; Taylor and Pruiksma 2014). Efforts also might be made to set behavioral goals for cutting back on stimulating activities or monitoring and controlling the rate of speech.

Cognitive restructuring methods can be used to help hypomanic individuals identify and modify distorted thinking (Newman et al. 2002). Examples of these types of interventions are 1) spotting cognitive errors (e.g., magnifying one's sense of competence or power, ignoring risks, overgeneralizing from one positive feature to a more grandiose view of self), 2) using thought recording techniques to recognize expansive or irritating cognitions, and 3) listing advantages and disadvantages of holding on to an overly positive belief or prediction.

The seventh goal of CBT for bipolar disorder is to **help patients with long-term illness management**, including making lifestyle changes, facing and coping with stigma, and dealing more effectively with stressful life problems. In these capacities, CBT is distinguished from more supportive models of therapy by continued use of mood and activity monitoring, a stepwise approach to problem solving, and cognitive methods such as weighing the evidence to guide decision making.

## Personality Disorders

Perhaps 30%–60% of patients with mood and anxiety disorders also meet criteria for one or more of the personality disorders listed in DSM-5 (American Psychiatric Association 2013; Grant et al. 2005). Although not all studies are in agreement, personality disorders typically have negative prognostic implications and decrease the probability of response to treatment for mood and anxiety disorders, slow the temporal course of recovery, or increase the likelihood of relapse (Thase 1996). Interestingly, findings from several early studies of major depressive disorder suggest that comorbid personality disorder may not adversely affect response to CBT (Shea et al. 1990; Stuart et al. 1992). Although these studies excluded patients with the most severe personality disorders, the findings do suggest that the structured methods used in CBT may be particularly well suited for patients with personality disorders.

The presence of a personality disorder is usually evident by the beginning of young adult life. However, personality pathology is not a static process and may be exaggerated by anxiety (e.g., increased avoidance), depression (e.g., increased dependence or exacerbation of borderline traits), or hypomania (e.g., increased narcissistic or histrionic traits). If your patient is presenting for treatment of depression or anxiety, it is often useful to defer definitive assessment of personality disorders until after at least partial resolution of the mood or anxiety disorder. On occasion, compelling clinical evidence of a personality disorder is not apparent until after treatment has been initiated. In such cases, your treatment plan may need to be revised.

The CBT model for treatment of personality disorders focuses on the interactions between the individual's organizing beliefs or schemas that guide behavior, dysfunctional (and typically excessive) interpersonal strategies, and environmental influences (A.T. Beck et al. 2015; J.S. Beck 2011). Personality disorders are viewed as being influenced by adverse developmental experiences. Young and colleagues (2003) outlined five thematic areas: 1) disconnection and rejection, 2) impaired autonomy and performance, 3) impaired limits, 4) other-directedness, and 5) overvigilance and inhibition.

Therapy of personality disorders generally uses many of the same methods developed for treatment of mood and anxiety disorders, but with a greater emphasis on schema work and on developing more effective coping strategies (J.S. Beck 2011). Other differences between CBT for treatment of personality disorders and CBT for treatment of depression and anxiety are the following: 1) the duration of therapy is usually much longer (i.e., a year or more); 2) more attention is paid to the therapeutic relationship and to transference reactions in working toward change; and 3) repeated practice of CBT methods is needed to modify chronic problems with self-concept, relationships with others, and emotional regulation and social skills.

Outlined in Table 10–3 are some of the predominant core beliefs, compensatory beliefs, and associated behavioral strategies common to specific personality disorders. Once a problematic schema or core belief is identified, CBT strategies such as examining the evidence and considering alternative explanations can be implemented.

## Dialectical Behavior Therapy

Linehan's (1993) dialectical behavior therapy (DBT) is one of the principal adaptations of CBT for personality disorders. DBT is distinguished by four key features: 1) the individual's acceptance and validation of his behavior in the moment, 2) emphasis on identifying and treating therapy-interfering behaviors, 3) use of the therapeutic relationship as an essential vehicle for behavior change, and 4) a focus on dialectical processes (defined below in this section). Evidence from randomized controlled clinical trials (Bohus et al. 2004; Linehan and Wilks 2015; Linehan et al. 1991; Robins and Chapman 2004) demonstrates that DBT can effectively reduce self-injurious and parasuicidal behavior, a finding that has

**Table 10–3.** Personality disorders: beliefs and strategies

| Personality disorder | Core belief about self | Belief about others | Assumptions | Behavioral strategy |
|---|---|---|---|---|
| **Avoidant** | I'm undesirable. | Other people will reject me. | If people know the real me, they'll reject me.<br>If I put on a facade, they may accept me. | Avoid intimacy |
| **Dependent** | I'm helpless. | Other people should take care of me. | If I rely on myself, I'll fail.<br>If I depend on others, I'll survive. | Rely on other people |
| **Obsessive-compulsive** | My world could go out of control. | Other people can be irresponsible. | If I'm not in total control, my world could fall apart.<br>If I impose tight rules and structure, things will turn out OK. | Control myself and others |
| **Paranoid** | I'm vulnerable. | Other people are malicious. | If I trust other people, they will harm me.<br>If I am on my guard, I can protect myself. | Be suspicious |
| **Antisocial** | I can do what I want. | Other people don't matter. | If I exploit others, I'll get what I want. | Exploit others |
| **Narcissistic** | I'm superior. (An underlying belief can be "I'm inferior.") | Other people are inferior. (An underlying core belief can be "Others are superior.") | If others regard me in a nonspecial way, it means they consider me inferior.<br>If I achieve my entitlements, it shows I'm special. | Demand special treatment |

**Table 10–3.** Personality disorders: beliefs and strategies *(continued)*

| Personality disorder | Core belief about self | Belief about others | Assumptions | Behavioral strategy |
|---|---|---|---|---|
| **Histrionic** | I'm nothing. | Other people may not value me for myself alone. | If I am not entertaining, others won't be attracted to me.<br>If I am dramatic, I'll get others' attention and approval. | Entertain |
| **Schizoid** | I'm a social misfit. | Other people have nothing to offer me. | If I keep my distance from others, I'll make out better.<br>If I try to have relationships, they won't work out. | Distance self from others |
| **Schizotypal** | I am defective. | Other people are threatening. | If I sense that others are feeling negatively toward me, it must be true.<br>If I'm wary of others, I can divine their true intentions. | Assume hidden motives |
| **Borderline personality disorder** | I'm defective.<br>I'm helpless.<br>I'm vulnerable.<br>I'm bad. | Other people will abandon me. People can't be trusted. | If I depend on myself, I won't survive.<br>If I trust others, they'll abandon me.<br>If I depend on others, I'll survive but ultimately be abandoned. | Vacillate in extremes of behavior |

*Source.* Adapted from Beck JS: "Cognitive Approaches to Personality Disorders," in *American Psychiatric Press Review of Psychiatry*, Vol. 16. Edited by Dickstein LJ, Riba MB, Oldham JM. Washington, DC, American Psychiatric Press, 1997, pp. 73–106. Copyright © 1997 American Psychiatric Press. Used with permission.

encouraged an expanding use of these methods in clinical practice. Also, DBT has been successfully adapted for work with patients with substance abuse and eating disorders in addition to personality disorders (Linehan and Wilks 2015; Linehan et al. 2002; Palmer et al. 2003).

Beyond helping to name the therapy, the term *dialectical* describes the core philosophical underpinnings of this approach. Linehan (1993) chose this term to describe a holistic approach to psychopathology, drawing heavily on both Western and Eastern philosophies. Rather than viewing dysfunctional behavior as simply a symptom of an illness, the DBT approach follows the principle that even very problematic behavior serves certain functions. For example, splitting between various helpers or care providers may minimize (at least in the short run) the chances for receiving unwelcome, critical feedback and may maximize the chances of obtaining a desired outcome. A similar strategy is sometimes referred to in the business world as "playing both ends against the middle." Progress in therapy involves helping patients to recognize their ultimate goals and to be able to consider, and eventually implement, alternate, more socially acceptable methods to accomplish these goals.

DBT also is directed at coaching the patient on ways of gaining a better sense of balance between competing goals; for example, between acceptance and change, flexibility and stability, or eliciting nurturance and obtaining autonomy. Mindfulness practices are commonly used to help achieve these goals (see section "Mindfulness-Based Cognitive Therapy" earlier in this chapter). The concept of *mindfulness* in DBT refers to teaching patients to better focus on the activity of the moment (i.e., to observe, describe, and participate), rather than being overwhelmed by strong emotions (Linehan 1993). Therapists also draw upon the behavioral methods from CBT (described in Chapter 7, "Behavioral Methods II: Reducing Anxiety and Breaking Patterns of Avoidance"), such as relaxation training, thought stopping, and breathing training, to assist patients with managing painful emotions. In addition, social skills training strategies, including cognitive and behavioral rehearsal, are employed to help patients learn more effective methods to cope with interpersonal disputes.

## Substance Use Disorders

Evidence regarding the utility of cognitive and behavioral therapies for substance use disorders (SUDs) has grown since the first studies were conducted in the 1980s and 1990s (e.g., Carroll et al. 1994; Woody et al. 1984). Although not all studies have yielded unequivocally positive outcomes (e.g., see Crits-Christoph et al. 1999; Project MATCH Re-

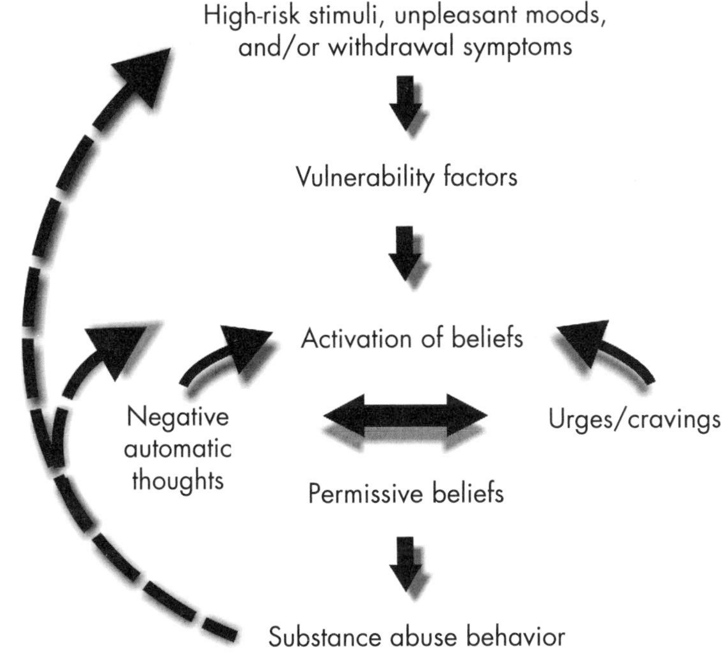


**Figure 10–2.** Cognitive-behavioral model of substance abuse.
*Source.* Adapted from Thase 1997.

search Group 1998), the weight of the evidence supports the use of CBT as part of a comprehensive treatment program for alcohol use disorder and other SUDs (Carroll 2014). As illustrated in Figure 10–2, the CBT model of substance abuse recognizes the highly interdependent and reciprocal nature of the affects, behaviors, and cognitions associated with problematic drug or alcohol use. Although there are important sociodemographic, physiological, and clinical differences among the various SUDs, the cognitive-behavioral model posits that a common underlying process links the act of using intoxicating substances with underlying beliefs, cue-elicited urges and cravings, and negative automatic thoughts (A.T. Beck et al. 1993; Thase 1997).

Several important tasks precede the initiation of formal therapy with CBT for substance abuse. First, if the SUD is characterized by a potentially dangerous withdrawal syndrome, enrollment in a medically supervised detoxification program may be necessary. Second, the patient's readiness for change should be assessed (Prochaska and DiClemente 1992). Motivation for therapy should be understood as occurring on a continuum, ranging from the stages of precontemplation (e.g., "I don't have a problem—I simply got caught driving after drinking a little too much"), contemplation, preparation, and finally to action. The methods of motivational interviewing (Miller et al. 2004; Strang and McCambridge 2004) are particularly well suited to help patients move from the precontemplation and contemplation stages to the preparation and action stages. A third precondition is to establish a sobriety contract. Specifically, patients should commit to not coming to sessions under the influence of drugs or alcohol, and therapists need to learn to be comfortable saying "no—not today" when this contract is violated.

An important aspect of the CBT model is to help the patient recognize that urges and cravings to drink alcohol or use drugs are often associated with activation of relevant beliefs about drug or alcohol abuse. Cognitions related to substance abuse can occur almost instantaneously in response to personally relevant cues (i.e., the "persons, places and things," as made popular by Alcoholics Anonymous). Although the distinction is somewhat artificial, urges can be conceptualized as the cognitive and behavioral predispositions to use drugs or alcohol, whereas cravings are the affective and physiological experiences that accompany the urges. In addition to situational cues, such as driving past a bar or seeing a television advertisement, urges and cravings also can be triggered by daydreams, memories, or dysphoric emotions (most commonly anger, anxiety, sadness, or even boredom). Examples of beliefs relevant to the onset and maintenance of SUDs are provided in Table 10–4.

As the frequency and intensity of substance abuse increases, further cognitive changes can play a role in the evolution of the disorder. For example, there may be a tendency to devalue beliefs about more conventional mainstream goals and pursuits, including the desirability of maintaining the love, support, and approval of significant others. Similarly, beliefs about the adverse consequences of drugs and alcohol tend to be minimized, and attitudes pertaining to the positive effects of drinking or drug use are exaggerated. Secondary or *permissive* beliefs also tend to develop (e.g., "I can get high this one last time and can restart working on my sobriety program tomorrow" and "Once I start using, I can't stop—so I might as well go ahead and enjoy the high"). Such beliefs help to explain the all-too-common tendency for a single use or lapse to spiral into a full-blown relapse.

Therapy thus proceeds down two simultaneous tracks: 1) achieving and maintaining sobriety, and 2) identifying and modifying the relevant beliefs and behaviors that predispose to and maintain problematic sub-

**Table 10–4.** Examples of beliefs about substance abuse

| |
|---|
| I can't control my cravings. |
| The only thing I can do to cope with craving is to use. |
| I can't learn to stop drinking—it's part of who I am. |
| People who stop using have willpower, which I lack. |
| Life is boring without getting high. |
| I've already ruined my life, so I should go ahead and get high. |
| I can always quit later—I'm not ready to stop yet. |

stance use (see A.T. Beck et al. 1993). As success is gained in these areas, additional longer-range therapy goals may be addressed, including lifestyle and vocational changes. The cornerstone of successful CBT for substance abuse is relapse prevention (Marlatt and Gordon 1985). Relapse prevention strategies include both behavioral strategies to minimize the likelihood of encountering urges and cravings, and cognitive restructuring exercises to counter distorted negative thoughts about drinking or drug use. Also, it is usually a good idea to encourage patients to participate in self-help programs such as Alcoholics Anonymous.

## Eating Disorders

CBT has become accepted as one of the primary methods of treatment for eating disorders, and many reviews and meta-analyses have concluded that strong evidence exists for the effectiveness of CBT for bulimia nervosa and binge-eating disorder (Hay et al. 2014; Hofmann et al. 2012; McElroy et al. 2015; Vocks et al. 2010). However, the effectiveness of CBT for anorexia nervosa has not yet been established (Hay et al. 2015), and a multidimensional approach including medical, nutritional, and cognitive-behavioral treatment elements is recommended (Hay et al. 2014, 2015).

The CBT model for treating eating disorders is based on the notion that dysfunctional beliefs about slimness, and resulting dissatisfaction with body shape and weight, drive and maintain abnormal eating behavior and associated features such as purging and abuse of laxatives, diuretics, and diet pills. Contemporary societal standards that reinforce unrealistic goals regarding slimness interact with individual vulnerabilities (e.g., perfectionism, difficulty regulating affects, propensity for depression) in the development of these conditions.

Before working with an individual with an eating disorder, you may find it helpful to review the results of the classic study by Keys and colleagues

(Keys 1950; Taylor and Keys 1950), which examined the effects of semistarvation on the attitudes and behaviors of healthy young men. Although these volunteers had virtually no risk of spontaneously developing an eating disorder, during the course of marked caloric restriction and significant weight loss, they developed preoccupations with food, diminished libido, mood and sleep disturbances, and cold intolerance. When the experimental caloric restriction ended, binge-eating behavior, food hoarding, and disturbed hunger and satiety cues developed. Most of the subjects regained more weight than they had lost, and it took weeks for them to fully stabilize. These observations underscore the fact that whatever the individual's vulnerability, the process of starvation and disordered eating behavior can play a significant role in maintaining an eating disorder.

The CBT approach is necessarily multimodal and includes nutritional counseling in addition to psychoeducation, self-monitoring, and cognitive and behavioral interventions. It is generally a good idea to work with an experienced dietician. An initial goal of treatment is to collaboratively determine a target weight range and meal plan. It is imperative that a realistic goal be identified and a consistent method for monitoring weight be implemented. Usually a weekly weight measurement is sufficient. A meal plan generally consists of three regular meals and at least two snacks, with calories divided to minimize hunger cues. In the course of negotiating these terms of treatment, you will have ample opportunity to discuss the patient's concerns that the plan will backfire. Moreover, sharing facts about the futility of common strategies presumed to facilitate weight loss, such as purging or using laxatives, is an important aspect of psychoeducation.

Self-monitoring initially entails keeping track of mealtimes and problem eating behavior, as well as potential environmental cues and triggers. Subsequently, three-column worksheets are used to help establish the links between negative thoughts, dysphoric affects, and problem eating behavior. Various strategies are used to either change or, if necessary, avoid responses to cues. Response prevention (see Chapter 7, "Behavioral Methods II: Reducing Anxiety and Breaking Patterns of Avoidance") is an important tool to help patients learn to prolong the interval between the urge (i.e., to binge, purge, or restrict) and the problematic behavior. Cognitive restructuring exercises are then employed to help patients cope with distorted negative thoughts about the consequences of not engaging in disordered eating behavior.

## Schizophrenia

Schizophrenia is associated with a significantly greater likelihood of disability and a lower probability of the occurrence of periods of sustained and complete remission than most other severe psychiatric disorders, including bipolar I disorder. The chronic nature of this severe illness has provided impetus for the development of adjunctive psychosocial therapies. This need has persisted despite the introduction of a newer generation of antipsychotic drugs.

CBT for schizophrenia was established by the mid-1990s (Beck and Rector 2000; Garety et al. 1994; Kingdon and Turkington 2004). There is now solid evidence from a series of clinical trials that CBT can have significant effects in improving treatment outcome for schizophrenia (Burns et al. 2014; Mehl et al. 2015; Rector and Beck 2001; Sensky et al. 2000; Turkington et al. 2004; Turner et al. 2014). Although not all studies have found effectiveness for CBT, meta-analyses have concluded that CBT has a moderate impact on positive symptoms of schizophrenia (Burns et al. 2014; Jauhar et al. 2014; Mehl et al. 2015; Turner et al. 2014) and a significant, but less robust effect, on negative symptoms (Jauhar et al. 2014; Turner et al. 2014; Velthorst et al. 2015). The CBT approach for schizophrenia is detailed and illustrated with videos in *Cognitive-Behavior Therapy for Severe Mental Illness: An Illustrated Guide* (Wright et al. 2009).

Just as when using CBT in treatment of bipolar disorder, therapy should be initiated after the patient has begun to stabilize on psychotropic medication. Sessions may be brief at the beginning. In some cases, two or three 20-minute sessions for a week or two may be more helpful than a single 45- or 50-minute session. It is also reasonable to anticipate that an optimal course of therapy will be longer than would be indicated for major depressive disorder or panic disorder.

Beyond establishing a therapeutic relationship, initial goals usually include psychoeducation about the disorder (including eliciting the patient's beliefs about the nature of schizophrenia and its treatment), increased involvement in activities, and improved adherence to pharmacotherapy regimens. As therapy progresses, attention shifts to identifying and modifying delusions and helping patients reduce or cope with hallucinations. Delusions can be viewed as an extreme form of cognitive errors described in earlier chapters of this book. The individual draws inferences on the basis of an incomplete assessment of facts and ignores or minimizes disconfirming evidence. If a collaborative therapeutic relationship can be established, the patient may be able to benefit from using logical analysis methods such as examining the evidence and searching for alternative solutions.

Figure 10–3 shows an example of an exercise in examining the evidence completed by a 27-year-old man with schizophrenia. Ted had been doing volunteer work in the office of a community care center and had developed delusions about this environment. One of the triggers for

Troubling thought: The Mafia or a foreign intelligence agency has infiltrated this office and is controlling everything.

| Evidence for this troubling thought: | Evidence against this troubling thought: |
|---|---|
| 1. Computer messages are suspicious. | 1. Computer messages are sent to everyone's computer. They are just witty sayings or jokes. They probably don't mean anything. |
| 2. Two employees were fired last week. | 2. The people who got fired were always missing work. |
| 3. There seem to be listening devices implanted in the TV monitors. | 3. I took apart a TV and couldn't find anything suspicious. I tend to get paranoid. |
| 4. I don't have any close friends at the center. People rarely talk to me. | 4. It is true that I don't have many friends, but that doesn't mean that there is a plot to take over the center. I like doing this job, and everyone has treated me well. |

Alternative thoughts: I know that I have a chemical imbalance that makes me get paranoid. Sitting in front of a computer for a couple hours a day has made me more suspicious. This job is worth my trying to calm my fears.

**Figure 10–3.** Examining the evidence for delusions: Ted's example.

these delusions was the appearance of a daily message on his computer screen. Although the daily message—typically a humorous quotation—was sent to every computer in the facility, Ted interpreted the messages in a delusional way. He had begun to think that there was a plot by the Mafia or a foreign intelligence agency to take over the community care center. The technique of examining the evidence helped him recognize the distortions in his thinking and develop an alternative way of seeing the situation. In this case, Ted was encouraged to label the delusion as a *troubling thought* and to then apply standard CBT methods to test this cognition.

In treating hallucinations, it is usually helpful to introduce a *normalizing rationale*—namely, that nearly everyone can experience hallucinations under extreme circumstances (e.g., drug intoxication or marked sleep deprivation; Kingdon and Turkington 2004; Wright et al. 2009). This concept can help persons with schizophrenia feel less stigmatized and be willing to look at possible environmental influences that could be aggravating hallucinations or to explore alternative explanations for hallucinations (to replace concepts such as "It's the devil"; "God is talking to me"; or "A woman's voice is torturing me"). The general goals in treating hallucinations with CBT are to help patients 1) accept a rational explanatory model for hallucinations (e.g., the normalizing rationale or a biological vulnerability), and 2) develop methods of reducing or limiting the impact of hallucinations.

| Actions that make the voices softer or make them go away: | Actions that stimulate the voices or make them louder: |
|---|---|
| 1. Listening to soothing music | 1. Arguments with my boyfriend or family members |
| 2. Doing craft projects | 2. Sleeping poorly |
| 3. Imagining that the voices are going into a closet in my house, a blanket is placed over the voices, and the door is locked | 3. Forgetting to take medication |
| 4. Doing volunteer work at my church | 4. Watching violent or disturbing movies or TV shows |
| 5. Reading a magazine or a book | |
| 6. Telling myself I have a chemical imbalance and I don't need to pay attention to the voices | |
| 7. Going to group therapy at the day treatment center | |

**Figure 10–4.** Actions that make voices better or worse: Barbara's example.

One of the most helpful strategies for working with hallucinations is to generate a list of behaviors that either quiet the voices or make them less intrusive or commanding. The patient might also benefit from making a list of activities that worsen the voices. She can then develop a behavioral plan to increase helpful behaviors and decrease activities that amplify the hallucinations. An example of such a list of behaviors is presented in Figure 10–4. Barbara, a 38-year-old woman with schizophrenia, made this list of behaviors that helped her manage voices. She was able to identify a number of useful strategies, including diversionary activities, coaching herself on the nature of her illness (e.g., "I have a chemical imbalance, and I don't need to pay attention to the voices"), and an imagery technique that she designed herself without prompting from her therapist. Her plan also included efforts to learn how to better manage the situations and issues that appeared to aggravate her hallucinations.

Negative symptoms can be approached with activity scheduling, graded task assignments, behavioral rehearsal, skills training, and related strategies. However, experts in the treatment of schizophrenia with CBT often recommend a "go-slow" approach in which the patient is given plenty of time to begin making changes in symptoms such as social isolation, withdrawal, and lack of initiative (Kingdon and Turkington 2004; Wright et al. 2009). Keep in mind that even though negative symptoms may well reflect underlying neuropathology, individuals who have experienced more debilitating forms of brain injury, including stroke or multiple sclerosis, can learn to use compensatory coping strategies in systematic approaches to rehabilitation.

## Summary

Cognitive-behavioral methods have been developed and tested for a broad range of severe psychiatric disorders such as treatment-resistant depression, bipolar disorder, personality disorders, and schizophrenia. In addition, CBT techniques are a first-line treatment for bulimia nervosa and can provide useful tools for management of substance use problems. Although many of the standard cognitive and behavioral methods for depression and anxiety also can be used in the treatment of conditions that are more difficult to treat, specific modifications are recommended for advanced applications of CBT. In addition, we have outlined basic concepts of related therapies (i.e., WBT, MBCT, and DBT) that can offer alternate approaches if desired.

In this chapter, we described empirical research that supports the use of CBT for chronic and severe mental illnesses, and we briefly detailed some of the strategies that can be used to meet the challenges of working with these conditions. In Chapter 11, "Building Competence in Cognitive-Behavior Therapy," we suggest additional readings, workshops, and clinical supervision that can help build expertise in using CBT for severe psychiatric disorders.

## References

Akincigil A, Bowblis JR, Levin C, et al: Adherence to antidepressant treatment among privately insured patients diagnosed with depression. Med Care 45(4):363–369, 2007 17496721

American Psychiatric Association: Practice guideline for major depressive disorder in adults. Am J Psychiatry 150(4) (suppl):1–26, 1993 8465906

American Psychiatric Association: Diagnostic and Statistical Manual of Mental Disorders, 5th Edition. Arlington, VA, American Psychiatric Association, 2013

Basco MR, Rush AJ: Cognitive-Behavioral Therapy for Bipolar Disorder, 2nd Edition. New York, Guilford, 2007

Beck AT, Rector NA: Cognitive therapy of schizophrenia: a new therapy for the new millennium. Am J Psychother 54(3):291–300, 2000 11008627

Beck AT, Rush AJ, Shaw BF, et al: Cognitive Therapy of Depression. New York, Guilford, 1979

Beck AT, Wright FD, Newman CF, et al: Cognitive Therapy of Substance Abuse. New York, Guilford, 1993

Beck AT, Davis DD, Freeman A: Cognitive Therapy of Personality Disorders, 3rd Edition. New York, Guilford, 2015

Beck JS: Cognitive Behavior Therapy: Basics and Beyond, 2nd Edition. New York, Guilford, 2011

Bohus M, Haaf B, Simms T, et al: Effectiveness of inpatient dialectical behavioral therapy for borderline personality disorder: a controlled trial. Behav Res Ther 42(5):487–499, 2004 15033496

Burns AMN, Erickson DH, Brenner CA: Cognitive-behavioral therapy for medication-resistant psychosis: a meta-analytic review. Psychiatr Serv 65(7):874–880, 2014 24686725

Carroll KM: Lost in translation? Moving contingency management and cognitive behavioral therapy into clinical practice. Ann N Y Acad Sci 1327:94–111, 2014 25204847

Carroll KM, Rounsaville BJ, Gordon LT, et al: Psychotherapy and pharmacotherapy for ambulatory cocaine abusers. Arch Gen Psychiatry 51(3):177–187, 1994 8122955

Crits-Christoph P, Siqueland L, Blaine J, et al: Psychosocial treatments for cocaine dependence: National Institute on Drug Abuse Collaborative Cocaine Treatment Study. Arch Gen Psychiatry 56(6):493–502, 1999 10359461

DeRubeis RJ, Gelfand LA, Tang TZ, Simons AD: Medications versus cognitive behavior therapy for severely depressed outpatients: mega-analysis of four randomized comparisons. Am J Psychiatry 156(7):1007–1013, 1999 10401443

Elkin I, Shea MT, Watkins JT, et al: National Institute of Mental Health Treatment of Depression Collaborative Research Program: general effectiveness of treatments. Arch Gen Psychiatry 46(11):971–982, discussion 983, 1989 2684085

Fava GA: Well-Being Therapy: Treatment Manual and Clinical Applications. New York, Karger, 2016

Fava GA, Ruini C: Development and characteristics of a well-being enhancing psychotherapeutic strategy: well-being therapy. J Behav Ther Exp Psychiatry 34(1):45–63, 2003 12763392

Fava GA, Grandi S, Zielezny M, et al: Cognitive behavioral treatment of residual symptoms in primary major depressive disorder. Am J Psychiatry 151(9):1295–1299, 1994 8067483

Fava GA, Savron G, Grandi S, Rafanelli C: Cognitive-behavioral management of drug-resistant major depressive disorder. J Clin Psychiatry 58(6):278–282, quiz 283–284, 1997 9228899

Fava GA, Rafanelli C, Cazzaro M, et al: Well-being therapy: a novel psychotherapeutic approach for residual symptoms of affective disorders. Psychol Med 28(2):475–480, 1998a 9572104

Fava GA, Rafanelli C, Grandi S, et al: Prevention of recurrent depression with cognitive behavioral therapy: preliminary findings. Arch Gen Psychiatry 55(9):816–820, 1998b 9736008

Fava GA, Ruini C, Rafanelli C, Grandi S: Cognitive behavior approach to loss of clinical effect during long-term antidepressant treatment: a pilot study. Am J Psychiatry 159(12):2094–2095, 2002 12450962

Frankl VE: Man's Search for Meaning. Boston, MA, Karger, 1959

Garety PA, Kuipers L, Fowler D, et al: Cognitive behavioural therapy for drug-resistant psychosis. Br J Med Psychol 67 (Pt 3):259–271, 1994 7803318

Grant BF, Hasin DS, Stinson FS, et al: Co-occurrence of 12-month mood and anxiety disorders and personality disorders in the US: results from the National Epidemiologic Survey on Alcohol and Related Conditions. J Psychiatr Res 39(1):1–9, 2005 15504418

Gregory VL Jr: Cognitive-behavioral therapy for depression in bipolar disorder: a meta-analysis. J Evid Based Soc Work 7(4):269–279, 2010 20799127

Hay P, Chinn D, Forbes D, et al; Royal Australian and New Zealand College of Psychiatrists: Royal Australian and New Zealand College of Psychiatrists clinical practice guidelines for the treatment of eating disorders. Aust N Z J Psychiatry 48(11):977–1008, 2014 25351912

Hay PJ, Claudino AM, Touyz S, Abd Elbaky G: Individual psychological therapy in the outpatient treatment of adults with anorexia nervosa. Cochrane Database Syst Rev 7(7):CD003909, 2015 26212713

Hofmann SG, Asnaani A, Vonk IJ, et al: The efficacy of cognitive behavioral therapy: a review of meta-analyses. Cognit Ther Res 36(5):427–440, 2012 23459093

Hollon SD, DeRubeis RJ, Fawcett J, et al: Effect of cognitive therapy with antidepressant medications vs antidepressants alone on the rate of recovery in major depressive disorder: a randomized clinical trial. JAMA Psychiatry 71(10):1157–1164, 2014 25142196

Huijbers MJ, Spinhoven P, Spijker J, et al: Discontinuation of antidepressant medication after mindfulness-based cognitive therapy for recurrent depression: randomised controlled non-inferiority trial. Br J Psychiatry 208(4):366–373, 2016 26892847

Isasi AG, Echeburúa E, Limiñana JM, González-Pinto A: How effective is a psychological intervention program for patients with refractory bipolar disorder? A randomized controlled trial. J Affect Disord 126(1–2):80–87, 2010 20444503

Ives-Deliperi VL, Howells F, Stein DJ, et al: The effects of mindfulness-based cognitive therapy in patients with bipolar disorder: a controlled functional MRI investigation. J Affect Disord 150(3):1152–1157, 2013 23790741

Jauhar S, McKenna PJ, Radua J, et al: Cognitive-behavioural therapy for the symptoms of schizophrenia: systematic review and meta-analysis with examination of potential bias. Br J Psychiatry 204(1):20–29, 2014 24385461

Jones SH, Smith G, Mulligan LD, et al: Recovery-focused cognitive-behavioural therapy for recent-onset bipolar disorder: randomised controlled pilot trial. Br J Psychiatry 206(1):58–66, 2015 25213157

Kabat-Zinn J: Full Catastrophe Living: How to Cope With Stress, Pain and Illness Using Mindfulness Meditation. New York, Dell, 1990

Keck PE Jr, McElroy SL, Strakowski SM, et al: Compliance with maintenance treatment in bipolar disorder. Psychopharmacol Bull 33(1):87–91, 1997 9133756

Keller MB, McCullough JP, Klein DN, et al: A comparison of nefazodone, the cognitive behavioral-analysis system of psychotherapy, and their combination for the treatment of chronic depression. N Engl J Med 342(20):1462–1470, 2000 10816183

Keys A: The residues of malnutrition and starvation. Science 112(2909):371–373, 1950 14781769

Kingdon DG, Turkington D: Cognitive Therapy of Schizophrenia. New York, Guilford, 2004

Kocsis JH, Gelenberg AJ, Rothbaum BO, et al; REVAMP Investigators: Cognitive behavioral analysis system of psychotherapy and brief supportive psychotherapy for augmentation of antidepressant nonresponse in chronic depression: the REVAMP Trial. Arch Gen Psychiatry 66(11):1178–1188, 2009 19884606

Kuyken W, Warren FC, Taylor RS, et al: Efficacy of mindfulness-based cognitive therapy in prevention of depressive relapse: an individual patient data meta-analysis from randomized trials. JAMA Psychiatry 73(6):565–574, 2016 27119968

Lam DH, Watkins ER, Hayward P, et al: A randomized controlled study of cognitive therapy for relapse prevention for bipolar affective disorder: outcome of the first year. Arch Gen Psychiatry 60(2):145–152, 2003 12578431

Linehan MM: Cognitive-Behavioral Treatment of Borderline Personality Disorder. New York, Guilford, 1993

Linehan MM, Wilks CR: The course and evolution of dialectical behavior therapy. Am J Psychother 69(2):97–110, 2015 26160617

Linehan MM, Armstrong HE, Suarez A, et al: Cognitive-behavioral treatment of chronically parasuicidal borderline patients. Arch Gen Psychiatry 48(12):1060–1064, 1991 1845222

Linehan MM, Dimeff LA, Reynolds SK, et al: Dialectical behavior therapy versus comprehensive validation therapy plus 12-step for the treatment of opioid dependent women meeting criteria for borderline personality disorder. Drug Alcohol Depend 67(1):13–26, 2002 12062776

Marlatt GA, Gordon JR (eds): Relapse Prevention: Maintenance Strategies in the Treatment of Addictive Behaviors. New York, Guilford, 1985

McCullough JP: Psychotherapy for dysthymia: a naturalistic study of ten patients. J Nerv Ment Dis 179(12):734–740, 1991 1744631

McCullough JP Jr: Skills Training Manual for Diagnosing and Treating Chronic Depression: Cognitive Behavioral Analysis System of Psychotherapy. New York, Guilford, 2001

McElroy SL, Guerdjikova AI, Mori N, et al: Overview of the treatment of binge eating disorder. CNS Spectr 20(6):546–556, 2015 26594849

Mehl S, Werner D, Lincoln TM: Does cognitive behavior therapy for psychosis (CBTp) show a sustainable effect on delusions? A meta-analysis. Front Psychol 6:1450, 2015 26500570

Miklowitz DJ, Otto MW, Frank E, et al: Intensive psychosocial intervention enhances functioning in patients with bipolar depression: results from a 9-month randomized controlled trial. Am J Psychiatry 164(9):1340–1347, 2007a 17728418

Miklowitz DJ, Otto MW, Frank E, et al: Psychosocial treatments for bipolar depression: a 1-year randomized trial from the Systematic Treatment Enhancement Program. Arch Gen Psychiatry 64(4):419–426, 2007b 17404119

Miller WR, Yahne CE, Moyers TB, et al: A randomized trial of methods to help clinicians learn motivational interviewing. J Consult Clin Psychol 72(6):1050–1062, 2004 15612851

Newman CF, Leahy RL, Beck AT, et al: Bipolar Disorder: A Cognitive Therapy Approach. Washington, DC, American Psychological Association, 2002

Palmer RL, Birchall H, Damani S, et al: A dialectical behavior therapy program for people with an eating disorder and borderline personality disorder—description and outcome. Int J Eat Disord 33(3):281–286, 2003 12655624

Parikh SV, Zaretsky A, Beaulieu S, et al: A randomized controlled trial of psychoeducation or cognitive-behavioral therapy in bipolar disorder: a Canadian Network for Mood and Anxiety Treatments (CANMAT) study [CME]. J Clin Psychiatry 73(6):803–810, 2012 22795205

Prochaska JO, DiClemente CC: The transtheoretical approach, in Handbook of Psychotherapy Integration. Edited by Norcross JC, Goldfried MR. New York, Basic Books, 1992, pp 301–334

Project MATCH Research Group: Matching alcoholism treatments to client heterogeneity: treatment main effects and matching effects on drinking during treatment. J Stud Alcohol 59(6):631–639, 1998 9811084

Rector NA, Beck AT: Cognitive behavioral therapy for schizophrenia: an empirical review. J Nerv Ment Dis 189(5):278–287, 2001 11379970

Robins CJ, Chapman AL: Dialectical behavior therapy: current status, recent developments, and future directions. J Pers Disord 18(1):73–89, 2004 15061345

Rush AJ, Weissenburger JE: Melancholic symptom features and DSM-IV. Am J Psychiatry 151(4):489–498, 1994 8147445

Rush AJ, Trivedi MH, Wisniewski SR, et al: Acute and longer-term outcomes in depressed outpatients requiring one or several treatment steps: a STAR*D report. Am J Psychiatry 163(11):1905–1917, 2006 17074942

Scott J, Paykel E, Morriss R, et al: Cognitive-behavioural therapy for severe and recurrent bipolar disorders: randomised controlled trial. Br J Psychiatry 188:313–320, 2006 16582056

Segal ZV, Williams JMG, Teasdale JD: Mindfulness-Based Cognitive Therapy for Depression: A New Approach to Preventing Relapse. New York, Guilford, 2002

Sensky T, Turkington D, Kingdon D, et al: A randomized controlled trial of cognitive-behavioral therapy for persistent symptoms in schizophrenia resistant to medication. Arch Gen Psychiatry 57(2):165–172, 2000 10665619

Shea MT, Pilkonis PA, Beckham E, et al: Personality disorders and treatment outcome in the NIMH Treatment of Depression Collaborative Research Program. Am J Psychiatry 147(6):711–718, 1990 2343912

Siebern AT, Manber R: New developments in cognitive behavioral therapy as the first-line treatment of insomnia. Psychol Res Behav Manag 4:21–28, 2011 22114532

Strang J, McCambridge J: Can the practitioner correctly predict outcome in motivational interviewing? J Subst Abuse Treat 27(1):83–88, 2004 15223098

Stuart S, Simons AD, Thase ME, Pilkonis P: Are personality assessments valid in acute major depression? J Affect Disord 24(4):281–289, 1992 1578084

Szentagotai A, David D: The efficacy of cognitive-behavioral therapy in bipolar disorder: a quantitative meta-analysis. J Clin Psychiatry 71(1):66–72, 2010 19852904

Taylor HL, Keys A: Adaptation to caloric restriction. Science 112(2904):215–218, 1950 15442306

Taylor DJ, Pruiksma KE: Cognitive and behavioural therapy for insomnia (CBT-I) in psychiatric populations: a systematic review. Int Rev Psychiatry 26(2):205–213, 2014 24892895

Thase ME: The role of Axis II comorbidity in the management of patients with treatment-resistant depression. Psychiatr Clin North Am 19(2):287–309, 1996 8827191

Thase ME: Cognitive-behavioral therapy for substance abuse, in American Psychiatric Press Review of Psychiatry, Vol 16. Edited by Dickstein LJ, Riba MB, Oldham JM. Washington, DC, American Psychiatric Press, 1997, pp 45–71

Thase ME, Friedman ES: Is psychotherapy an effective treatment for melancholia and other severe depressive states? J Affect Disord 54(1–2):1–19, 1999 10403142

Thase ME, Howland R: Refractory depression: relevance of psychosocial factors and therapies. Psychiatr Ann 24:232–240, 1994

Thase ME, Simons AD, Cahalane J, et al: Severity of depression and response to cognitive behavior therapy. Am J Psychiatry 148(6):784–789, 1991 2035722

Thase ME, Greenhouse JB, Frank E, et al: Treatment of major depression with psychotherapy or psychotherapy-pharmacotherapy combinations. Arch Gen Psychiatry 54(11):1009–1015, 1997 9366657

Thase ME, Friedman ES, Biggs MM, et al: Cognitive therapy versus medication in augmentation and switch strategies as second-step treatments: a STAR*D report. Am J Psychiatry 164(5):739–752, 2007 17475733

Turkington D, Dudley R, Warman DM, Beck AT: Cognitive-behavioral therapy for schizophrenia: a review. J Psychiatr Pract 10(1):5–16, 2004 15334983

Turner DT, van der Gaag M, Karyotaki E, Cuijpers P: Psychological interventions for psychosis: a meta-analysis of comparative outcome studies. Am J Psychiatry 171(5):523–538, 2014 24525715

Velthorst E, Koeter M, van der Gaag M, et al: Adapted cognitive-behavioural therapy required for targeting negative symptoms in schizophrenia: meta-analysis and meta-regression. Psychol Med 45(3):453–465, 2015 24993642

Vocks S, Tuschen-Caffier B, Pietrowsky R, et al: Meta-analysis of the effectiveness of psychological and pharmacological treatments for binge eating disorder. Int J Eat Disord 43(3):205–217, 2010 19402028

Watkins ER, Mullan E, Wingrove J, et al: Rumination-focused cognitive-behavioural therapy for residual depression: phase II randomised controlled trial. Br J Psychiatry 199(4):317–322, 2011 21778171

Weitz ES, Hollon SD, Twisk J, et al: Baseline depression severity as moderator of depression outcomes between cognitive behavioral therapy vs pharmacotherapy: an individual patient data meta-analysis. JAMA Psychiatry 72(11):1102–1109, 2015 26397232

Wiles N, Thomas L, Abel A, et al: Cognitive behavioural therapy as an adjunct to pharmacotherapy for primary care based patients with treatment resistant depression: results of the CoBalT randomised controlled trial. Lancet 381(9864):375–384, 2013 23219570

Williams JMG, Teasdale JD, Segal ZV, Kabat-Zinn J: The Mindful Way Through Depression: Freeing Yourself From Chronic Unhappiness. New York, Guilford, 2007

Wong DFK: Cognitive behavioral treatment groups for people with chronic depression in Hong Kong: a randomized wait-list control design. Depress Anxiety 25(2):142–148, 2008 17340612

Woody GE, McLellan AT, Luborsky L, et al: Severity of psychiatric symptoms as a predictor of benefits from psychotherapy: the Veterans Administration–Penn study. Am J Psychiatry 141(10):1172–1177, 1984 6486249

Wright JH, Turkington D, Kingdon DG, Basco MR: Cognitive-Behavior Therapy for Severe Mental Illness: An Illustrated Guide. Washington, DC, American Psychiatric Publishing, 2009

Wright JH, Sudak DM, Turkington D, Thase ME: High-Yield Cognitive-Behavior Therapy for Brief Sessions: An Illustrated Guide. Washington, DC, American Psychiatric Publishing, 2010

Young JE, Klosko JS, Weishaar ME: Schema Therapy: A Practitioner's Guide. New York, Guilford, 2003

# 11

# Building Competence in Cognitive-Behavior Therapy

If you've had a basic course in cognitive-behavior therapy (CBT), worked your way through this book, and used the learning exercises to practice therapy skills, you probably have made significant strides toward becoming a competent cognitive-behavior therapist. However, it is likely that additional training and experience will be needed to help you master this approach (Rakovshik and McManus 2010). There are three principal reasons why we recommend that you strive to obtain full competence in CBT. First, you are likely to have better treatment outcomes (Rakovshik and McManus 2010; Strunk et al. 2010; Westbrook et al. 2008), Second, therapist knowledge and expertise are very important to patients. Along

---

Items mentioned in this chapter that are available in Appendix 1, "Worksheets and Checklists," are also available as a free download in larger format on the American Psychiatric Association Publishing Web site: https://www.appi.org/wright.

with excellent listening skills, accurate empathy, and other general therapy attributes, your capability to deliver the specific methods of CBT can mean a great deal to the people you treat. Third, you may have greater satisfaction in your daily work—a phenomenon we have experienced as we have become more proficient in CBT and are able to offer more help to patients. In this chapter, we detail competency guidelines, outline methods of measuring your progress in learning CBT, suggest some ways to continue your development as a therapist, and offer tips on avoiding therapist fatigue and burnout.

## Core Competencies in CBT

The American Association of Directors of Psychiatric Residency Training (AADPRT; www.aadprt.org) has emphasized the importance of achieving competence in psychotherapy and has issued guidelines for assessing knowledge, skills, and attitudes of trainees who are learning CBT. These AADPRT competency standards for psychiatry residents (Sudak et al. 2001) are summarized in Table 11–1. Because the standards are quite broad, they can be useful to educators and trainees in CBT from a variety of disciplines.

The main value of the AADPRT competency standards is in laying out specific goals for learning this form of therapy. To get a sense of where you are in your path to learning CBT, we suggest that you perform the next learning exercise.

**Learning Exercise 11–1.** Self-Assessment of Competence in CBT

1. Review each item in Table 11–1.

2. Assess your knowledge, skills, and attitudes in CBT by giving yourself a score of excellent (E), satisfactory (S), or unsatisfactory (U) for each item. The standard for your self-assessment should not be at the master therapist level but at the level of a clinician who has completed residency courses, graduate training programs, or other concentrated educational programs in CBT.

3. If you noted problems in knowledge, skills, or attitudes for any items, think of a plan to upgrade your competence. Ideas might include rereading sections of this book, reviewing class notes, getting additional supervision, and studying other materials.

**Table 11–1.** Competency standards for cognitive-behavior therapy (CBT)

| Knowledge | Skills | Attitudes |
|---|---|---|
| *The clinician will demonstrate an understanding of* | *The clinician will be able to* | *The clinician will be* |
| ___1. The cognitive-behavioral model. | ___1. Assess and conceptualize patients with the CBT model. | ___1. Empathic, respectful, nonjudgmental, and collaborative. |
| ___2. Concepts of automatic thoughts, cognitive errors, schemas, and behavioral principles. | ___2. Establish and maintain a collaborative therapeutic relationship. | ___2. Sensitive to sociocultural, socioeconomic, and educational issues. |
| ___3. Cognitive-behavioral formulations for common disorders. | ___3. Educate the patient about the CBT model. | ___3. Open to review of audio or video recordings or direct observations of treatment sessions. |
| ___4. Indications for CBT. | ___4. Educate the patient about schemas and help him or her understand the origin of these beliefs. | |
| ___5. Rationale for structuring sessions, collaboration, and problem solving. | ___5. Structure sessions, including setting agendas, reviewing and assigning homework, working on key problems, and using feedback. | |
| ___6. Basic principles for psychoeducation. | ___6. Utilize activity scheduling and graded task assignments. | |
| ___7. Basic principles for behavioral methods. | ___7. Utilize relaxation training and graded exposure techniques. | |
| ___8. Basic principles for cognitive techniques such as modifying automatic thoughts and schemas. | ___8. Employ thought recording techniques. | |
| ___9. The importance of continued education in CBT. | ___9. Use relapse prevention techniques. | |
| | ___10. Recognize his or her own thoughts and feelings stimulated by the therapy. | |
| | ___11. Write a CBT formulation. | |
| | ___12. Seek appropriate consultation when needed. | |

*Source.* Adapted from Sudak DM, Wright JH, Beck JS, et al: "AADPRT Cognitive Behavioral Therapy Competencies." Farmington, CT, American Association of Directors of Psychiatric Residency Training, 2001.

## Becoming a Competent Cognitive-Behavior Therapist

Most experienced educators in CBT believe that a combination of learning experiences is required (Sudak et al. 2003, 2009). For graduate students, residents, or other clinicians in training, these experiences usually include 1) a basic course (the Academy of Cognitive Therapy recommends at least 40 hours of course work); 2) assigned readings (at least a core text on CBT theory and methods, such as this book, and other targeted readings for special topics); 3) written case formulations; 4) experiential role-plays to practice the implementation of CBT skills; 5) case supervision (either in individual or group format, or both); 6) use of video- or audio-recorded sessions that are reviewed and rated by an experienced cognitive-behavior therapist; and 7) significant practice in treating patients with CBT (treatment of 10 cases or more with varied diagnoses, including depression and different types of anxiety disorders).

A number of options are available for clinicians who believe they need additional education to become skilled in CBT. The most rigorous and well-established training programs for practicing clinicians are provided by the Beck Institute in Philadelphia, Pennsylvania (www.beckinstitute.org). On-site fellowships and extramural fellowships are available. In these programs, the clinician typically receives extensive didactic instruction in addition to individual case consultation.

An alternate method for training practicing clinicians is for an organization or agency to arrange a customized educational program. For example, one of us (J.H.W.) developed a yearlong curriculum for therapists at a large community mental health center. None of the clinicians attending the program had had any substantive prior training in CBT. As part of the program, four senior therapists enrolled in the extramural fellowship at the Beck Institute and then became assistants to the author in conducting the training for a group of more than 40 clinicians. The kickoff session for this training was an 8-hour workshop conducted by the author and Judith Beck, Ph.D., from the Beck Institute. This workshop was followed by weekly classes taught by the author, four additional intensive workshops, and weekly supervision provided by the extramural fellows. By the end of this year of training, the extramural fellows were able to continue the education of the other therapists at the agency by providing ongoing case supervision. Although significant resources were required to implement this training program, it was successful in educating a large number of clinicians in CBT.

Other practicing clinicians have obtained basic competence in CBT by participating in workshops at major scientific meetings, viewing videos of master therapists, attending retreats or camps designed to teach CBT (e.g., boot camps and other training workshops taught by Christine Padesky, Ph.D., and associates; www.padesky.com), and obtaining individual supervision in CBT (see Appendix 2, "Cognitive-Behavior Therapy Resources"). The Academy of Cognitive Therapy (ACT), a certifying organization in CBT, lists on its Web site educational opportunities and provides a directory of certified cognitive-behavior therapists who may be able to offer supervision or other training consultation (www.academyofct.org).

## Measuring Your Progress

CBT is noted for having a long tradition of assessing the skills of clinicians and providing constructive feedback. When learning CBT, it is important to carefully evaluate and identify specific skills that require improvement, as well as to develop specific learning objectives to assess progress. Several rating scales, checklists, and tests are available (Sudak et al. 2003). Here we describe four instruments that you may find helpful for evaluating your progress in learning CBT.

### Cognitive Therapy Scale

The principal measure used to give feedback on proficiency in CBT is the Cognitive Therapy Scale (CTS; see this chapter's appendix), developed by Young and Beck 1980 (Vallis et al. 1986). The CTS contains 11 items (e.g., agenda setting and structuring, collaboration, pacing and efficient use of time, guided discovery, focusing on key cognitions and behaviors, skill in applying CBT techniques, and homework) that are used to rate a therapist's performance on critical functions of CBT. Up to 6 points are awarded for each item on the CTS, thus yielding a maximum score of 66. An overall score of 40 usually is considered to represent satisfactory performance in CBT. The ACT requires that applicants for certification achieve a score of at least 40 on CTS ratings of a recorded interview. In addition, a score of 40 on the CTS is commonly used as a measure for qualifying as a cognitive-behavior therapist for research investigations that study the effectiveness of this approach (Wright et al. 2005).

The CTS can help you learn about your strengths and weaknesses in doing CBT and can stimulate ideas for making improvements. In the next learning exercise, you are asked to rate one of your sessions on the CTS and to discuss these ratings with a colleague or supervisor.

**Learning Exercise 11–2.** Using the Cognitive Therapy Scale

1. Record one of your CBT sessions on video or audio. This session should preferably be with an actual patient. However, a role-play session can be used for this exercise.

2. Perform a self-rating on this session using the CTS. Also ask a supervisor or a colleague to rate the session.

3. Discuss the ratings with your supervisor or colleague.

4. Identify your strengths in the session.

5. If you or your colleague or supervisor identified areas where you could improve your performance, list ideas you have for doing things differently.

6. Perform further ratings of video- or audio-recorded sessions on a regular basis until you can routinely score 40 or above on this scale.

## Cognitive Formulation Rating Scale

The ACT has developed specific guidelines for writing case conceptualizations to meet their criteria for certification in CBT. Detailed instructions for formulating cases and planning treatment can be found at the ACT Web site (http://www.academyofct.org). An example of a written case formulation also is provided on the Web site. A number of training programs in CBT have adopted the ACT guidelines and scoring system for case conceptualizations and require completion of one or more written formulations.

The system for formulating cases that we present in Chapter 3, "Assessment and Formulation," is based directly on the ACT guidelines. Therefore, you should already know the basics of developing case conceptualizations that meet ACT standards. Each component of a case conceptualization is scored by the ACT on a scale of 0–2 (0=not present, 1=present but inadequate, 2=present and adequate). Three general areas of performance are scored: 1) case history (two items), 2) formulation (five items), and 3) treatment plan and course of therapy (five items). The ACT standard for a passing score is 20 out of a possible 24 points. The scoring criteria are available on the ACT Web site.

We have found that writing out case formulations is one of the most worthwhile exercises for learning CBT. If you take the time to carefully think through formulations and get feedback from supervisors or other experienced cognitive-behavior therapists, you can build considerable sophistication and skill in this treatment approach. Although writing conceptualizations takes some effort, the rewards can be great.

**Learning Exercise 11–3.** Practicing Case Formulations

1. Download the instructions for writing a case conceptualization from the ACT Web site (www.academyofct.org). Also review the example of a written formulation and the scoring criteria provided on the Web site.

2. Use the case formulation worksheet to organize your key observations and plans.[1] Then follow the ACT guidelines to write a full case conceptualization.

3. Use the ACT scoring criteria to perform a self-rating of your written case conceptualization.

4. Ask a supervisor or experienced cognitive-behavior therapist to score your conceptualization and to discuss your ideas for understanding and treating this case.

## Cognitive Therapy Awareness Scale

Although the Cognitive Therapy Awareness Scale (CTAS) was originally developed to assess knowledge of CBT principles in patients treated with this form of therapy (Wright et al. 2002), it has subsequently been used in training programs as a pre- and posttest of awareness of basic concepts and terms. The CTAS is not a comprehensive measure of CBT knowledge, but it can be used to gauge progress in learning about key theories and methods. The scale includes 40 true-or-false questions on topics such as automatic thoughts, cognitive errors, schemas, thought recording, activity scheduling, and identifying cognitive distortions.

One point is awarded for each correct response to the 40 questions in the CTAS. Thus, a score of about 20 might be expected if the person taking the test had no prior knowledge of CBT. The maximum score on this

---

[1]For a blank copy of the worksheet, see Appendix 1, "Worksheets and Checklists." For more information about the worksheet, including examples of completed worksheets, see Chapter 3, "Assessment and Formulation."

scale is 40. Studies of the CTAS in patient populations have shown significant increases in scores after treatment with CBT (Wright et al. 2002, 2005). For example, in an investigation of 96 patients who received computer-assisted CBT for depression or anxiety, mean scores improved from 24.2 before treatment to 32.5 after use of the computer program (Wright et al. 2002). Studies of the CTAS for assessing trainee knowledge of CBT also have shown significant positive changes (Fujisawa et al. 2011; Macrodimitris et al. 2010, 2011; Reilly and McDanel 2005). Our experience in using this scale with psychiatry residents suggests that mean scores before a basic course in CBT typically range from the mid-20s to the lower 30s. As expected, CTAS scores usually increase substantially after completion of course work, readings, and other educational experiences in CBT. The CTAS is published in Wright et al. 2002.

### Cognitive-Behavior Therapy Supervision Checklist

If you are receiving or providing supervision in CBT, you may be interested in using the Cognitive-Behavior Therapy Supervision Checklist, a form developed by several members of the AADPRT competency standards work group (Sudak et al. 2001). This checklist is divided into two sections: 1) competencies that should be demonstrated in each session (e.g., "maintains collaborative empirical alliance," "demonstrates ability to use guided discovery," and "effectively sets agenda and structures session"), and 2) competencies that may be demonstrated over a course of therapy or therapies (e.g., "sets goals and plans treatment based on CBT formulation," "educates patient about CBT model and/or therapy interventions," and "can utilize activity or pleasant events scheduling"). The Cognitive-Behavior Therapy Supervision Checklist is available in Appendix 1, "Worksheets and Checklists."

## Continued Experience and Training in CBT

To retain your skills in CBT, it will be important to practice cognitive-behavioral interventions regularly and to take advantage of postgraduate education opportunities. Also, if you wish to add depth and range to your abilities, you will need to explore options for further learning. Our experiences in training and supervising clinicians in CBT suggest that skills can atrophy if they are not used regularly and stimulated by ongoing educational activities.

Earlier in this chapter, we suggested that attending workshops at scientific meetings, viewing videos of accomplished cognitive-behavior therapists, and going to educational retreats or camps can be used to build basic competency (see "Becoming a Competent Cognitive-Behavior Therapist"). These same experiences can play a useful role in helping clinicians maintain their CBT skills and develop new areas of expertise. For example, courses or workshops on CBT methods for treatment-resistant depression, schizophrenia, eating disorders, posttraumatic stress disorder, chronic pain, personality disorders, and other conditions are commonly offered at national and international conferences (e.g., annual meetings of the American Psychiatric Association, the American Psychological Association, and the Association for Behavioral and Cognitive Therapies; see Appendix 2, "Cognitive-Behavior Therapy Resources").

Readings in CBT also can help you learn new ways to apply these methods. A list of books that can expand your knowledge of CBT is provided in Appendix 2, "Cognitive-Behavior Therapy Resources." We have included classic texts such as those by A.T. Beck and colleagues on depression, anxiety disorders, and personality disorders, in addition to volumes on diverse topics such as marital and group therapies, treatment of psychosis, and advanced CBT techniques.

Another way to work on improving CBT proficiency is to apply for certification from the ACT. Some of the certification criteria for this organization, including submission of recorded material for rating on the CTS and writing a case formulation that follows the ACT guidelines, are discussed earlier in this chapter (see section "Cognitive Therapy Scale" and Learning Exercise 11–2). Studying and preparing for an ACT certification submission can be a valuable tactic for sharpening your ability to perform CBT. Certified members of the ACT also have access to a number of superb continuing-education opportunities, including subscribing to e-mail communications lists, receiving updates on new developments in CBT, and attending special lectures by leading clinicians and researchers.

Our final suggestion for continuing your growth as a cognitive-behavior therapist is to attend an ongoing seminar or CBT supervision group. These types of group learning experiences may be offered routinely at CBT centers, educational institutions, and other clinical and research settings. A weekly supervision group might provide reviews and ratings of recorded sessions, role-play demonstrations, and learning modules designed to help clinicians expand their abilities in specific CBT applications (e.g., treatment-resistant depression, personality disorders, chronic pain). Although the level of experience in CBT could range from novice to expert, responsibility for bringing material to meetings and contributing to the educational process nevertheless could rotate among all participants. If you do not have such a group available in your community, you might consider starting one. Many cognitive-behavior therapists value these ongoing supervision groups because they provide a stimulating and collegial forum for learning.

## Therapist Fatigue or Burnout

Energy, concentration, hopefulness for good outcomes, staying power with difficult patients, and many other therapist capacities can be undermined by burnout—a problem that can impair the competent delivery of effective CBT.

Burnout is a risk for all therapists, regardless of level of experience. When you are new to CBT and are not fully confident in your skills, you can feel frustrated with patients who are not making progress. A temporary feeling of burnout can make you want to give up on patients, or give up on being a therapist altogether. If you can persevere through the training process until you have refined your skills and gained confidence, the temporary feeling of burnout is likely to dissipate. However, the mentally intensive nature of psychotherapy may lead to periodic fatigue with this form of work.

There are several things you can do to prevent or limit burnout in performing psychotherapy. Troubleshooting Guide 6 gives some ideas for avoiding this problem, while staying enthusiastic and engaged over a long career as a cognitive-behavior therapist.

### Troubleshooting Guide 6
**Avoiding Burnout**

1. **Are you taking care of your basic needs?** Busy therapists who are accustomed to working hard can drive themselves so relentlessly that they neglect their own personal daily needs. Telltale signs of this problem include running late in the morning so you don't take time for breakfast, overscheduling or being late between sessions so that there are no breaks between patients, and agreeing to see patients during a lunch hour. To be effective as a therapist, you must be mentally sharp, focused, and not distracted by competing physical and mental stressors. If you want to give your patients your best, schedule time to take care of yourself.

## Troubleshooting Guide 6 *(continued)*
### Avoiding Burnout

2. **Are you exceeding reasonable workload limits?** There is wide variety in the number of hours of clinical practice therapists can conduct each day or each week without becoming overly fatigued. You have exceeded your limit when you find that you are too exhausted to be effective, too tired to do anything after work, disinterested in hearing about the problems of your family members or friends, or self-medicating after work to decompress from the day. Another indicator that you have exceeded your limit is when you no longer enjoy your work. Find your limits and create a daily schedule that allows you to function within these boundaries.

3. **Is there a healthy balance between your dedication to work and other parts of your life?** Develop a hobby or interest that adds variety to your schedule. Have other things to look forward to in your week in addition to your patients. Devote time to other things that are meaningful to you.

4. **Are you getting enough rest?** Improve your sleep habits. Find relaxing activities that recharge your energy level. Schedule a long weekend or a vacation away from work to rest your mind and refuel your spirit. When you are not working, engage in activities that use a different set of cognitive skills or that are more physical in nature. This change will give the empathic-listening and problem-solving parts of your brain a short rest. Avoid thinking about work during this time off.

5. **Is supervision needed?** If you think your fatigue is focused on a specific patient, talk to a supervisor or colleagues about your work. If you are experiencing countertransference, discuss this issue in supervision and develop a strategy to manage the response. Perhaps you find certain illnesses or clusters of symptoms difficult or tedious to manage or do not yet possess the skills to treat them. For example, some clinicians do not like working with people who have substance abuse problems or personality disorders. If you find this kind of work unpleasant or uninteresting, find colleagues who specialize in these areas and refer patients to them.

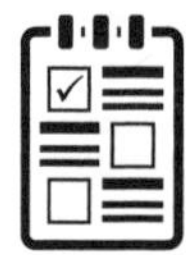

**Troubleshooting Guide 6 *(continued)***
**Avoiding Burnout**

6. **Would it help to learn something new?** Fatigue or burnout can be associated with doing the same thing repetitively. In CBT, there is a risk that methods for specific disorders can become so structured and similar to one another that you may find yourself becoming bored with the routine. If this is the case, learn something new. Take a class, read a book, or talk with other clinicians about their therapeutic approaches. As long as you stay within the conceptual model of CBT, there is an abundance of creative ways in which the methods can be applied. Examples include a) implementing a new technique (e.g., dialectical behavior therapy for borderline personality disorder, mindfulness-based cognitive therapy for depression, cognitive restructuring for psychoses; see Chapter 10, "Treating Chronic, Severe, or Complex Disorders"), b) using computer programs for CBT (see Chapter 4, "Structuring and Educating"), c) employing teaching devices such as marker boards or drawing materials, and d) suggesting self-help reading materials that encourage patients to bring alternative ideas to treatment sessions.

## Summary

In this chapter, we described several useful ways of assessing proficiency and suggested methods for expanding knowledge and building expertise. Efforts to continue developing skills in this therapy approach can have many benefits. Being able to deliver treatment competently and consistently should help you achieve good results. In addition, specific CBT methods are now available for virtually all psychiatric disorders for which psychotherapy is indicated. Studying these methods can help you increase your abilities to treat diverse groups of patients effectively. Although there is a risk for burnout along the path toward competency in CBT, there are many steps you can take to avoid this problem and gain enduring satisfaction and enjoyment in your work. We hope that further education in this form of therapy will give you a deeper understanding of the cognitive-behavioral paradigm and its power to change patients' lives.

# References

Fujisawa D, Nakagawa A, Kikuchi T, et al: Reliability and validity of the Japanese version of the Cognitive Therapy Awareness Scale: a scale to measure competencies in cognitive therapy. Psychiatry Clin Neurosci 65(1):64–69, 2011 21265937

Macrodimitris SD, Hamilton KE, Backs-Dermott BJ, et al: CBT basics: a group approach to teaching fundamental cognitive-behavioral skills. J Cogn Psychother 24(2):132–146, 2010

Macrodimitris S, Wershler J, Hatfield M, et al: Group cognitive-behavioral therapy for patients with epilepsy and comorbid depression and anxiety. Epilepsy Behav 20(1):83–88, 2011 21131237

Rakovshik SG, McManus F: Establishing evidence-based training in cognitive behavioral therapy: a review of current empirical findings and theoretical guidance. Clin Psychol Rev 30(5):496–516, 2010 20488599

Reilly CE, McDanel H: Cognitive therapy: a training model for advanced practice nurses. J Psychosoc Nurs Ment Health Serv 43(5):27–31, 2005 15960032

Strunk DR, Brotman MA, DeRubeis RJ, Hollon SD: Therapist competence in cognitive therapy for depression: predicting subsequent symptom change. J Consult Clin Psychol 78(3):429–437, 2010 20515218

Sudak DM: Training and cognitive behavioral therapy in psychiatry residence: an overview for educators. Behav Modif 33(1):124–137, 2009 18723836

Sudak DM, Wright JH, Bienenfeld D, et al: AADPRT Cognitive Behavioral Therapy Competencies. Farmington, CT, American Association of Directors of Psychiatric Residency Training, 2001

Sudak DM, Beck JS, Wright J: Cognitive behavioral therapy: a blueprint for attaining and assessing psychiatry resident competency. Acad Psychiatry 27(3):154–159, 2003 12969838

Vallis TM, Shaw BF, Dobson KS: The Cognitive Therapy Scale: psychometric properties. J Consult Clin Psychol 54(3):381–385, 1986 3722567

Westbrook D, Sedgwick-Taylor A, Bennett-Levy J, et al: A pilot evaluation of a brief CBT training course: impact on trainees' satisfaction, clinical kkills and patient outcomes. Behav Cogn Psychother 36:569–579, 2008

Wright JH, Wright AS, Salmon P, et al: Development and initial testing of a multimedia program for computer-assisted cognitive therapy. Am J Psychother 56(1):76–86, 2002 11977785

Wright JH, Wright AS, Albano AM, et al: Computer-assisted cognitive therapy for depression: maintaining efficacy while reducing therapist time. Am J Psychiatry 162(6):1158–1164, 2005 15930065

Young J, Beck AT: Cognitive Therapy Scale Rating Manual. Philadelphia, PA, Center for Cognitive Therapy, 1980

# Appendix 11–A
# Cognitive Therapy Scale

Therapist: ______________________ Patient: ________________

Date of Session: ______________________ Session No.: ______________

**Directions:** Rate performance on a scale from 0 to 6, and record the rating on the line next to the item number. Descriptions are provided for even-numbered scale points. If you believe the rating falls between two of the descriptors, select the intervening odd number (1, 3, 5).

If the descriptions for an item occasionally do not seem to apply to the session you are rating, feel free to disregard them and use the more general scale below:

| 0 | 1 | 2 | 3 | 4 | 5 | 6 |
|---|---|---|---|---|---|---|
| Poor | Barely adequate | Mediocre | Satisfactory | Good | Very good | Excellent |

## Part I. General Therapeutic Skills

### ___1. Agenda

0 Therapist did not set agenda.

2 Therapist set agenda that was vague or incomplete.

4 Therapist worked with patient to set a mutually satisfactory agenda that included specific target problems (e.g., anxiety at work, dissatisfaction with marriage).

6 Therapist worked with patient to set an appropriate agenda with target problems, suitable for the available time. Established priorities and then followed agenda.

---

## ___2. Feedback

0 Therapist did not ask for feedback to determine the patient's understanding of, or response to, the session.
2 Therapist elicited some feedback from the patient but did not ask enough questions to be sure the patient understood the therapist's line of reasoning during the session or to ascertain whether the patient was satisfied with the session.
4 Therapist asked enough questions to be sure that the patient understood the therapist's line of reasoning throughout the session and to determine the patient's reactions to the session. The therapist adjusted his or her behavior in response to the feedback, when appropriate.
6 Therapist was especially adept at eliciting and responding to verbal and nonverbal feedback throughout the session (e.g., elicited reactions to session, regularly checked for understanding, helped summarize main points at end of session).

## ___3. Understanding

0 Therapist repeatedly failed to understand what the patient explicitly said and thus consistently missed the point. Poor empathic skills.
2 Therapist was usually able to reflect or rephrase what the patient explicitly said, but repeatedly failed to respond to more subtle communication. Limited ability to listen and empathize.
4 Therapist generally seemed to grasp the patient's "internal reality" as reflected by both what was explicitly said and what the patient communicated in more subtle ways. Good ability to listen and empathize.
6 Therapist seemed to understand the patient's "internal reality" thoroughly and was adept at communicating this understanding through appropriate verbal and nonverbal responses to the patient (e.g., the tone of the therapist's response conveyed a sympathetic understanding of the patient's "message"). Excellent listening and empathic skills.

## ___4. Interpersonal Effectiveness

0 Therapist had poor interpersonal skills. Seemed hostile, demeaning, or in some other way destructive to the patient.
2 Therapist did not seem destructive but had significant interpersonal problems. At times, therapist appeared unnecessarily impatient, aloof, or insincere or had difficulty conveying confidence and competence.
4 Therapist displayed a satisfactory degree of warmth, concern, confidence, genuineness, and professionalism. No significant interpersonal problems.
6 Therapist displayed optimal levels of warmth, concern, confidence, genuineness, and professionalism, appropriate for this particular patient in this session.

### ___5. Collaboration

0 Therapist did not attempt to set up a collaboration with the patient.
2 Therapist attempted to collaborate with the patient but had difficulty either defining a problem that the patient considered important or establishing rapport.
4 Therapist was able to collaborate with the patient, focus on a problem that both the patient and therapist considered important, and establish rapport.
6 Collaboration seemed excellent; the therapist encouraged the patient as much as possible to take an active role during the session (e.g., by offering choices) so they could function as a team.

### ___6. Pacing and Efficient Use of Time

0 Therapist made no attempt to structure therapy time. Session seemed aimless.
2 Session had some direction, but the therapist had significant problems with structuring or pacing (e.g., too little structure, inflexible about structure, too slowly paced, too rapidly paced).
4 Therapist was reasonably successful at using time efficiently. Therapist maintained appropriate control over flow of discussion and pacing.
6 Therapist used time efficiently by tactfully limiting peripheral and unproductive discussion and by pacing the session as rapidly as was appropriate for the patient.

## Part II. Conceptualization, Strategy, and Technique

### ___7. Guided Discovery

0 Therapist relied primarily on debate, persuasion, or "lecturing." Therapist seemed to be cross-examining the patient, putting the patient on the defensive, or forcing his or her point of view on the patient.
2 Therapist relied too heavily on persuasion and debate, rather than guided discovery. However, therapist's style was supportive enough that patient did not seem to feel attacked or defensive.
4 Therapist, for the most part, helped the patient see new perspectives through guided discovery (e.g., examining evidence, considering alternatives, weighing advantages and disadvantages) rather than through debate. Used questioning appropriately.
6 Therapist was especially adept at using guided discovery during the session to explore problems and help the patient draw his or her own conclusions. Achieved an excellent balance between skillful questioning and other modes of intervention.

## ___8. Focusing on Key Cognitions or Behaviors

0 Therapist did not attempt to elicit specific thoughts, assumptions, images, meanings, or behaviors.

2 Therapist used appropriate techniques to elicit cognitions or behaviors; however, the therapist had difficulty finding a focus, or focused on cognitions and behaviors that were irrelevant to the patient's key problems.

4 Therapist focused on specific cognitions or behaviors relevant to the target problem. However, the therapist could have focused on more central cognitions or behaviors that offered greater promise for progress.

6 Therapist very skillfully focused on key thoughts, assumptions, behaviors, etc., that were most relevant to the problem area and offered considerable promise for progress.

## ___9. Strategy for Change

(*Note:* For this item, focus on the quality of the therapist's strategy for change, not on how effectively the strategy was implemented or whether change actually occurred.)

0 Therapist did not select cognitive-behavioral techniques.

2 Therapist selected cognitive-behavioral techniques; however, the overall strategy for bringing about change either seemed vague or did not seem promising in helping the patient.

4 Therapist seemed to have a generally coherent strategy for change that showed reasonable promise and incorporated cognitive-behavioral techniques.

6 Therapist followed a consistent strategy for change that seemed very promising, and incorporated the most appropriate cognitive-behavioral techniques.

## ___10. Application of Cognitive-Behavioral Techniques

(*Note:* For this item, focus on how skillfully the techniques were applied, not on how appropriate they were for the target problem or whether change actually occurred.)

0 Therapist did not apply any cognitive-behavioral techniques.

2 Therapist used cognitive-behavioral techniques, but there were significant flaws in the way they were applied.

4 Therapist applied cognitive-behavioral techniques with moderate skill.

6 Therapist very skillfully and resourcefully employed cognitive-behavioral techniques.

## ___11. Homework

0 Therapist did not attempt to incorporate homework relevant to cognitive therapy.

2 Therapist had significant difficulties incorporating homework (e.g., did not review previous homework, did not explain homework in sufficient detail, assigned inappropriate homework).

4 Therapist reviewed previous homework and assigned "standard" cognitive therapy homework generally relevant to issues dealt with in session. Homework was explained in sufficient detail.

6 Therapist reviewed previous homework and carefully assigned homework drawn from cognitive therapy for the coming week. Assignment seemed custom-tailored to help patient incorporate new perspectives, test hypotheses, experiment with new behaviors discussed during session, etc.

## ___Total Score

# Appendix I
# Worksheets and Checklists

## Contents



---

Appendix 1 is available as a free download in its entirety and in larger format on the American Psychiatric Association Publishing Web site: https://www.appi.org/wright.

[a]Adapted with permission from Wright JH, Wright AS, Beck AT: *Good Days Ahead*. Moraga, CA, Empower Interactive, 2016.  Permission is granted for readers to use these items in clinical practice.

# Cognitive-Behavior Therapy Case Formulation Worksheet

| Patient Name: | | Date: |
|---|---|---|
| Diagnoses/Symptoms: | | |
| Formative Influences: | | |
| Situational Issues: | | |
| Biological, Genetic, and Medical Factors: | | |
| Strengths/Assets: | | |
| Treatment Goals: | | |
| **Event 1** | **Event 2** | **Event 3** |
| | | |
| **Automatic Thoughts** | **Automatic Thoughts** | **Automatic Thoughts** |
| | | |
| **Emotions** | **Emotions** | **Emotions** |
| | | |
| **Behaviors** | **Behaviors** | **Behaviors** |
| | | |
| Schemas: | | |
| Working Hypothesis: | | |
| Treatment Plan: | | |

*Note.* Available at: https://www.appi.org/wright.

## Automatic Thoughts Checklist

**Instructions:** Place a check mark beside each negative automatic thought that you have had in the past 2 weeks.

_____ I should be doing better in life.

_____ He/she doesn't understand me.

_____ I've let him/her down.

_____ I just can't enjoy things anymore.

_____ Why am I so weak?

_____ I always keep messing things up.

_____ My life's going nowhere.

_____ I can't handle it.

_____ I'm failing.

_____ It's too much for me.

_____ I don't have much of a future.

_____ Things are out of control.

_____ I feel like giving up.

_____ Something bad is sure to happen.

_____ There must be something wrong with me.

*Note.* Available at: https://www.appi.org/wright.

## Thought Change Record

| Situation | Automatic thought(s) | Emotion(s) | Rational response | Outcome |
|---|---|---|---|---|
| a. *Describe* event leading to emotion *or*<br>b. Stream of thoughts leading to emotion *or*<br>c. Physiological sensations. | a. *Write* automatic thought(s) that preceded emotion(s).<br>b. *Rate* belief in automatic thought(s), 0%–100%. | a. *Specify* sad, anxious, angry, etc.<br>b. *Rate* degree of emotion, 1%–100%. | a. *Identify* cognitive errors.<br>b. *Write* rational response to automatic thought(s).<br>c. *Rate* belief in rational response, 0%–100%. | a. *Specify and rate* subsequent emotion(s), 0%–100%.<br>b. *Describe* changes in behavior. |
| | | | | |

*Source.* Adapted from Beck AT, Rush AJ, Shaw BF, et al.: *Cognitive Therapy of Depression*. New York, Guilford, 1979, pp. 164–165. Reprinted with permission of Guilford Press. Available at: https://www.appi.org/wright.

## Definitions of Cognitive Errors

**Selective abstraction** (sometimes called *ignoring the evidence* or *the mental filter*) A conclusion is drawn after looking at only a small portion of the available information. Salient data are screened out or ignored in order to confirm the person's biased view of the situation.

> *Example:* A depressed man with low self-esteem doesn't receive a holiday card from an old friend. He thinks, "I'm losing all my friends; nobody cares about me anymore." He is ignoring the evidence that he has received a number of other cards, his old friend has sent him a card every year for the past 15 years, his friend has been busy this past year with a move and a new job, and he still has good relationships with other friends.

**Arbitrary inference** Coming to a conclusion in the face of contradictory evidence or in the absence of evidence.

> *Example:* A woman with fear of elevators is asked to predict the chances that an elevator will fall if she rides in it. She replies that the chances are 10% or more that the elevator will fall to the ground and she will be injured. Many people have tried to convince her that the chances of a catastrophic elevator accident are negligible.

**Overgeneralization** A conclusion is made about one or more isolated incidents and then is extended illogically to cover broad areas of functioning.

> *Example:* A depressed college student gets a B on a test. He considers this unsatisfactory. He overgeneralizes when he has these automatic thoughts: "I'm in trouble in this class.... I'm falling short everywhere in my life.... I can't do anything right."

**Magnification and minimization** The significance of an attribute, event, or sensation is exaggerated or minimized.

> *Example:* A woman with panic disorder starts to feel light-headed during the onset of a panic attack. She thinks, "I'll faint.... I might have a heart attack or a stroke."

**Personalization** External events are related to oneself when there is little evidence for doing so. Excessive responsibility or blame is taken for negative events.

*Example:* There has been an economic downturn, and a previously successful business is now struggling to meet the annual budget. Layoffs are being considered. A host of factors have led to the budget crisis, but one of the managers thinks, "It's all my fault....I should have seen this coming and done something about it....I've failed everyone in the company."

**Absolutistic thinking** (also called *all-or-nothing thinking*) Judgments about oneself, personal experiences, or others are placed into one of two categories: all bad or all good; total failure or complete success; completely flawed or absolutely perfect.

*Example:* Dan, a man with depression, compares himself with Ed, a friend who appears to have a good marriage and whose children are doing well in school. Although the friend has a fair amount of domestic happiness, his life is far from ideal. Ed has troubles at work, financial strains, and physical ailments, among other difficulties. Dan is engaging in absolutistic thinking when he tells himself, "Ed has everything going for him....I have nothing."

*Note.* Available at: https://www.appi.org/wright.

# Examining the Evidence for Automatic Thoughts Worksheet

**Instructions:**

1. Identify a negative or troubling automatic thought.
2. Then list all the evidence that you can find that either supports ("evidence for") or disproves ("evidence against") the automatic thought.
3. After trying to find cognitive errors in the "evidence for" column, you can write revised or alternative thoughts at the bottom of the page.

**Automatic thought:**

| Evidence for automatic thought: | Evidence against automatic thought: |
|---|---|
| 1. | 1. |
| 2. | 2. |
| 3. | 3. |
| 4. | 4. |
| 5. | 5. |

**Cognitive errors:**

**Alternative thoughts:**

*Note.* Available at: https://www.appi.org/wright.

## Weekly Activity Schedule

**Instructions:** Write down your activities for each hour and then rate them on a scale of 0–10 for mastery **(m)** or degree of accomplishment and for pleasure **(p)** or amount of enjoyment you experienced. A rating of 0 would mean that you had no sense of mastery or pleasure. A rating of 10 would mean that you experienced maximum mastery or pleasure.

| | Sunday | Monday | Tuesday | Wednesday | Thursday | Friday | Saturday |
|---|---|---|---|---|---|---|---|
| 8:00 A.M. | | | | | | | |
| 9:00 A.M. | | | | | | | |
| 10:00 A.M. | | | | | | | |
| 11:00 A.M. | | | | | | | |
| 12:00 P.M. | | | | | | | |
| 1:00 P.M. | | | | | | | |
| 2:00 P.M. | | | | | | | |
| 3:00 P.M. | | | | | | | |
| 4:00 P.M. | | | | | | | |
| 5:00 P.M. | | | | | | | |
| 6:00 P.M. | | | | | | | |
| 7:00 P.M. | | | | | | | |
| 8:00 P.M. | | | | | | | |
| 9:00 P.M. | | | | | | | |

*Note.* Available at: https://www.appi.org/wright.

# Schema Inventory

**Instructions:** Use this checklist to search for possible underlying rules of thinking. Place a check mark beside each schema that you think you may have.

**Healthy Schemas**

___ No matter what happens, I can manage somehow.
___ If I work hard at something, I can master it.
___ I'm a survivor.
___ Others trust me.
___ I'm a solid person.
___ People respect me.
___ They can knock me down, but they can't knock me out.
___ I care about other people.
___ If I prepare in advance, I usually do better.
___ I deserve to be respected.
___ I like to be challenged.
___ There's not much that can scare me.
___ I'm intelligent.
___ I can figure things out.
___ I'm friendly.
___ I can handle stress.
___ The tougher the problem, the tougher I become.
___ I can learn from my mistakes and be a better person.
___ I'm a good spouse (and/or parent, child, friend, lover).
___ Everything will work out all right.

**Maladaptive Schemas**

___ I must be perfect to be accepted.
___ If I choose to do something, I must succeed.
___ I'm stupid.
___ Without a woman (man), I'm nothing.
___ I'm a fake.
___ Never show weakness.
___ I'm unlovable.
___ If I make one mistake, I'll lose everything.
___ I'll never be comfortable around others.
___ I can never finish anything.
___ No matter what I do, I won't succeed.
___ The world is too frightening for me.
___ Others can't be trusted.
___ I must always be in control.
___ I'm unattractive.
___ Never show your emotions.
___ Other people will take advantage of me.
___ I'm lazy.
___ If people really knew me, they wouldn't like me.
___ To be accepted, I must always please others.

*Note.* Available at: https://www.appi.org/wright.

## Examining the Evidence for Schemas Worksheet

Instructions:

1. Identify a negative or maladaptive schema that you would like to change. Write it down on this form.
2. Write down any evidence that either supports or disproves this schema.
3. Look for cognitive errors in the evidence for the maladaptive schema.
4. Finally, note your ideas for changing the schema and your plans for putting these ideas into action.

Schema I want to change:

| Evidence for this schema: | Evidence against this schema: |
|---|---|
| 1. | 1. |
| 2. | 2. |
| 3. | 3. |
| 4. | 4. |
| 5. | 5. |

Cognitive errors:

Now that I've examined the evidence, my degree of belief in the schema is:

Ideas I have for modifications to this schema:

Actions I will take now to change my schema and act in a healthier way:

*Note.* Available at: https://www.appi.org/wright.

## Well-Being Log: Building and Sustaining Well-Being

| Situation | Experiences and feelings of well-being | Intensity (0–100) | Interfering thoughts and/or behaviors | Observer |
|---|---|---|---|---|
| | | | | |

*Note.* Available at: https://www.appi.org/wright.

## Safety Plan Worksheet

| Step 1: Warning signs: | | | |
|---|---|---|---|
| 1. | ______ | | |
| 2. | ______ | | |
| 3. | ______ | | |
| **Step 2: Internal coping strategies—Things I can do to take my mind off my problems without contacting another person:** | | | |
| 1. | ______ | | |
| 2. | ______ | | |
| 3. | ______ | | |
| **Step 3: People and social settings that provide distraction:** | | | |
| 1. | Name______ | | Phone______ |
| 2. | Name______ | | Phone______ |
| 3. | Place______ | 4. | Place______ |
| **Step 4: People whom I can ask for help:** | | | |
| 1. | Name______ | | Phone______ |
| 2. | Name______ | | Phone______ |
| 3. | Name______ | | Phone______ |
| **Step 5: Professionals or agencies I can contact during a crisis:** | | | |
| 1. | Clinician/Agency Name______ | | Phone______ |
| | Clinician Pager or Emergency Contact #______ | | |
| 2. | Clinician/Agency Name ______ | | Phone______ |
| | Clinician Pager or Emergency Contact #______ | | |
| 3. | Local Emergency Department______ | | |
| | Emergency Department Address______ | | |
| | Emergency Department Phone______ | | |
| 4. | Suicide Prevention Lifeline Phone: **1-800-273-TALK (8255)** | | |
| 5. | Other:______ | | |

*Note.* Available at: https://www.appi.org/wright.

| **Step 6: Making the environment safe:** | | | |
|---|---|---|---|
| 1. | ______ | | |
| 2. | ______ | | |
| 3. | ______ | | |
| **Step 7: Reasons for living—The things that are most important to me and worth living for are:** | | | |
| 1. | ______ | 4. | ______ |
| 2. | ______ | 5. | ______ |
| 3. | ______ | 6. | ______ |

*Source.* Reproduced with permission (© 2008, 2012, 2016 Barbara Stanley, Ph.D., and Gregory K. Brown, Ph.D.). To register to use this form and for additional training resources, go to: www.suicidesafetyplan.com.

*Note.* Available at: https://www.appi.org/wright.

# Cognitive-Behavior Therapy Supervision Checklist[a]

Therapist ________________________________________
Supervisor __________________ Date ________________________

**Instructions:** Use this checklist to monitor and evaluate competencies in CBT. Listed in Part A are competencies that should typically be demonstrated in each session. Part B contains competencies that may be demonstrated over a course of therapy or therapies. The checklist is not intended for evaluation of performance in first or last sessions.

**Part A: Competencies that should typically be demonstrated in each session**

| Competency | Superior | Satisfactory | Needs improvement | Did not attempt or N/A |
|---|---|---|---|---|
| 1. Maintains collaborative empirical alliance | | | | |
| 2. Expresses appropriate empathy, genuineness | | | | |
| 3. Demonstrates accurate understanding | | | | |
| 4. Maintains appropriate professionalism and boundaries | | | | |
| 5. Elicits and gives appropriate feedback | | | | |
| 6. Demonstrates knowledge of CBT model | | | | |
| 7. Demonstrates ability to use guided discovery | | | | |
| 8. Effectively sets agenda and structures session | | | | |
| 9. Reviews and assigns useful homework | | | | |
| 10. Identifies automatic thoughts and/or beliefs (schemas) | | | | |
| 11. Modifies automatic thoughts and/or beliefs (schemas) | | | | |

*Note.* Available at: https://www.appi.org/wright.

| Competency | Superior | Satisfactory | Needs improvement | Did not attempt or N/A |
|---|---|---|---|---|
| 12. Utilizes behavioral intervention or assists patient with problem solving | | | | |
| 13. Applies CBT methods in flexible manner that meets needs of patient | | | | |

**Part B: Competencies that may be demonstrated over a course of therapy or therapies**

| Competency | Superior | Satisfactory | Needs improvement | Did not attempt or N/A |
|---|---|---|---|---|
| 1. Sets goals and plans treatment based on CBT formulation | | | | |
| 2. Educates patient about CBT model and/or therapy interventions | | | | |
| 3. Demonstrates ability to use thought record or other structured method of responding to dysfunctional cognitions | | | | |
| 4. Can utilize activity or pleasant events scheduling | | | | |
| 5. Can utilize exposure and response prevention or graded task assignment | | | | |
| 6. Can utilize relaxation and/or stress management techniques | | | | |
| 7. Can utilize CBT relapse prevention methods | | | | |
| **Comments:** | | | | |

[a]Checklist developed by Donna Sudak, M.D., Jesse H. Wright, M.D., Ph.D., David Bienenfeld, M.D., and Judith Beck, Ph.D., 2001.

*Note.* Available at: https://www.appi.org/wright.

# Appendix 2
# Cognitive-Behavior Therapy Resources

## Self-Help Books

Basco MR: Never Good Enough: How to Use Perfectionism to Your Advantage Without Letting It Ruin Your Life. New York, Free Press, 1999

Burns DD: Feeling Good: The New Mood Therapy, Revised. New York, HarperCollins, 2008

Clark DA, Beck AT: The Anxiety and Worry Workbook: The Cognitive Behavioral Solution. New York, Guilford, 2012

Craske MG, Barlow DH: Mastery of Your Anxiety and Panic, 4th Edition. Oxford, UK, Oxford University Press, 2006

Foa EB, Wilson R: Stop Obsessing! How to Overcome Your Obsessions and Compulsions, Revised Edition. New York, Bantam, 2001

Greenberger D, Padesky CA: Mind Over Mood: Change How You Feel by Changing the Way You Think, 2nd Edition. New York, Guilford, 2015

Hayes SC, Smith S: Get Out of Your Mind and Into Your Life: The New Acceptance and Commitment Therapy (A New Harbinger Self-Help Workbook). Oakland, CA, New Harbinger Publications, 2005

Kabat-Zinn J: Full Catastrophe Living: Using the Wisdom of Your Body to Fight Stress, Pain, and Illness. New York, Hyperion, 1990

Kabat-Zinn J: Wherever You Go, There You Are: Mindfulness Meditation in Everyday Life. New York, Hyperion, 2005

Leahy RL: The Worry Cure: Seven Steps to Stop Worry From Stopping You. New York, Three Rivers Press, 2005

Linehan MM: DBT Skills Training Manual, 2nd Edition. New York, Guilford, 2015
Siegel RD: The Mindfulness Solution. New York, Guilford, 2010
Williams M, Teasdale JD, Segal ZV, Kabat-Zinn J: The Mindful Way Through Depression. New York, Touchstone, 2002
Wright JH, McCray LW: Breaking Free From Depression: Pathways to Wellness. New York, Guilford, 2012

## Computer Programs

Beating the Blues: U Squared Interactive. Available at: http://beatingthebluesus.com
FearFighter. CCBT Ltd. Available at: http://fearfighter.cbtprogram.com
Good Days Ahead. Empower Interactive. Available at: http://empower-interactive.com
MoodGYM. Australian National University. Available at: http://moodgym.anu.edu.au
Virtual reality programs by Rothbaum B et al. Decatur, GA, Virtually Better, 1996. Available at: http://virtuallybetter.com

## Web Sites

Academy of Cognitive Therapy: www.academyofct.org
American Psychiatric Association: www.psychiatry.org
American Psychological Association: www.apa.org
Association for Behavioral and Cognitive Therapies: www.abct.org
Beck Institute: https://beckinstitute.org
Dialectical behavior therapy: www.linehaninstitute.org
Mindfulness-based cognitive therapy: http://mbct.com
Safety planning resources: www.suicidesafetyplan.com
University of Louisville Depression Center: https://louisville.edu/depression

## Videos of Master Cognitive-Behavior Therapists

Aaron T. Beck, M.D.: Advances in Cognitive Therapy. DVD. Bala Cynwyd, PA, Beck Institute for Cognitive Therapy and Research. Available at: https://beckinstitute.org
Aaron T. Beck, M.D.: Cognitive Therapy of Depression: Interview #1 (Patient With Hopelessness Problem). DVD. Bala Cynwyd, PA, Beck Institute for Cognitive Therapy and Research. Available at: https://beckinstitute.org

Aaron T. Beck, M.D.: Demonstration of the Cognitive Therapy of Depression: Interview #1 (Patient With Family Problem). DVD. Bala Cynwyd, PA, Beck Institute for Cognitive Therapy and Research. Available at: https://beckinstitute.org

Judith S. Beck, Ph.D.: Brief Therapy Inside Out: Cognitive Therapy of Depression. DVD. Bala Cynwyd, PA, Beck Institute for Cognitive Therapy and Research. Available at: https://beckinstitute.org

David M. Clark, Ph.D.: Cognitive Therapy for Panic Disorder. Available at: www.apa.org.pubs/videos

Michelle G. Craske, Ph.D.: Treating Clients With Generalized Anxiety Disorder. Available at: www.apa.org.pubs/videos

Keith S. Dobson, Ph.D.: Cognitive-Behavioral Treatment Strategies. Available at: www.apa.org.pubs/videos

Arthur Freeman, Ed.D.: CBT for Personality Disorders. Available at: https://www.psychotherapy.net

Steven Hayes: Facing the Struggle. Available at: https://www.psychotherapy.net

Marsha Linehan, Ph.D.: Dialectical Behavior Therapy. Available at: https://www.psychotherapy.net

Donald Meichenbaum, Ph.D.: Mixed Anxiety and Depression: A Cognitive-Behavioral Approach. Available at: https://www.psychotherapy.net

Christine Padesky, Ph.D.: Cognitive Therapy for Panic Disorder. Huntington Beach, CA. Available at: http://store.padesky.com

Christine Padesky, Ph.D.: Constructing New Core Beliefs. Huntington Beach, CA. Available at: http://store.padesky.com

Christine Padesky, Ph.D.: Guided Discovery Using Socratic Dialogue. Huntington Beach, CA. Available at: http://store.padesky.com

Jacqueline Persons, Ph.D.: Cognitive-Behavior Therapy. Available at: www.apa.org.pubs/videos

Zindel V. Segal, Ph.D.: Mindfulness-Based Cognitive Therapy for Depression. Available at: www.apa.org.pubs/videos

Jeffrey E. Young, Ph.D.: Schema Therapy. Available at: www.apa.org.pubs/videos

## Professional Organizations With Special Interest in Cognitive-Behavior Therapy

Academy of Cognitive Therapy (www.academyofct.org)

Association for Behavioral and Cognitive Therapies (www.abct.org)

British Association for Behavioural and Cognitive Psychotherapies (www.babcp.com)

European Association for Behavioural and Cognitive Therapies (www.eabct.eu)

International Association for Cognitive Psychotherapy (www.the-iacp.com)

## Recommended Reading

Alford BA, Beck AT: The Integrative Power of Cognitive Therapy. New York, Guilford, 1997

Barlow DH, Cerney JA: Psychological Treatment of Panic. New York, Guilford, 1988

Basco MR, Rush AJ: Cognitive-Behavioral Therapy for Bipolar Disorder, 2nd Edition. New York, Guilford, 2005

Beck AT: Love Is Never Enough: How Couples Can Overcome Misunderstandings, Resolve Conflicts, and Solve Relationship Problems Through Cognitive Therapy. New York, Harper & Row, 1988

Beck AT, Rush AJ, Shaw BF, et al: Cognitive Therapy of Depression. New York, Guilford, 1979

Beck AT, Davis DD, Freeman A: Cognitive Therapy of Personality Disorders, 3rd Edition. New York, Guilford, 2015

Beck JS: Cognitive Therapy: Basics and Beyond, 2nd Edition. New York, Guilford, 2011

Brown GK, Wright JH, Thase ME, Beck AT: Cognitive therapy for suicide prevention, in The American Psychiatric Publishing Textbook of Suicide Assessment and Management, 2nd Edition. Edited by Simon RI, Hales RE. Washington, DC, American Psychiatric Publishing, 2012, pp 233–249

Clark DA, Beck AT: Cognitive Therapy of Anxiety Disorders: Science and Practice. New York, Guilford, 2010

Clark DA, Beck AT, Alford BA: Scientific Foundations of Cognitive Theory and Therapy of Depression. New York, Wiley, 1999

Dattilio FM: Cognitive-Behavioral Therapy With Couples and Families. New York, Guilford, 2010

Fava GA: Well-Being Therapy: Treatment Manual and Clinical Applications. Basel, Switzerland, Karger, 2016

Frankl VE: Man's Search for Meaning: An Introduction to Logotherapy, 4th Edition. Boston, MA, Beacon Press, 1992

Guidano VF, Liotti G: Cognitive Processes and Emotional Disorders: A Structural Approach to Psychotherapy. New York, Guilford, 1983

Hayes SC, Strosahl K, Wilson KG: Acceptance and Commitment Therapy: The Process and Practice of Mindful Change, 2nd Edition. New York, Guilford, 2012

Kingdon DG, Turkington D: Cognitive Therapy of Schizophrenia. New York, Guilford, 2005

Leahy RL (ed): Contemporary Cognitive Therapy: Theory, Research, and Practice. New York, Guilford, 2004

Linehan MM: Cognitive-Behavioral Treatment of Borderline Personality Disorder. New York, Guilford, 1993

Mahoney MJ, Freeman A (eds): Cognition and Psychotherapy. New York, Plenum, 1985

McCullough JP Jr: Skills Training Manual for Diagnosing and Treating Chronic Depression: Cognitive Behavioral Analysis System of Psychotherapy. New York, Guilford, 2001

Meichenbaum DB: Cognitive-Behavior Modification: An Integrative Approach. New York, Plenum, 1977

Persons JB: Cognitive Therapy in Practice: A Case Formulation Approach. New York, WW Norton, 1989

Safran JD, Segal ZV: Interpersonal Process in Cognitive Therapy. New York, Basic Books, 1990

Salkovskis PM (ed): Frontiers of Cognitive Therapy. New York, Guilford, 1996

Siegel RD: The Mindfulness Solution. New York, Guilford, 2010

Turk DC, Meichenbaum D, Genest M: Pain and Behavioral Medicine: A Cognitive-Behavioral Perspective. New York, Guilford, 1983

Wright JH, Thase ME, Beck AT, et al (eds): Cognitive Therapy With Inpatients: Developing a Cognitive Milieu. New York, Guilford, 1993

Wright JH, Turkington D, Kingdon DG, Basco MR: Cognitive-Behavior Therapy for Severe Mental Illness: An Illustrated Guide. Washington, DC, American Psychiatric Publishing, 2009

Wright JH, Sudak DM, Turkington D, Thase ME: High-Yield Cognitive-Behavior Therapy for Brief Sessions: An Illustrated Guide. Washington, DC, American Psychiatric Publishing, 2010

Young JE, Klosko JS, Weishaar ME: Schema Therapy: A Practitioner's Guide. New York, Guilford, 2003

# Index

*Page numbers printed in* **boldface** *type refer to tables or figures.*